*The Harvard-MIT Division of
Health Sciences and Technology*

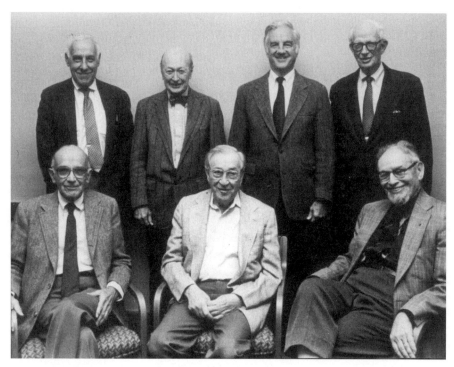

Planning Meeting for "HST History" November 1992. *From left to right:*
Seated: Irving M. London, Jerome B. Wiesner, Walter A. Rosenblith.
Standing: William S. Beck, Robert H. Ebert, Derek Bok, Walter H.
Abelmann.

The Harvard-MIT Division of Health Sciences and Technology

The First 25 Years 1970–1995

WALTER H. ABELMANN, M.D.
EDITOR

CAMBRIDGE, MASSACHUSETTS:
Published by the Harvard-MIT Division of Health Sciences and Technology
Distributed by the Harvard University Press
2004

*Dedicated to the
Faculty and Students
whose creativity,
enthusiasm, and hard work
made it all possible.*

CONTRIBUTORS

HMS = Harvard Medical School
HST = Division of Health Sciences and Technology
MIT = Massachusetts Institute of Technology

Walter H. Abelmann, M.D.
Professor of Medicine, Emeritus, HMS
Senior Physician, Beth Israel Hospital
Director of Alumni Affairs, HST
Acting Co-Director, HST, 1990–1992

Derek Bok, J.D., L.L.D.
President Emeritus, Professor of Law,
300th Anniversary University Professor,
Harvard University

Robert H. Ebert, M.D.
Dean, HMS 1965–1977
Deceased, January 29, 1996

Howard W. Johnson
President Emeritus, Professor Emeritus, MIT

Richard J. Kitz, M.D.
Henry Isaiah Dorr Professor of Research and Teaching in
Anesthetics and Anaesthesia, HMS
Faculty Dean for Clinical Affairs, HMS
Co-Director, HST, 1985–1990

Walter L. Koltun, Ph.D.
Assistant Director for Resources, HST, 1970–1994

Irving M. London, M.D.
Grover M. Hermann Professor of Health Sciences and
Technology in the Harvard-MIT Division, Emeritus
Professor of Biology, MIT
Director, HST 1970–1985

Roger G. Mark, M.D., Ph.D.
Grover M. Hermann Professor of Health Sciences and
Technology in the Harvard/MIT Division
Co-Director, HST, 1985–1996

Michael Rosenblatt, M.D.
Ebert Professor of Molecular Medicine, HMS
Co-Director, HST, 1992–1998

Walter A. Rosenblith, Ph.D.
Institute Professor, Emeritus, MIT
Chairman, MIT Faculty, 1967–1969
Associate Provost, MIT, 1969–1971
Provost, MIT, 1971–1980
Deceased May 1, 2002

TABLE OF CONTENTS

Conclusions/Perspective   221

Appendices

ILLUSTRATIONS

Frontispiece. Planning Meeting for "HST History" November 1992. From left to right: *Seated:* Irving M. London, Jerome B. Wiesner, Walter A. Rosenblith. *Standing:* William S. Beck, Robert H. Ebert, Derek Bok, Walter H. Abelmann.

Located between pages 150 and 151

4. *Above,* Harvey Goldman, M.D., with Adel M. Malek, M.D., Ph.D., 1994, and Ralph de la Torre, M.D., 1992, in HST 030 Human Pathology, 1988; *below,* Frederick J. Schoen, M.D., Ph.D., with Volney L. Sheen, M.D., 1997, Charlene M. Chiang, M.D., 1996, Thomas J. Mullen, Ph.D., 1998, Nada Boustany, Ph.D., 1997, Robert Hurford, M.D., 1994, and Tai Sing Lee, Ph.D., 1993, in HST 030, Human Pathology, 1990.

5. *Above,* Abul K. Abbas, M.D., in HST 175, Cellular and Molecular Immunology, ca. 1988; *below,* Samuel A. Latt, M.D., Ph.D., George Q. Daley, M.D., 1991, and other students in HMS 700, Genetics, 1987.

6. *Above,* Paul M. Gallop, Ph.D., HST 141, Molecular Basis of Some Clinical Disorders, in his laboratory at Children's Hospital, ca. 1988; *below,* Walter H. Abelmann, M.D., in HST 090 Cardiovascular Pathophysiology, ca. 1988.

7. *Above,* Walter H. Olson, Ph.D., and Roger G. Mark, M.D., Ph.D., in the Biomedical Engineering Center, ca. 1979; *below,* Richard J. Cohen, M.D., Ph.D., 1976, in his laboratory, ca. 1985.

8. *Above,* William S. Beck, M.D., with students in HST 080, Hematology, ca. 1979; *below,* Martin C. Carey, M.D., D.Sc., in HST 120, Gastro- entrology, 1984.

9. *Above,* Cecil H. (Pete) Coggins, M.D., with Nada Boustany, Ph.D., 1997, at the HST Forum of 1991; *below,* Arnold N. Weinberg, M.D., and John M. Moses, M.D., with Kenneth S. Hu, M.D., 1994, and Jack Tsao, M.D., Ph.D., 1997, in HST 220, Introduction to Patient Care and the Profession that Cares in 1990.

10. *Left,* W. Hallowell Churchill, Jr., M.D., with students in HST 200, Introduction to Clinical Medicine at Brigham and Women's Hospital, ca. 1990; *right,* Annabelle Okada, M.D., 1988, in HST 200, Introduction to Clinical Medicine, in 1986.

11. *Above,* Martha L. Gray, Ph.D., 1986, in HST 201, Introduction to Clinical Medicine and Medical Engineering, ca. 1982; *below,* James Oliver, M.D., Ph.D., 1994.

12. *Above,* John T. Fallon, M.D., Ph.D., HST 090, Cardiovascular Pathophysiology, 1980s; *below,* Herman N. Eisen, M.D., Immunology, 1970s.

13. *Above,* Ronald A. Arky, M.D., HST 060, Endocrinology, 1980s; *below,* Cassandra Hall Walcott, M.D., 1992.

FOREWORD

Derek Bok, J.D., L.L.D.

Every Harvard President early in his term begins to think that there should be much more collaboration with Massachusetts Institute of Technology (MIT). It is, after all, a remarkable thing to have two of the world's most renowned research universities only two subway stops apart. Think of the cost savings achieved by eliminating duplicating programs. Think of the opportunities for strengthening academic programs by combining the intellectual resources of the two institutions. How attractive it would be to have Harvard give the humanities courses for MIT while MIT provides the engineering courses for Harvard students.

Somewhere during the middle years of a President's career, these early thoughts recede from view. Certainly, they did for me even though I will always count my relations with Jerry Wiesner and Walter Rosenblith among the happiest I experienced during twenty years of academic administration. Of course, informal research collaborations between individual Harvard and MIT professors abound. Most of them are not even known to the top administrators of either institution, and their number and variety invariably come as a surprise whenever some internal census brings them to light. Hundreds of students also take advantage of the courses offered by both institutions as a result of the happy existence of an agreement that allows students from each university to enroll in courses in the other without charge. In contrast to all this spontaneous, informal cross-pollination, however, formal collaborative programs and curricula are notable chiefly for their absence.

Just why this should be so is not entirely clear. Perhaps it is because it is so hard to establish governing procedures that will accommodate the separate administrative structures of both institutions. Meshing the two administrations is all the more difficult since Harvard is famously decentralized while MIT is rather the opposite. Moreover, faculties are conservative; they do not like to give up control over academic programs. As a result, every important decision must satisfy two sets of professors and administrators, hardly a recipe for prompt, efficient decision-making. In view of these formidable obstacles, the relevant question may not be why there are not more joint institutional arrangements but why the Harvard-MIT Program in Health Sciences and Technology (HST) has managed to survive. To my knowledge, it is now the only formal collaborative program (aside from ROTC) that exists between the two universities.

How did this single program endure when so many others have failed to materialize or disappear after a few years of existence? The answer is surely not because large sums of money were made available to attract faculty members, like bees sensing honey, from either end of Cambridge. The HST program did not begin with a large gift for endowment nor did it prove to be much of a magnet to draw large gifts from wealthy alumni.

Two reasons, I believe, were far more important to the program's existence. First of all, there were professors from both institutions who believed enough in the promise of marrying biology and the physical sciences and engineering that they were willing to spend substantial amounts of time and energy bringing their convictions into being. However worthy the purpose, however ample the funding, however enthusiastic the top university leadership, no academic enterprise can succeed without committed faculty participants. In addition to the participating professors, the HST program was always able to attract extremely gifted students. In my experience, excellent students are the best possible glue to hold collaborative ventures together, whether they be collaborations between separate faculties and departments or collaborations between different institutions.

Whatever the reason, HST has clearly endured, and that in itself is remarkable. Has it achieved its original purposes? I believe that the answer is a definite yes insofar as educating students is concerned. As the following pages attest, the students have continued to be exceptionally able. By all accounts, they look back on the HST experience with great appreciation and have gone on to achieve success in their chosen fields. The Program has proved especially important with the introduction of a new Harvard Medical School curriculum which, with all its virtues, is thought to place a less than heavy emphasis on basic science. Complementing this "new pathway" in the Medical School, the HST program offers an M.D. degree with a strong emphasis on science for the benefit of students who prefer this orientation.

I am less sure how successful the HST program has been in helping to develop new breakthroughs in bio-engineering or other forms of research that combine bio-medical science with engineering and the physical sciences. Others will be far better equipped than I to evaluate the Harvard-MIT program from this perspective. Of one thing, however, I am sure. Much collaboration across disciplinary boundaries will take place among Harvard and MIT researchers whether or not there are formal structures to embrace them. Thus, the HST program is not essential to allow such cooperative work to take place. In contrast, the educational opportunities HST provides could not have developed without the creation of a formal collaborative program.

In the end, therefore, the Health Sciences and Technology Program represents a special achievement in the history of two great universities. Its very uniqueness commands respect. In my experience, the great challenge in presiding over a university filled with extremely talented, highly independent scholars is to create a whole that is somewhere close to the sum of its constituent parts. The HST program, happily, seems to represent a whole that is even greater than the sum of those distinguished faculty members who work within it. That fact alone deserves our gratitude and appreciation.

INTRODUCTION

Howard W. Johnson

The long years of the late sixties and early seventies were times of turmoil and dispute on a rare scale on the campuses of the United States
and elsewhere around the world. Issues like the Vietnam War, civil
rights, gender inequities, inter-generational disaffection, and other societal disagreements created large fissures in the society at large and
within most institutions. The universities and colleges were hardly
immune, of course. In fact, the universities were the foci of many of
these issues, often splitting faculties, students, administrators, and
alumni.

Despite or because of those unsettled times, some major new educational and research programs emerged. At the Massachusetts Institute of Technology and at Harvard University, there were major
innovations in curriculum and new cooperative institutional arrangements. No better model of the most productive kind of inter-university innovation can be found than the Harvard-MIT Health Sciences
and Technology (HST) program. This program, begun in the late sixties, dealt with important challenges facing medical education and research in new ways. Enough time has now elapsed to assess the record of the outstanding men and women who were admitted to the

program and who have now graduated from HST. In general, they have gone on to distinguish themselves in practice and in research. The research programs have been exceptionally productive. Since many of the graduates are still quite young, it seems clear that the yield of their research will multiply as the years go by. It is instructive to examine the HST program as a model of how such experiments develop, improve, overcome difficulties, and become part of the institutional fabric of two major universities. It is probably important to remember this history and to understand the problems that developed in maintaining program quality.

One place to begin the story of this modern chapter in the long and distinguished history of medical education and research in Cambridge and in Boston is to cite the remembered visit of Dr. James Shannon, Director of the National Institutes of Health, in 1966 when he came to ask a new administration at MIT to establish a brand-new school of medicine. The President's Commission on Heart Disease, Cancer, and Stroke had made its first report in December 1964, and had outlined an all-out national program to conquer or ameliorate these leading diseases of contemporary society. The timing was just right for such initiatives. Biomedical engineering and life sciences were expanding at MIT and elsewhere in the preceding years. In December 1965, the Whitaker Building for the life sciences had just been dedicated. Dr. Shannon turned to my colleagues and to me at MIT in 1966 because, as he said, NIH was convinced that mere expansion of the number of physicians would not suffice. A new kind of physician was needed who could integrate and exploit the full power of modern science and technology in the practice of medicine. Dr. Shannon was convinced that MIT was the right place to break with the past in the education of medical doctors. For example, in the preceding twenty years MIT had been first among the universities without a medical school in the number of NIH fellowships awarded in the U.S. For that and other reasons, he felt MIT was a natural place to start. We were strongly tempted to accept Dr. Shannon's proposal. A faculty review of the project confirmed that more than 100 research projects at MIT involved collaboration with nearby medical schools and hospitals, chiefly with the Harvard Medical School, and that MIT students and faculty were much in need of expanded clinical associations to further their growing involvement in the life and health sciences and biomedical engineering.

In the end, the MIT administration and the faculty committee had serious doubts about the idea. Not least was the issue of funding such an effort. We were close enough to our sister institutions to understand the high cost of maintaining a medical school, and we knew that the Institute, at any moment of time, is stretched to the limit in its resources. That seems to be the one constant in research university life. At the end of the spirited review, we decided, reluctantly, to decline Dr. Shannon's proposition. Independently, and at about the same time, Dean Robert H. Ebert, the head of the Harvard Medical School, had begun searching for ways to bring the advances of emerging technology to bear upon the education of physicians. Provost Jerome B. Wiesner, Associate Provost Walter A. Rosenblith, and I began to explore the possibilities of some kind of formal relationship with Harvard Medical School that would serve both institutions.

In January 1967, at the urging of Dr. Ebert and Dr. Wiesner, President Nathan M. Pusey of Harvard and I appointed a Joint Committee on Engineering and Living Systems to consider the desirability and feasibility of establishing joint programs of education, research, development and service in the fields of health and medicine. We defined the objectives: "The major new task of the two institutions is to realize the benefits of science in relation to these human needs—to provide a human focus for technology." The rest moved quickly. The subsequent committee processes and debates moved to the point so that in 1969, with funds granted by the Commonwealth Fund, planning for a joint Harvard-MIT School in Health Sciences and Technology began under the leadership of Dr. Irving London. If one had to cite a single important step along the way in determining the future success of the program, it would be the appointment of Dr. London.

The concept of the first part of the new program—to turn out well-trained medical doctors who had deep training in the biological and physical sciences—was a clearly worthwhile and understandable concept. The implementation in the faculties and the trustee bodies was a good deal more difficult. The approval process by both faculties and by the governing bodies of the two institutions was finally achieved but not without debate and compromise. If passage of a new curriculum within a great faculty is difficult, the passage by three faculties of a new program of education and research is surely more than three times as difficult. In this situation, the MIT faculty and the faculties of the Harvard Medical School and the Harvard School of Public Health all had to approve the program. But finally, agreement was reached, and the program was launched in 1970.

The equally important medical engineering and medical physics program, envisioned from the beginning as a new way of educating physical scientists and engineers who had deep medical training, took more time to develop. This second part of the program was the vital counterpart of the medical doctor program. Many of the HST students would go on to qualify for both the M.D. and the Ph.D. degrees.

Beginning in 1971-72, both Harvard and MIT had new presidents—Jerome Wiesner at MIT and Derek Bok at Harvard—who gave renewed priority to the new program. It is important to add that the enthusiastic and mature support of the many students involved was significant in achieving progress.

A final large requirement in making the programs viable was securing adequate funding for the program. At MIT, for example, not only were the teaching and research programs in need of new funding, but the new facilities were a critical necessity. A key gift for a new structure to house the program came from MIT trustees, Uncas and Helen Whitaker, but support for all aspects of the programs remained a vital need.

This book is a welcome history of all these developments. The chapters are written by several of the Harvard and MIT founders of the program whose prodigious efforts made the idea a success. It is a history worthy of the review of all those who want to understand contemporary education in medicine, science, and engineering.

PREFACE

Walter H. Abelmann, M.D.

The twenty-fifth anniversary of the founding of a novel enterprise is
an appropriate time to look back at its inception, evolution, *modus
operandi* and accomplishments. The time may be too early for a
definite historical assessment and critique. On the other hand, a point
in time when most key individuals who participated in the founding
and development are still accessible permits the combination of historiography with oral history, which gives the enterprise a personal
slant.

When the present endeavor was conceived, in anticipation of the
celebration of the twenty-fifth anniversary of the Harvard-MIT Division of Health Sciences and Technology (HST) in December 1995,
the detailed nature and format of this volume were not defined. At a
meeting of Drs. Robert H. Ebert, Irving M. London, Walter A.
Rosenblith and Walter H. Abelmann, held on October 15, 1992 (see
frontispiece), it was decided that it would be preferable that the editor should have personal experience with the HST program, that key
individuals should be invited to contribute and that the result should
be of value to the two universities and the departments involved, as
well as to other institutions that might consider similar, or even dif-

ferent, inter-institutional collaborations in both research and education. In addition, it was expected that the eventual volume would be of interest to students and alumni, as well as present and past members of the faculty. From the outset, then, this volume was planned as an institutional biography, rather than a comprehensive documentary history.

In Walter Rosenblith's words, at the October 15, 1992 meeting, "Each person should write his personal story and reminiscences. Essays should focus not only on successes, but also on problems encountered in bringing together an innovative program."

At the same meeting, Robert Ebert stated that the volume should address "the institutionalization of the program and its problems."

Chapter 1 comprises a concise review of past collaborations between Harvard University and the Massachusetts Institute of Technology (MIT). In Chapter 2, the then Provost of MIT recounts the confluence of his background in engineering and medical sciences that led to his role in the birth of HST. In Chapter 3, the then Dean of the Harvard Medical School (HMS) describes the early efforts on the part of Harvard to participate in a joint, interdisciplinary, inter-university, interdepartmental program.

Chapter 4, written by the first director of the program, describes in detail the early years 1970–85. Chapters 5 and 6 give overviews of the later years.

Chapter 7 highlights the difficulties encountered in financing the program. Chapter 8, based upon recorded, in-depth interviews of twenty-four present and past members of the faculty and administration of HST, presents an overview of the "HST Experience," focusing primarily upon the M.D. program. Chapter 9 describes the Medical Engineering and Medical Physics Program (MEMP), inaugurated in 1978.

The following two chapters, 10 and 11, address the evaluation of the M.D. and MEMP programs, respectively. They look at both process and outcome evaluation and include narrative comments by students.

The appendices provide a time-line, a comprehensive listing of courses offered, typical curricula, a roster of HST faculty, lists of graduates and their M.D. and Ph.D. theses, and a list of major research projects.

Thirty-five photographs illustrate aspects of the educational and research programs, which will be appreciated especially by present and former members of the faculty and the student body.

Acknowledgements

Thanks are due to many individuals who have responded to our requests for records, files and archival material, to those who have consented to be interviewed, and to those who have assisted in processing the chapters, notes and appendices that comprise this volume. Special thanks are due Paul A. Kirby for transcribing the taped interviews (Chapter 8); to Barbara Jaskela and Carol Campbell for preparation of the manuscript; to Barbara Ebert for editing and referencing Chapter 3; to Richard J. Wolfe, formerly Curator of Rare Books and Manuscripts of the Francis A. Countway Library, for advice and assistance in the publication process; to the reference archivists at MIT; to Clark Elliott, Associate Curator for Archives, Administration and Research of the Harvard University Archives; and to Keiko Oh, Director, Inter-Institutional and Student Financial Affairs in HST. The photographs used for the illustrations were largely the work of L. Barry Hetherington, Martha Stewart and Margo Woodruff. The Commonwealth Fund, Bank of Boston, The Gillette Company and The Raytheon Company provided financial support for this work.

Chapter 1

EARLY COLLABORATIVE EFFORTS OF HARVARD AND MIT

Walter H. Abelmann, M.D.

Although this chapter intends to focus primarily on early collaborative efforts of Harvard University and the Massachusetts Institute of Technology (MIT) in the Health Sciences, it may be of interest to cast a brief look at the earliest joint ventures of the two universities.

In 1869, Charles W. Eliot, then Professor of Chemistry at MIT, was elected president of Harvard University. Harvard's Lawrence Scientific School became one of his early interests.[1] The Lawrence School had been relatively unsuccessful and had been quickly eclipsed by MIT. Serious negotiations of a merger of Harvard and MIT ensued but failed. Following renewed merger attempts by Eliot in 1878 and 1890, which also did not succeed, Harvard's Lawrence School was placed under the Faculty of Arts and Sciences. In 1891, Nathaniel Southgate Shaler was appointed Dean of the Lawrence School and proceeded to strengthen it. To this end, he secured a bequest of $24 million from his friend, the industrialist, Gordon McKay. This permitted Eliot and the then president of MIT, Henry Pritchett, to re-open consideration of an alliance if not merger.[2] In 1905, there were serious proposals for a new MIT campus on the site presently occupied by the Harvard Business School. This, however, was blocked by the courts because of restrictions in the original bequest of that land.

1

In 1906, Eliot replaced the Lawrence Scientific School with the Graduate School of Applied Sciences.

The concept of merger continued to simmer, and in 1914 Presidents Lowell and Maclaurin signed an agreement to combine Harvard's and MIT's engineering programs.[3] The agreement called for Harvard to transfer to MIT a major share of the income from the McKay endowment for instruction in engineering. Subsequently, three classes of engineers graduated with joint Harvard-MIT degrees. In 1917, however, the Supreme Court of Massachusetts declared the agreement void!

Let us now turn to the health fields. Although collaborative medical research between individual members of the faculties of Harvard and MIT may be traced back much earlier, the first formal association of the two universities in the health field occurred in 1912 when the Harvard-MIT School for Health Officers was established by MIT's Professor William Thompson Sedgwick, who was soon joined by Harvard's Milton J. Rosenau, Professor of Preventive Medicine, and George C. Whipple, Gordon McKay Professor of Sanitary Engineering.[4] The objective of this school, which was the first such program in the United States, was the education of public health officers in the fields of preventive medicine and sanitary engineering. MIT contributed its interest in food technology and sanitary bacteriology whereas Harvard focused on sanitary engineering and medical aspects of environmental and industrial public health. Harvard's growing interest in public health led to the founding of a Division of Industrial Hygiene in 1918. In 1921, the International Health Board of the Rockefeller Foundation proposed that Harvard establish a School of Public Health. C.K. Drinker and Richard Strong took on this challenge, and in 1922, the Harvard-MIT School of Health Officers became the Harvard School of Public Health.

World War II kindled an expansion of interest in research at the interface of physiology and biological sciences. A new Department of Biophysics was founded at Harvard in 1946, under the leadership of Professor Arthur K. Solomon, to be joined by Professor Bertram Vallee in 1951. In 1952, a physics research laboratory was established at the Massachusetts General Hospital and directed by Gordon Brownell, Associate Professor of Nuclear Engineering at MIT.

Nineteen fifty-six saw the ground breaking for The Cambridge Electron Accelerator, four years after the first proposal had been submitted to the Atomic Energy Commission (AEC), jointly by Harvard University and the Massachusetts Institute of Technology.[5] Operation of the facility began in 1961 and continued until the funding by the AEC was discontinued in 1975.[6] Another joint initiative was created in 1956, when a group of otolaryngologists at the Harvard-affiliated Massachusetts Eye and Ear Infirmary (MEEI), led by Dr. Leroy Schall, Chief of Otolaryngology and Professor of Otolaryngology at the Harvard Medical School, with the help of President James Killian of MIT, established a basic science laboratory at the MEEI. This laboratory was established jointly with the Research Laboratory of Electronics at MIT[7] and staffed by scientists and engineers from MIT. This became the Eaton-Peabody Laboratory of Auditory Physiology, under the direction of Dr. Nelson Y-S Kiang, previously a member of Professor Walter Rosenblith's group at MIT.[8]

In the late 1950's, the Department of Preventive Medicine at the Harvard Medical School and the Research Laboratory of Electronics at MIT developed a collaborative program in medicine and mathematics.[9] Professor Murray Eden, a biomathematician at MIT, was appointed Visiting Lecturer at the Harvard Medical School. A course in biomathematics was then offered, dealing with the application of mathematical theory to biology and medicine, aimed at the highly motivated student with a good background in mathematics. The 1950's also saw the creation of the Division of Biomathematics in the Department of Medicine at the Peter Bent Brigham Hospital (now part of the Brigham and Women's Hospital) and, in Harvard's Faculty of Arts and Sciences, the establishment of the Division of Engineering and Applied Physics, with affiliation with the Faculties of Medicine and Public Health.[10]

Multiple Harvard-MIT collaborative activities, both in research and in education, resulted from these enterprises. Many basic research endeavors, as well as applied research at the interface between quantitative and biological sciences ensued, often involving close collaboration between Harvard and MIT. Examples are Professor Edward Merrill's investigations of polymer and surface chemistry in biological systems,[11] Professor Ascher Shapiro's studies on cardiac assist devices[12] and the hydrodynamics of peristaltic flow in the human ureter,[13] and Professor Lawrence R. Young's research dealing with the vestibular system and its role in the performance of pilots and astronauts.[14] Professor Robert W. Mann's development of the "Boston Arm,"[15] in collaboration with the Harvard Medical School and the Massachusetts General Hospital, must also be mentioned. Collaborative educational ventures resulted as well, such as the inclusion of courses in biomathematics in the curriculum at the Harvard

Medical School by Professor David Rutstein in the Department of Preventive Medicine, with participation of members of the MIT faculty.

A major collaborative effort in the area of regional and urban health information systems was started in 1959 as the Harvard-MIT Joint Center for Urban Studies with major support from the Ford Foundation. Its mission was "to further the educational purposes of both institutions by stimulating and facilitating basic research and applied studies in urban and regional affairs." This Center did not offer courses or confer degrees. In its first seven years, fourteen books and thirty monographs were published, including *Beyond the Melting Pot* by Nathan Glazer and Daniel Patrick Moynihan.[16] The Center continued to be active and productive into the eighties. As Presidents Derek C. Bok of Harvard and Jerome B. Wiesner of MIT wrote in 1980, the Center "as an established part of the Harvard/MIT community, continues to provide the unique environment where scholars meet to explore problems that cut across disciplinary boundaries, and where governmental and private leaders join them in an effort to define and clarify major intellectual and policy issues."[17]

In 1964, Gordon S. Brown, the Dean of Engineering, appointed an *ad hoc* committee on Biomedical Engineering, which later became the MIT Committee on Engineering and Living Systems.[18] This committee was charged to prepare an inventory of research and course offerings in biomedical engineering to determine the extent of faculty commitment and the potential for future growth of the field. The report "Graduate Studies at the Massachusetts Institute of Technology in Engineering and Living Systems" by Philip A. Drinker listed more than eighty-seven members of the MIT faculty and staff, from eleven departments, who were involved in research in biomedical engineering in 1968.[19]

In 1966, Dr. James A. Shannon, Director of the National Institutes of Health, and Dr. Colin MacLeod, Deputy Director of the Office of Science and Technology in the White House, approached the President of MIT, Howard Johnson, and the Provost, Jerome Wiesner, with the proposal to establish a medical school, to which he and the federal government were prepared to provide support in the amount of $50 million or more.[20] This offer was prompted by the view that "the United States was lacking a medical school that benefitted from a close relationship with research and teaching in technology."[21] This opportunity was explored in depth by the leadership of MIT with the trustees, members of the faculty, and potential donors. While there was a great deal of interest on the part of both the faculty and students in greater involvement in health sciences and their application to medicine, it was decided—for many cogent reasons—that MIT should not establish a fourth medical school in the city of Boston.

About the same time, Professor Jerome B. Wiesner, Provost of MIT, learned that discussions were taking place at the Harvard Medical School about the formation of a Department of Engineering and Technology. Thus, the stage was set for a joint venture by the two universities.[21]

Notes

1. W.J. Hughes, "Engineering and Other Applied Sciences in the Harvard Engineering School and Its Predecessors 1847–1929," Chapter 26 in S.E. Morrison, ed., *Development of Harvard University since the Inauguration of President Eliot 1869–1929* (Cambridge, MA: Harvard University Press, 1930), pp. 413–422; B. Sinclair, "Harvard, MIT, and the Ideal Technical Education," in C.A. Elliott and M.W. Rossitor, eds., *Science at Harvard University* (Bethlehem, PA: Lehigh University Press, 1992), pp. 76–95.

2. W.J. Hughes, "Engineering and Other Applied Sciences in the Harvard Engineering School and Its Predecessors 1847–1929," also, J.R. Killian, *The Education of a College President* (Cambridge, MA: The MIT Press, 1985), pp. 76–95.

3. *Harvard and Tech in Co-operation,* The Harvard-Tech Supplement published with the *Harvard Alumni Bulletin* 45, no. 14 (January 7, 1914), 4 pp.; S.E. Morison, *Three Centuries of Harvard 1636–1936* (Cambridge, MA: Harvard University Press, 1936) p. 471.

4. J. A. Curran, *Founders of the Harvard School of Public Health, with Biographical Notes, 1909–1946* (New York: The Josiah Macy, Jr. Foundation, 1970).

5. *Technology Review,* 61 (1956/9): 145; *Harvard Crimson,* October 27, 1961; Letter from Norman F. Ramsey to M. Stanley Livingston, Director of the Cambridge Electron Accelerator, September 5, 1962, Institute Archives and Special Collection, MIT Libraries, Cambridge, MA. 14N-118 MC244 Box 1.

6. Personal communication to the author from Professor Karl Strauch, the last Director of the Cambridge Electron Accelerator, April 22, 1997.

7. D.D. Rutstein and M. Eden, *Engineering and Living Systems: Interfaces and Opportunities* (Cambridge, MA: The MIT Press, 1970).

8. In 1992, under the leadership of Professor Nelson Y-S Kiang, the Speech and Hearing Sciences Doctoral Program was established, leading to a Ph.D. in Speech and Hearing Sciences awarded by MIT through the Harvard-MIT Division of Health Sciences and Technology.

9. D.D. Rutstein, *The Coming Revolution in Medicine* (Cambridge, MA: The MIT Press, 1967), p. 180.

10. Ibid.
11. J.C. Bray and E.W. Merrill, "Polyvinyl Alcohol Hydrogels for Synthetic Articular Cartilage Material," *Journal of Biomedical Materials Research* 7 (1973): 431–443; E.W. Salzman, S. Berger, E.W. Merrill and P.S.L. Wong, "Thrombosis Induced by Artificial Surfaces," *Thrombosis et Diathesis Haemorragica* Suppl., 59 (1974): 107–122.
12. V.S. Murthy, T.A. McMahon, M.Y. Jaffrin and A.H. Shapiro, "The Intra-aortic Balloon for Left Heart Assistance: An Analytic Model," Biomechanics 4 (1971): 351–367.
13. A. H. Shapiro, M. Y. Jaffrin and S. L. Weinberg, "Peristaltic Pumping with Long Wavelengths at Low Reynolds Number," *Journal of Fluid Mechanics*, 37, no. 4 (1969): 700–825.
14. L.R. Young, C.M. Oman, D.G.D. Watt, K.E. Money, B.K. Lichtenberg, R.V. Kenyon and A.P. Arrott, "Sensory Adaptation to Weightlessness and Readaptation to One-g: An Overview," *Experimental Brain Research*, 64 (1986): 291–298; L.R. Young, M. Shelhamer and S. Modestino, "MIT/Canadian Vestibular Experiments on the Spacelab-1 Mission: 2. Visual Vestibular Tilt Interaction in Weightlessness," *Experimental Brain Research*, 64 (1986): 299–307.
15. R. W. Mann, "Kinesthetic Sensing for EMG Controlled 'Boston Arm'," *IEEE Transactions on Man-Machine Systems*, MMS-11 (1970), 110–115.
16. N. Glazer and D.P. Moynihan, *Beyond the Melting Pot* (Cambridge, MA: The MIT Press, 1963).
17. D.C. Bok and J.B. Wiesner, Foreword to Announcement, Joint Center for Urban Studies, 1980.
18. D.D. Rutstein and M. Eden, *Engineering and Living Systems: Interfaces and Opportunities*.
19. Ibid.
20. B. Sinclair, "Harvard, MIT, and the Ideal Technical Education."
21. J.R. Killian, *The Education of a College President.*

Chapter 2

EARLY PLANNING FOR HST BY MIT

Walter A. Rosenblith, Ph.D.

As I think back to the period of formation of the Harvard-MIT Division of Health Sciences and Technology (HST), I ask myself what were the factors that led to or allowed its formation and, perhaps immodestly, what I may have contributed. As Chairman of the MIT Faculty during the years from 1967 to 1969, and Associate Provost from 1969 to 1971, I was deeply involved in faculty discussions (curricula, new programs, student unrest, etc.). This, together with my other MIT activities and those related to the National Academy of Sciences, allowed me to be of some assistance to Presidents Howard W. Johnson and Jerome B. Wiesner in relation to the formation of HST. Thus, it might be useful for me to attempt to convey my own perspective on the events leading up to its creation.

It is important to understand that I came to MIT in 1951 with a rather international background. I was born in Vienna, Austria and moved to Berlin when I was ten. My family and I moved to Paris in the early 1930's at the time when Hitler was coming to power in Germany. There, I took courses in physics, mathematics, psychology, and history at the Sorbonne. Later I became more practical and obtained first a degree in Radio Engineering at the University of Bordeaux and an advanced degree at the Ecole Supérieure d'Electricité (one of the "grandes ecoles") in Paris.

As a non-citizen in France, I found it difficult to obtain a job in engineering. However, I obtained employment with a professor of medicine who was interested in the area of occupational medicine. He gave me the task of using relatively new electronic equipment to study the effects of extraordinarily loud noises on boilermakers who had worked in such an environment for prolonged periods of time. I was able to measure the levels of intense noise in the factory and obtain audiograms of several hundred workers.

During the summer of 1939 I was sent to the United States to learn about related research here. I visited a number of factories and the Bell Laboratories, but before I had finished my task, World War II broke out. My passport labeled me as "ex-Austrian." Being neither a French citizen nor a legal immigrant in the U.S., I was unable to obtain gainful employment; but I was able to obtain fellowships or their equivalent, first in the Department of Physics at New York University, then at the Cold Spring Harbor Biological Laboratories, where I measured the velocity of electric impulses in electric eels. Next, I obtained a graduate fellowship at the University of California at Los Angeles (UCLA) where the Physics Department had a strong group in acoustics.

During the war my fellowship became a junior teaching appointment at UCLA and, in 1943, I became an Assistant Professor of Physics at the South Dakota School of Mines (the "Mines") in Rapid City. They quickly sent me to a special program at MIT (run by Professor Gordon S. Brown) in order to learn more about how to teach courses in servomechanisms. At both UCLA and the Mines, I taught physics and communication engineering to special groups of Navy and Army students and later to civilians at the Mines. I obtained U.S. citizenship in 1946 while living in South Dakota. In 1947, I had the good fortune of being offered a position as Senior Research Associate at the Harvard Psycho-Acoustic Laboratory (PAL). After the war, PAL's highly reputed research staff was focused on basic research involving the auditory system (psychophysics, neurophysiology and speech communication).

In the late 1940's the Boston-Cambridge intellectual scene was greatly influenced by the ideas of the famous MIT mathematician Norbert Wiener, who had just published his book *Cybernetics or Control and Communication in the Animal and the Machine*.[1] I was invited to join the Wiener "Supper Seminar" and benefited from meeting colleagues from Harvard, Harvard Medical School and MIT.

During World War II, MIT's Radiation Laboratory (which had up to four thousand staff members from several fields of science and branches of engineering) played a key role in the development of radar. This turned out to be an outstanding model of interdisciplinary problem solving. At the end of the war, MIT tried to renew and expand its staff in both established departments and new laboratories. I was offered a position as Associate Professor in Electrical Engineering (EE) affiliated with two major laboratories—Acoustics and the Research Laboratory of Electronics (RLE). After some discussion, my title in EE was to be Associate Professor of Communication Biophysics, which was rather unusual, but in line with the tradition that EE had of acting as an incubator for new ventures.

Up to this point, I have dealt mainly with my own academic path as it might be relevant to my role in the formation of the HST program. Now I will try to outline certain aspects of the intellectual climate after World War II, both at MIT and in the country more generally, which, together with the thoughtful and thorough chapters written by my colleagues at both institutions, should aid in understanding how HST came about.

During World War II, this country's major efforts were in the production of weapons and relevant research and development. After the war, many scientific disciplines sought to incorporate up-to-date technology at their own research frontiers. This task was made easy by the fact that a large number of scientists and engineers had participated in major national projects—radar, computers, materials projects and the Manhattan Project. In the 1950's and 1960's, most R and D efforts related to space and weapons. During the same period, important discoveries in molecular biology were attracting the attention of the younger generation.

Around the time that I joined MIT (1951), concerns of the public and in particular of the Navy regarding effects of jet noise became widespread. The medical division of the National Research Council (NRC) put together a task force to study this problem. My early paper on industrial noise and industrial hearing loss[2] and my consultancies to several medical groups concerned with these problems were probably what led to my becoming the Chairperson of this task force. The task force visited several medical laboratories and spent a week at sea on an aircraft carrier. Our report led to a continuing and interdisciplinary NRC committee devoted to these issues.

Meanwhile, I tried to build a laboratory, the Communications Biophysics Laboratory (CBL), within RLE that would combine the area of auditory psychophysics with computerized study of the electric activity in the auditory nervous system and, more generally, of the brain. As the laboratory grew, there were colleagues, graduate students, post docs (many of them from other countries) and staff (including Ph.D. students from various departments) from several fields and disciplines. It also involved personnel from MIT's Lincoln Laboratory in the development of appropriate computers.

The Office of Scientific Research of the U.S. Air Force supported CBL in organizing an international symposium on sensory communication. I traveled extensively in Europe visiting laboratories in order to select, with the aid of an international organizing committee, outstanding scientists to be invited. Half a dozen European countries were represented, as were Japan and Mexico. During the week of the symposium, many of the participants visited relevant laboratories at MIT and other research institutions. The symposium proceedings appeared as a book, *Sensory Communication*,[3] which became a "classic." This whole process acquainted me with broad areas of physiology, which became targets for me and my colleagues in CBL to examine with the aid of the kind of computers then becoming available.

My whole career to this point had exposed me to various disciplines—physics, engineering, biology and medicine. These exposures left me well able to appreciate the need for new academic and research organizations. But the national climate was also changing. In December 1960, President-elect Kennedy appointed a pre-inaugural task force to suggest priorities in the areas of health and social security. That task force report had considerable influence on public policy in the next decade. One of its principal recommendations was that the President of the National Academy of Sciences (NAS) should arrange for the establishment of a National Academy of Medicine comparable to the NAS,[4] and it was recommended that such a new institution should recognize and honor the leaders in health research, teaching, patient care, and administration. It should also ensure a continuing body competent to advise the government and the public in questions of health.

In the middle of the 1960's, the NAS President established a new structure, a Board of Medicine. He selected the board's members, most of whom were physicians, with a few social scientists, one lawyer, and myself as the only engineer. The next half dozen years were occupied by intra-Academy institutional problems. The NAS complex had not yet settled its relations with the recently formed Academy of Engineering, which did not make the problems of dealing with yet another institution, one in the area of health and medicine, any easier. In 1970 the new body was accepted into the NAS complex as the Institute of Medicine (IOM). The charter members were primarily members of the former Board of Medicine to which were added half a dozen outstanding physicians. After overcoming many obstacles, the IOM has become a growing and increasingly prestigious body.[5]

Also in the early 1960's, then MIT President Julius A. Stratton invited me to join him in a meeting with Doctor James Shannon, the Director of the National Institutes of Health (NIH), who had come to visit MIT because he had been impressed with the number of research projects that the NIH was supporting at MIT. His question: Why were so many health related projects supported at a technical institute? Elsewhere in this volume the important succeeding visit by Doctor Shannon (after Howard W. Johnson had become MIT's President) is reported in great detail. In short, he came to offer MIT considerable resources to establish a medical school at MIT. MIT, wisely I feel, decided that this was not an appropriate step to take. However, as noted in relation to Shannon's earlier visit, this was the period during which many of my colleagues in mechanical, electrical, chemical and even nuclear engineering worked on projects that involved cooperation with medical people. One example was Professor Robert W. Mann and his students who developed "the Boston Arm."[6] And I might also note that then Provost Jerome B. Wiesner (an engineer) was deeply concerned with prosthetic devices that might ameliorate problems of blindness and deafness.

In 1967, MIT Press published a book, *The Coming Revolution in Medicine*,[7] by Dr. David D. Rutstein, a distinguished Professor of Preventive Medicine and Head of the Department of Preventive Medicine at the Harvard Medical School. The foreword was written by MIT's then Dean of the School of Engineering, Gordon S. Brown, who had appointed me several years earlier to chair a faculty committee on "Engineering and Living Systems." These events are indicative of changes that were taking place with respect to the boundaries between engineering and fields related to health and medicine.

In Chapter 1, Dr. Abelmann reviews early stages of Harvard/MIT cooperation mainly related to sanitary engineering and public health.

My curiosity led me to explore President Killian's "Memoirs"[8] regarding the outlook of MIT's leaders about possible interactions between engineering and biomedicine. In the mid-thirties, MIT's President Karl Compton (a distinguished physicist) and Vanever Bush had proposed a program in biological engineering. President Compton expressed his view that progress in biological engineering would benefit from multi-disciplinary approaches. Dr. Abelmann also enumerated some of the cooperative arrangements between MIT faculty members and opposite numbers in medical institutions. Some entailed research projects that needed complementary skills and others joint teaching. But it was in the post-war period that these arrangements gained in both scope and scale.

Thus, the intellectual climate in the country at large and at MIT in particular provided fertile ground in which to plant the seeds of what became HST. In this short paper it would be impossible to describe the many faculty groups and meetings that were in some sense forerunners of HST. Suffice it to say that in March 1970 (the year the IOM was founded), the faculty of the Harvard Medical School, under the leadership of Dean R. H. Ebert, approved the plan for a joint Harvard-MIT program. The MIT faculty had already held several regularly scheduled faculty meetings during which topics and issues related to what ultimately came to be known as the Joint Harvard-MIT Division on Health Sciences and Technology or HST were discussed. In these discussions, quite a few voices from different schools and departments were heard. During this whole period, my colleague Professor Murray Eden served as an effective link between the Harvard Medical School faculty and ours.

In April 1970 I had the privilege (as Associate Provost) of introducing the resolution that the MIT faculty voted on, expressing in the process the hope that this proposal would provide an opportunity for MIT to respond in a human, rational, and effective manner to the needs and expectations of our citizens. The faculty voted in favor of the novel venture, and now the seed could sprout.

On the Board of Medicine, I had become acquainted with Doctor Irving London; I was very impressed with his broad knowledge, his research and his willingness to look at new institutional forms that had to be created at the frontiers where medicine, the physical sciences and engineering meet. When it was time to find a Director for this new enterprise, I was enthusiastic in supporting the selection of Dr. London. His appointment turned out to be most fortunate. He has guided HST into its present fruitful and prospering position.

Notes

1. N. Wiener, *Cybernetics or Control and Communication in the Animal and the Machine* (New York: The Technology Press, John Wiley & Sons, 1948).
2. W.A. Rosenblith, *Industrial Noise and Industrial Deafness, Journal of Acoustical Society* 13 (1941): 80–85.
3. W.A. Rosenblith, Ed., *Sensory Communication: Contributions to the Symposium on Principles of Sensory Communications* (Cambridge, Mass: MIT Press, 1961).
4. The National Academy of Sciences was chartered by Congress in 1863, two years before the founding of MIT. It was to be an advisor to the federal government with respect to scientific and technological decisions. The Academy complex grew over the next century and today is called "The National Academies," Advisers to the Nation on Science, Engineering and Medicine, composed of the National Academy of Science, the National Academy of Engineering, the Institute of Medicine and the National Research Council.
5. E.D. Berkowitz, *History of the Institute of Medicine* (Washington, D.C.: National Academy Press, 1998).
6. R.W. Mann, *"Kinesthetic Sensing for the EMG Controlled 'Boston Arm',"* *IEEE Transaction on Man-Machine Systems*, MMS 11 (1970): 110–115.
7. D.D. Rutstein, *The Coming Revolution in Medicine* (Cambridge, Mass: The MIT Press, 1967).
8. J.R. Killian, Jr., *The Education of a College President: A Memoir* (Cambridge, Mass: The MIT Press, 1985).

Chapter 3

EARLY PLANNING FOR HST BY HARVARD

Robert H. Ebert, M.D.

This book tells the story of how a collaborative program between two major universities came into being, why it happened when it did, the difficulties encountered and the problem of institutionalizing a program responsible to two separate governing boards. As one of the storytellers involved at the beginning, I will relate what happened from my own viewpoint, while trying to record accurately what happened based on a review of all the archival material I could find at the Harvard Medical School Countway Library. I hope it will be useful to other universities contemplating inter-institutional collaboration. Perhaps it will to the degree that there are communalities of organization and authority for decision-making among all American universities. But a word of caution is in order. Harvard's organization is unique, a fact that made the initiation of planning easier and institutionalization more difficult. I know of no other American university with schools and faculties as relatively autonomous as Harvard's. The philosophy of "every tub on its own bottom" means that each school is responsible for its own budget, derived from its own portion of the university endowment and whatever other monies it can garner from tuition, grants and gifts. As a consequence, the dean of each school is given considerable freedom in what he or she may initiate in the way of programs, provided he or she can pay for them. (I speak of the time when I was Dean of the Faculty of Medicine, not of the present. I understand there is now an effort to integrate the activities of Harvard's various schools and faculties, a laudable goal.) Thus, it was relatively easy for me to initiate discussions with MIT without any formal authorization by the university administration. I did, of course, keep President Pusey informed; but there was nothing in writing until planning was under way. However, autonomy cuts both ways. It facilitates action, but it encourages a competitive environment between schools with overlapping interests—in this case, the Medical School and the School of Public Health. As we shall see, that competition slowed the process of institutionalization, making it more difficult for Harvard to agree on a final organization than for MIT.

The Social Environment

Whenever a university considers the development of a new program, particularly one that will require new resources, it becomes especially sensitive to the current social environment. Walter Abelmann recently told me that in his opinion the time was exactly right in the mid-1960's for the initiation of a joint program by two major universities. I believe he was right, but we made it just in time. In another few years it might have been too late, for 1966–1969 were the last years of an era that began at the end of World War II, an era of expansive optimism.

For those of us who have lived as adults through the period of history beginning in 1939 and ending in 1969, there are memories of fear, resolve, triumph and optimism. There was fear at the start of World War II that Nazi Germany with the support of other fascist countries (and, temporarily, Communist Russia) would subjugate the free world. This was followed after the attack on Pearl Harbor by the resolve to commit all of our national resources to the defeat of the Axis powers. And at the end of World War II there was the feeling that good had triumphed over evil. There was also the belief that this country could accomplish anything it set out to do, no matter how difficult.

There was even faith in government, something difficult to imagine today, a belief that working together, the public and private sectors could accomplish a scientific revolution in any area we wished. The so-called Manhattan Project was the paradigm for government and university scientists working together to accomplish the seemingly impossible, the harnessing of nuclear power to create a super bomb. I can vouch for its destructive power, having helped care for victims of the bomb in Nagasaki. But there was also the hope that nuclear power could be used for the good of mankind. Most important of all was the message to the American public and their representatives in Congress. If we could produce an atomic bomb by a concerted effort during a time of war, why not tackle disease with the same vigor and resources in a time of peace. The nation's universities and medical schools became the vehicles for fulfilling the promise of science in the war against disease.

Even the Korean War, the Cold War with Russia, the rise of Communism in China and the constant threat of nuclear war did not dampen the feeling of national optimism. We would still triumph in the long term. Nor was there the view that social programs initiated by the Federal Government were too expensive. Legislation creating Medicare, Medicaid and a variety of social programs was passed during Lyndon Johnson's tenure as President despite our deeper and deeper involvement in the Vietnam War. We could still afford guns and butter. It was the right time to start an expansive new program, but not the best time to institutionalize it. A dramatic change in the social environment became evident in 1969.

Early Beginnings

David Rutstein, Chairman of Harvard's Department of Preventive Medicine, more than any other Harvard person was responsible for cultivating a relationship between Harvard and MIT that was finally to culminate in the present program. His enthusiasm for joining forces with MIT in order to foster bioengineering in the Harvard Medical School is reflected in a memorandum he wrote in June of 1964. He had just met with an *ad hoc* committee on biomedical engineering at MIT. Here is what he said:

> This meeting provided a real opportunity for the exchange of information on plans of Massachusetts Institute of Technology for the field of biomedical engineering. There is increasing activity year by year at the Massachusetts Institute of Technology in the field and one might guess that it will become an important activity for them and will demand joint planning on the part of both schools. One could look forward to

a smooth evolution by a joint program which would widen the opportunities of candidates in this field in which individual programs of each school would supplement the other . . . The desirability was also indicated of the eventual appointment of a joint committee on which both schools would be represented.[1]

Rutstein's perception of a growing interest in bioengineering at MIT was certainly correct. In May 1964, Gordon Brown, Dean of Engineering, asked a small number of his colleagues at MIT to give their opinion about where they thought bioengineering would be heading over the next five to ten years. Did they think there were major forces that would shape the future of bioengineering nationally, and, if so, what should the Engineering Council do to develop the field at MIT? He asked also for an inventory of teaching and research within the scope of what was loosely being called bioengineering. Was there sufficient interest among faculty and students to make a development effort worth while?[2]

Pressure came from another front as well. James Shannon, the powerful Director of the National Institutes of Health (NIH), believed that medical research and development required input from the engineering sciences in order to flourish fully. He further believed that a new medical school based at a university committed to engineering, such as MIT, could catalyze the development of a new field of bioengineering. To this end he visited with Jerome Wiesner, Dean of MIT's School of Science, and President Howard Johnson to suggest that MIT start such a medical school. He offered a grant of $50,000,000 to initiate the new school. (In those days Shannon had the power to deliver on such a promise.) Despite the magnitude of the offer, and the potential for a major development in bioengineering, the MIT administration decided not to start a medical school. Fifty million dollars would not fully fund the effort; there were other priorities. Certainly Boston did not need a fourth medical school. Perhaps collaboration with an existing medical school would be more prudent. Rejection of the medical school proposal, however, did not reflect any diminution in interest in bioengineering. Just the opposite. A new medical school might prove a distraction rather than a catalyst for a major bioengineering program.

Rutstein with his MIT partner, Professor Murray Eden, had already planted the idea of collaboration between the Harvard Medical School (HMS) and MIT. As early as March of 1964 the idea of a joint "biomedical technological resource" based in Harvard's Department of Physiology was explored with the HMS administration.[3] While the laboratory was never established, Rutstein and Eden were not discouraged. They continued to pursue other avenues for collaboration.

Response to Dean Brown's request was strongly positive. An inventory of bioengineering activities by MIT faculty members provided evidence for a substantial investment in the field. There was considerable enthusiasm for expanding research and education in bioengineering. The *ad hoc* committee referred to by Rutstein was succeeded by a committee on engineering and living systems, which in turn was the predecessor of the Harvard-MIT Joint Committee on Engineering and Living Systems established in 1967. More about that later.

Interest in bioengineering was not as intense at HMS as at MIT, in part because of the decentralized character of the Medical School and its teaching hospitals. When an inventory of collaborative bioengineering projects was finally put together in 1968, everyone was surprised to discover the magnitude of the interest. But even in 1964–65 there was visible evidence of an interest in biophysics and bioengineering. Arthur Solomon came to HMS in 1946 to establish a biophysics laboratory. Bert Vallee joined the faculty in 1951 to start a biophysics laboratory in the Department of Medicine at the Peter Bent Brigham Hospital. The Massachusetts General Hospital (MGH) developed a physics research laboratory under the direction of Gordon Brownell, who held a professorial appointment at MIT. The Eaton-Peabody Laboratory at the Massachusetts Eye and Ear Infirmary (MEEI) operated jointly with the MIT Research Laboratory of Electronics. Professor Gerald Austen at the MGH was interested in the development of synthetic surgical implants. The Department of Orthopedics worked on the development of more effective prostheses.

Interest of the Harvard Medical School faculty was divided, however. There was far greater interest among members of the clinical faculty in hospital departments than among members of the preclinical departments. The only other island of interest in bioengineering was in the Division of Applied Physics in the Faculty of Arts and Sciences at Harvard. Chairman Harvey Brooks was a participant in the earliest stages of joint planning.

I assumed the position of Dean of the Faculty of Medicine in July 1965 and quickly learned from Associate Dean Henry Meadow and Professor Rutstein of the interest of some members of the Medical School faculty in bioengineering. I was further informed about the growing interest in the field at MIT. Early in December I received a cordial letter from Jerome Wiesner, then Dean of the School of Science at MIT, in which he made the following comments:

> As you are undoubtedly aware, MIT, and particularly MIT's School of Engineering and Science, have had friendly and fruitful relations with several of your departments. These contacts have been in basic research fields, as well as such areas as biomathematics, biomedical instrumentation, use of computers, etc. In recent years the traffic in these interfaces seems to have increased. At MIT, a sizable body of engineering and applied science faculty and students with a strong interest in living systems has emerged. We are also aware of complementary interests at your institution. Therefore, it would seem appropriate for us to hold some preliminary discussions on likely directions and trends. Perhaps a small, joint committee could explore these matters after we have had an opportunity to talk about mutual interests.[4]

Although I cannot be certain of the timing, I believe this letter followed an informal conversation we had at a Cambridge social gathering during which we talked about these matters. I know that I was aware at this time of Shannon's proposal for an MIT medical school and the response.

I quickly followed up on Dr. Wiesner's letter, and beginning early 1966 a series of meetings were held with a number of people from both institutions. The principal planners were Wiesner, Walter Rosenblith and Eden from MIT and Rutstein, Meadow and Ebert from HMS. Early on Harvey Brooks indicated his interest in participating in any joint effort that might develop. In the course of these conversations it became evident that MIT needed access to a medical school if it were to fulfill the growing demand for work on living systems. I also became aware that there was substantial interest in bioengineering in the clinical faculty at Harvard. A fruitful collaboration appeared to be possible.

But I had another reason for wanting a joint program. I was well aware that Harvard's teaching hospitals did not need the Medical School's permission to forge collaborative relationships with MIT. They already existed. Since World War II the MGH in particular had cultivated a close working relationship with MIT. I felt that the Medical School was in a good position to coordinate activities with MIT, including those in the hospitals. Nor was I unaware of the potential competition with HMS had MIT decided to start a medical school. Rather than go to the expense of building a new teaching hospital, it would be natural to seek an affiliation with an existing hospital, possibly the MGH. There was no binding contract between Harvard and the MGH (nor with any other Harvard hospital) that would prevent the MGH from forming a second affiliation. Only tradition and the strong Harvard ties on the MGH Board of Trustees would prevent such an action. After spending a year at the MGH as Head of the Department of Medicine, I knew firsthand of the intense feeling of independence at that institution.

It was in everyone's interest to develop a collaborative relationship between Harvard Medical School and MIT. In addition, I found great pleasure in working with Wiesner and Rosenblith. Both were highly intelligent, creative people, who showed great understanding of the difficulties inherent in any effort to bring two universities together in a collaborative relationship. Yet they were determined to try.

Formal Planning Begins—First Phase

In early 1967 Harvard's President Pusey and MIT's President Johnson were asked to authorize the appointment of a joint Harvard-MIT Committee on Engineering and Living Systems. There is nothing in writing in my files about the appointment of the Committee until August 9, 1967, at which time I wrote to President Pusey about a proposed press release. In that letter I noted that most of the negotiations were carried on orally so that he would find no earlier letter from me in his own files. I reminded him that Harvey Brooks and I felt a cooperative effort should be explored and to this end had asked Alexander Leaf, Elkan Blout, Philip Drinker and David Rutstein to join the two of us for Harvard to meet with an MIT group consisting of Jerome Wiesner, Gordon Brown, Robert Alberti, Walter Rosenblith, Irwin Sizer and Murray Eden to form a Joint Committee on Engineering and Living Systems (JCELS). I mention this to emphasize the comparative freedom I had to act on the initiatives of the joint committee. Later in this chapter it will become evident that I did not have the same freedom when the time came to institutionalize a collaborative effort.

The charge to the committee was written by David Rutstein with editorial help from Murray Eden.[5] In the preamble the congruence of Harvard's and MIT's needs was noted as follows:

- Engineers have developed mathematical models for dealing with complex systems, but have little opportunity to apply these models to living systems. MIT faculty need better access to providers of medical care in an academic setting.

- Clinical medicine needs access to engineers expert in instrumentation and other engineering sciences. Biology and biochemistry are insufficient as the only basis for medical science. There needs to be greater use of the physical sciences and mathematics.

Based on these premises the preamble went on to discuss three areas in which collaboration could be fruitful: education, research and medical care.

- *Education.* There is little opportunity for medical students interested in the physical sciences, mathematics and engineering to exploit these interests in medical school. For MIT students there is insufficient opportunity to study living systems.
- *Research.* Four opportunities were noted:
  1. Systems analysis and operations research applied to medical care planning.
  2. Devices attached to patients.
  3. Automation of laboratory technologies.
  4. Collaboration in basic research.

- *Medical care.* Two areas were listed:
  1. Planning for medical manpower.
  2. Regional organization of medical care facilities.

The actual charge to the joint committee read as follows:

> The Joint Committee on Engineering and Living Systems of Harvard University and Massachusetts Institute of Technology is charged with the exploration of and recommendations concerning the development of collaborative efforts for planning of a long-range program and short-term studies in education, research and medical care. The Committee is also charged with maintaining administrative interrelationships on all joint activities.

I cannot find minutes of the first meeting of the Joint Committee, but at that meeting it was agreed to appoint several working subcommittees, the first of which was the subcommittee on medical care. That subcommittee held its first meeting on May 10, 1967, and reported to the full committee on May 25. At the May 25 meeting, Philip Drinker was appointed secretary and all subsequent meetings of the Joint Committee were faithfully reported by Dr. Drinker. At the next meeting of the Joint Committee on July 5, two other subcommittees were appointed—a subcommittee on research and one on education. Both were asked to consider the structure of a "collaborative institute which would bring academic and research personnel with different interests and projects together in one environment."[6] (This charge apparently came from the MIT summer study, which will be discussed a little later.) The more specific charges to the two subcommittees will be given when the deliberations of each of the subcommittees are presented.

The undertakings influenced the deliberations of the Joint Committee, the summer study sponsored by the MIT Committee on Engineering and Living Systems held June 13–23, 1967, at the American Academy of Arts and Sciences, and the study done by Harvard and MIT in response to a request for a proposal from the National Academy of Engineering. The latter was initiated and funded by James Shannon at the NIH. Before discussing the work of the Joint Committee, I will summarize these two initiatives.

The Summer Study on MIT's Future Role in the Life and Health Sciences June 13–23, 1967

At the May 25th meeting of JCELS, Murray Eden discussed plans for the summer study and invited all members of the Joint Committee to attend all or part of the sessions. Eden said the purpose of the meeting was " . . . to determine areas of concern and dedication among the MIT faculty in problems in engineering and living systems."[7] A number of Harvard members of the Joint Committee did attend along with other members of the Harvard Medical School faculty. There were guests from other area medical schools as well. James Shannon attended several sessions using his visit as an opportunity to announce his intention to commission a national study of bioengineering.

The conference was organized around a series of panels, each of which had a specific charge. The three most important were Panel B-1, medicine and public health; Panel B-2, mission-oriented research development and evaluation; and B-3, education. Members of Panels B-1 and B-2 were unanimous in their recommendations. There was less unanimity among members of Panel B-3. Here are the recommendations:

- Panel B-1 proposed a research and development institute jointly administered by Harvard and MIT that would consider problems of health and medical care planning and the delivery of care. The joint facility would use as its laboratory the provision of care in a complex urban setting. The staff would be largely full-time.

- Panel B-2 recommended an interdisciplinary laboratory for engineering and biology to be administered by MIT but with collaboration from other institutions. It would have two main functions: basic research at the interface of biology and engineering, and the development of new biomedical equipment.
- Panel B-3. Although there was disagreement among panel members about what should be done, there was general agreement about the needs. These were:
  1. Courses for engineers and biologists at MIT who wish to become medical scientists.
  2. A combined Harvard-MIT premedical and medical program.
  3. Postgraduate research and training programs.[8]

The summer study was discussed by the Joint Committee at both its July and September meetings. Eden reported that the summer study had been well attended by MIT faculty, who expressed considerable enthusiasm for the recommendations of the panels. There was some criticism, however, that the report of the panels lacked specificity.

The observations by Dr. Wiesner at the September meeting were particularly relevant to the deliberations of the Joint Committee. He asked how far should MIT go with medical education since there seemed to be general agreement at the summer study that some sort of joint Harvard-MIT education program should be developed. He added that the development of an interdisciplinary laboratory for research and development was an issue for MIT to address before any collaborative arrangements could be made with Harvard or any other institution.[9]

National Academy of Engineering Commissioned Study

Early in 1967 Dr. Shannon spoke to Wiesner and Ebert about his plan to ask several universities to study national trends in bioengineering. He subsequently asked the National Academy of Engineering (NAE) to administer an NIH grant provided to fund the studies.[10] In November of 1967 a letter was sent to Presidents Johnson and Pusey in which a request for a proposal was outlined by Dr. John Truxal, Chairman of the NAE Committee on the Interplay of Engineering with Biology and Medicine.[11] The charge to Truxal's committee was to determine how engineering, the physical, biological, medical, social and management sciences could collaborate in such a way as to improve the quality and distribution of medical care. The request for a proposal was referred to the Joint Harvard-MIT Committee and, at its December 6, 1967, meeting, it was decided to ask Eden and Rutstein to prepare a proposal to meet the deadline of January 2, 1968.[12]

In preparation of their proposal, Rutstein and Eden used the MIT summer study and the deliberations of the Joint Committee as the basis for the study. Twenty-six proposals were submitted to the NAE by January 2, many of which came from universities represented by members of Truxal's committee.[13] To avoid conflict of interest, a special selection committee was appointed. Selections were made in mid-January, and the Harvard-MIT proposal was one of six to be funded. An award of $37,000 was made for the duration of the study.

At the March 27, 1968 meeting of JCELS, Professor Eden announced a steering committee for the NAE contract study consisting of Drinker, Eden, Meadow, J. F. O'Connor and Rutstein. He listed fourteen task forces to be appointed with suggestions for membership. Ten of these related to research and development, ranging from skeletal prostheses to subcellular engineering. Two task forces dealt with medical care, one on macrosystems and one on microsystems. Two task forces dealt with education, bioengineering curricula and continuing education. (A complete list of task forces is given in the Notes.[14]) A preliminary report of the study was presented to the National Academy of Engineering in Washington on October 29, 1968.[15] Based on the comments made at that meeting, revisions were made, and a final report was submitted in December.

The task force reports dealing with education and medical care differed little from the deliberations of the JCELS and its subcommittees. The task forces dealing with specific areas of research and development did supplement the work of the research subcommittee, but the conclusions were pretty much the same. This being the case, I shall simply incorporate the findings of the NAE study into the conclusions of the JCELS and its subcommittees.

The importance of the NAE contract study was not in its recommendations. It was important because it bolstered the conviction of the members of the JCELS that their deliberations were in the mainstream of a national commitment to support the bringing together of engineering and medicine. It encouraged the belief that NIH money would be available for a joint Harvard-MIT school.

I will now return to a discussion of the deliberations of the JCELS. The Committee met regularly from May 1967 until June 1969. In the early sessions, most of the Committee's work was devoted to a discussion of subcommittee reports, the conclusions of the MIT summer study and the progress of the NAE contract. Later, time was spent discussing the structure of a Harvard-MIT "school" to administer a joint program. Finally, before the Committee was dissolved, a grant proposal to The Commonwealth Fund was prepared asking for money to support the final stages of planning. Once the grant was approved, the second stage of planning began.[16]

I shall first report on the deliberations of each of the subcommittees beginning with the subcommittee on medical care. I will then discuss the various structural proposals for a "school" presented to the JCELS, following which I will talk about The Commonwealth Fund proposal.

The *Subcommittee on Medical Care* began its deliberations May 10, 1967, with statements by Rosenblith and Rutstein to the effect that the application of technology in both the scientific and management areas could do much to improve the provision of health care. The committee was asked to consider how collaboration between MIT and Harvard could bring this about. The first meeting was devoted to reports from members of the committee about initiatives already under way or planned. Leona Baumgartner reviewed her study of health services offered by the City of Cambridge and her participation in planning for the expansion of the Cambridge City Hospital. She felt that the City of Cambridge offered an exciting potential site for a joint MIT-Harvard systems analysis. Rutstein, Seeler and Mann reported on MIT's interest in health problems of the Cambridge population. Octo Barnett discussed a variety of applications of computer technology to medical care problems. Osler Peterson reported on his work in regional planning. Jerome Pollack reported on the nascent Harvard Community Health Plan, noting that the prime incentives for starting the plan were to provide a laboratory for teaching and research.

After these presentations there was vigorous discussion by the eighteen members present (of the twenty-one member subcommittee). Some were enthusiastic about the use of Cambridge and the Cambridge City Hospital as a laboratory for analysis. Others favored the use of a more established teaching hospital. Despite differences in opinion, there was considerable optimism about the potential of a collaborative effort.[17] Certainly there was greater faith in academic planning for health services than exists today.

The subcommittee continued to meet at regular intervals, and its deliberations were discussed by members of the Joint Committee. It soon became apparent that translating the perceived potential of a joint enterprise into a defined program was going to be very difficult. Was it better to develop *ad hoc* projects, bringing together medical, managerial and engineering skills, or should there be a study of needs and how to fulfill them, using methods such as operations research? The debate never came to closure. No one seemed able to define in precise terms what should be done.

Almost by default in December 1967, the subcommittee on medical care decided to recommend to its parent committee that the City of Cambridge and the Cambridge City Hospital would be a good place to start. In November James Hartgering had been appointed Commissioner of Health and Hospitals of the City of Cambridge and Lecturer at the Harvard Medical School. The appointment had been anticipated by the subcommittee, the members of which believed that Hartgering would be sympathetic to the idea of using Cambridge as a community laboratory. It was suggested that he might even be willing to work with a deputy commissioner, nominated by the subcommittee, who would be given the responsibility for planning a study. Hartgering was interested in working with a joint Harvard-MIT team. Since the Cambridge City Hospital had affiliated with Harvard in 1964, he already had a working relationship with HMS. The next step would be easy. Or would it be?

Hartgering was asked to join the subcommittee on medical care in December 1967,[18] a move thought to be a way of facilitating the hoped-for relationship. But—two months in office taught Hartgering that Cambridge politicians were not about to relinquish authority to academia. In January 1968 he reported to the subcommittee that the City Hospital administration had little real autonomy and that planning was highly politicized.[19] He reported to the subcommittee periodically about his plans for satellite health centers, a new emergency service and a revamped school health program. But nothing was ever done to engage the subcommittee in a more specific plan for a joint Harvard-MIT program. The idea of using Cambridge as a community laboratory was never realized, partly because of politics, partly because no concrete plan was ever devised.

One other medical care proposal was considered by JCELS. Sherman, Reiffen and Rodman in December 1967 submitted a proposal for "An Ambulatory Health Care Program" to be a joint project of Lincoln Laboratory and the MIT Medical Department. It would start as a pilot at MIT, then expand to Cambridge. The idea was to develop computer-assisted history-taking, diagnosis and treatment. Some initial planning occurred, although no action was taken by the Joint Committee. It subsequently reappeared a year later as a joint project of Lincoln Laboratory and the Beth Israel Hospital, now called "Ambulatory Care Service."[20] I received a copy of the proposal in December 1968 signed by Howard Hiatt and Matthew Budd for the Beth Israel and Sherman and Reiffen for the Lincoln Laboratory. I was told the proposal was to be submitted to The Commonwealth Fund and the Hartford Foundation.[21]

When the Sherman-Reiffen-Rodman proposal was originally discussed at the JCELS, the observation was made that the greatest use of computers to date had been to automate old procedures. What was needed was a group of researchers who were not interested in institutionalizing the past. But the idea put forward at the MIT summer study to create a joint MIT-Harvard institute to work on problems of medical care never came to fruition.

Education Subcommittee. On November 21, 1966, more than seven months before the Education Subcommittee was appointed, I received a letter from Alexander Leaf, reporting on his conversation with Dean Irwin Sizer at MIT about a six-year B.S., M.D. program. Both Leaf and Sizer felt that the premedical program in biology at MIT could easily be combined with the medical degree program at Harvard, eliminating one year from each without sacrificing intellectual content. Leaf also called attention in a footnote to his letter that Rutstein was interested in developing a premed bioengineering curriculum.

This idea of a combined B.S.M.D. curriculum was actively pursued during the life of the subcommittee. Later it was proposed to develop a bioengineering-premedical curriculum to be combined with the M.D. program. These two themes merged in the final deliberations of the subcommittee. A third issue demanding attention was the need for MIT graduate students to have access to human biology if bioengineering was to flourish. Clearly it would be advantageous for MIT if courses could be taken at HMS, thus avoiding an expensive duplication of faculty.

The Education Subcommittee was appointed in July 1967 with Alexander Leaf and Irwin Sizer as co-chairmen.[22] Its broad charge was to look at all possible areas for collaboration in education between the two institutions. But special reference was made to a premedical-medical degree program to shorten the educational process and make it more efficient. It was also to look at opportunities for students at

MIT in engineering and the physical sciences to enroll in Harvard Medical School courses and for medical students to take MIT courses. Finally, the subcommittee was asked to look at potential opportunities for graduate students from both universities to participate in collaborative research and educational programs.

Much of the early meetings of the Education Subcommittee was devoted to the six-year B.S.M.D. program. When a specific proposal was made to the parent committee, it was criticized for being too inflexible. Dr. Wiesner in particular was against the loss of a flexible curriculum in the first year. The subcommittee also had difficulty in defining a core curriculum. When it reported this at the December 1967 meeting of the JCELS, there was further criticism by some members, who felt that the premedical part of the curriculum was too much oriented to biology. At that meeting Eden and Siebert agreed to develop a proposal for a bioengineering premedical curriculum.[23]

Even before this there had been discussions in the subcommittee about a bioengineering curriculum designed for premedical students. There was concern that watered-down courses in physics and mathematics would be designed for premedical students. But Professor Zacharias of MIT vigorously defended the concept. He argued that the teaching of the physical sciences to premedical students could be made just as rigorous as the courses designed for engineers, but he insisted that the material taught should have relevance to medicine. (Abraham Flexner made the same argument in 1910, when he described how medical students should be taught the basic medical sciences.) While agreeing with Zacharias' concept, some members of the subcommittee questioned the ability of the faculty to teach such courses.

On January 2, 1968, the Education Subcommittee approved a six-year B.S.M.D. program with three premedical years based on a proposal from MIT's Department of Biology and three years at HMS.[24] This was presented to the JCELS at its January 11 meeting where, after considerable discussion, the combined curriculum was accepted in principle. But the subcommittee was urged to consider this curriculum in relation to the bioengineering premedical curriculum presently being prepared.[25]

At subsequent meetings of both the subcommittee and the JCELS, there continued to be debate about the six-year program. Professor Blout reported on his conversation with faculty members in the Faculty of Arts and Sciences at Harvard. Comments ranged from "great" to "not radical enough."[26] Meanwhile, Murray Eden spoke to the

JCELS about the difficulties in developing a single bioengineering curriculum. At the March 27 meeting he described a problem-oriented curriculum in which students would do research and develop course work around the needs of their research projects.[27]

In the spring of 1968 both the HMS Curriculum Committee and the MIT Committee on Educational Policy approved the six-year program, but with the reservation that it seemed too restrictive. Based on these criticisms, the Education Subcommittee decided to abandon its original plan. On May 1, 1968, it reported to the JCELS that it was designing a more flexible curriculum.[28] Ten to twelve students would be chosen at the end of the second year at MIT to participate in a special B.S.M.D. program tailored to individual needs and interests. This raised the question of preferential admission to Harvard Medical School at the end of two years at MIT.

There continued to be a debate in the Education Subcommittee about the most appropriate curriculum for a combined program, during which it was decided that it was more important to have a truly innovative curriculum rather than one shortened to six years.

Finally, at its meeting on January 27, 1969, the subcommittee agreed to recommend a combined B.S.M.D. with one track for students interested in biology and a second for students who wished a bioengineering background. The latter track would use electrical engineering as the bioengineering preparation, it being argued that it was impossible to devise a single bioengineering curriculum. The opinion was expressed in the subcommittee that if this proposal was rejected, there was little reason for the subcommittee to continue.[29]

On January 29, the JCELS accepted the proposal based on the four principles enunciated in the written proposal:

1. Abolish the artificial separation of premedical and medical education.
2. Bring together faculties with different interests and backgrounds.
3. Allow students to intermingle knowledge and cultures from very different intellectual disciplines.
4. Develop a new breed of bioscientists and physician-engineers.[30]

Early admission to the medical school did not appear to be an insurmountable problem, but there was growing concern among members of Harvard's preclinical faculty that MIT was in effect developing a two-year medical school. The reason for this will become apparent when the second phase of planning is described.

Research Subcommittee. The Research Subcommittee was appointed in July 1967 with Murray Eden as the co-chairman for MIT. A Harvard co-chairman was not appointed until December. The subcommittee was asked (1) to examine, with the Medical Care Subcommittee, the feasibility of a joint research institute recommended by the MIT summer study, and (2) to study how to strengthen ongoing collaborative research efforts.[31]

The subcommittee did not meet until December 1967 by which time Judah Folkman, newly appointed Professor of Surgery at Children's Hospital, had been appointed the co-chairman. Elkan Blout reported at the January 11, 1968, meeting of the JCELS that at its first meeting the subcommittee had defined three areas of effort:

1. Support and develop areas of collaborative basic research;
2. Support new applications of existing technologies in medicine and biology; and
3. Assess the full scope of collaborative research between MIT and Harvard now under way.

To this latter end Joseph Parrish, the subcommittee's secretary, was asked to catalog all research in the Harvard medical area being done in collaboration with MIT faculty and to prepare a brochure similar to the one published by MIT in January 1967.[32]

Relatively few meetings of the Research Subcommittee were held. Reports to the JCELS dealt largely with the progress of Parrish's cataloging of collaborative research projects. He interviewed 140 individuals and discovered that most MIT collaborators were identified by personal contact. The majority were being supported by the NIH. Most Harvard investigators were unaware of other collaborative efforts. They expressed surprise at the extent of the collaboration between Harvard and MIT faculty. As suspected, most of the Harvard research was being done in the teaching hospitals. The major research areas were membrane studies, electronic instrumentation, radiobiology, mechanical engineering and life support systems, chemical engineering and antithrombogenic surface research. A research brochure describing more than 100 collaborative research projects was published in December 1968.

The Research Subcommittee appears to have done little else. I can find no record of joint meetings with the Medical Care Subcommittee to discuss a research institute. That idea appears to have been dropped. Judah Folkman and Professor Edward Merrill from MIT worked together on a broad collaborative program on antithrombogenic surfaces involving MIT workers and most Harvard hospitals. This project was subsequently funded by the NIH.

Other Activities of the Joint Committee on Engineering and Living Systems

By October of 1968 several things had become evident. There was sufficient interest among members of both faculties to continue planning; but without someone to direct planning, the process had become cumbersome and inefficient. Funds were needed to launch a more structured plan before it could be taken to both the MIT and HMS faculties for their approval and to the two universities' governing boards. At the October 24, 1968, meeting of the JCELS, there began to be serious discussions of how to address these issues. There was also the question of what kind of an organization was needed in order to establish a viable administrative arrangement involving both universities.

Mr. Meadow outlined several general principles to guide the development of a new organization. It should have major status in both universities but should be non-parasitic on either institution. The most appropriate designation for this new institution would be "school." Questions were asked about what powers the "school" would have. It was agreed that it should be able to make new faculty appointments, although there would be defined limits on the types of staff appointments. It would not grant degrees and, finally, some level of necessary funding should be established. Meadow urged that it not have a separate corporate identity so that either MIT or Harvard could receive funds earmarked for the school. This would not, however, preclude fund raising by the school.[33]

At subsequent meetings there was further discussion of governance. The school would be headed by a dean, who would also be the CEO. He would report to a governing board, the members of which would include the president of both universities, the provost of MIT, the dean of HMS and several other members chosen by the two presidents. The dean of the new school would have several advisory committees and possibly a visiting committee.

At the November 15, 1968, meeting of the JCELS, Professor Rosenblith reported that he and Irving London (Chairman of the Department of Medicine at Albert Einstein University) had had several visits with Quigg Newton and Colin MacLeod of The Commonwealth Fund and were told that the Fund was very interested in bioengineering. Subsequent visits by Wiesner and Ebert not only confirmed commitment to bioengineering but provided an invitation to submit a grant application for planning. This was an encouraging development, since a grant in the neighborhood of $500,000 would certainly facilitate planning. At the November meeting of the JCELS, the co-chairmen appointed a planning subcommittee of Eden, Meadow, Rosenblith, Rutstein and London to prepare a proposal. Irving London, although not a member of either faculty, was much interested in the joint effort. It was agreed that he should be retained as a consultant to the JCELS, be made a full member of the Planning Subcommittee and should be an author of the proposal.[34]

The Planning Subcommittee, working with dispatch, had a draft proposal ready for review by the JCELS at its December 2 meeting.[35] Some revisions were made, based on the discussions at that meeting. In a letter to Quigg Newton, President of The Commonwealth Fund, jointly signed by Provost Wiesner and me dated December 9, 1968, we said that we were submitting a grant proposal "with great enthusiasm." The letter indicated that Irving London had agreed to act as a major consultant to the program and would carry " . . . a substantial portion of the planning burden." The request was for $655,000.

In a letter to President Pusey dated December 27, 1968, asking for a letter of support for the grant proposal to be sent to Quigg Newton, I mentioned the need to bring someone on full time to coordinate planning. I said that Dr. London had been much involved in the discussions the past year and would, I believed, take on the job of coordinator. The Commonwealth Fund administration had a very high regard for Irving London and I knew would welcome his full-time involvement in planning. At the February 22 meeting of JCELS, Dr. Wiesner reported that he and Ebert had met with Newton, MacLeod and Terrence Keenan the day before and were told that an initial grant for $300,000 would be made to cover the summer study with additional funding to come after our plans were better defined.[36] The summer study had been planned by the committee as a way of accelerating the planning process.

A few days later I sent a memorandum to Henry Meadow saying that the Commonwealth Board wanted a more specific budget for the period following the summer study. The Board would reconsider the remainder of the grant at its May meeting. I said that Terry Keenan planned to come to Boston the first week in March to discuss the budget with him in preparation for the May meeting. I also said that Terry Keenan wanted to allay one of The Commonwealth Fund Board member's concern. Calvin Plimpton, also a member of the Board of the University of Massachusetts, wanted to be sure that we weren't starting another medical school.[37]

A new budget was submitted by Henry Meadow on March 10,

1969. Terry Keenan was reassured that we were not starting a new medical school. Everything was now in order for final action by The Commonwealth Fund Board. The Board approved an additional grant of $355,000, and Presidents Pusey and Jonnson were so informed in a letter dated May 29. By this time Irving London had agreed to become the full-time coordinator and to assume the position of dean and CEO of the new school if and when it was approved by the two governing boards. There is no doubt in my mind about the importance of Irving London's role. Had he not accepted the leadership role, I doubt that the present Harvard-MIT Division of Health Sciences and Technology would exist today. The Joint Committee on Engineering and Living Systems submitted its final report to the two presidents on July 1, 1969, and asked to be discharged, thus ending the first planning phase.[38]

Change in the Social Environment

The Vietnam War "radicalized" many college students, particularly in the elite universities. By 1969 there were eruptions on the campuses of several major universities, including Harvard. In the spring of 1969, University Hall in Harvard Yard was occupied by a group of students belonging to the SDS (Students for a Democratic Society). The majority of Harvard students did not take this action very seriously until it was decided to call in the Cambridge police one early morning in April. There was a confrontation, a few heads were bloodied, and University Hall was reclaimed. What was unexpected was the reaction of the majority of students. Overnight they were radicalized. Classes were suspended, students held rallies, and the faculty spent much of the remainder of the term debating what had happened and what should be done.

One might have expected the professional schools, particularly the medical school, to have been immune from this unrest. But one of the "causes" being pursued by SDS was the purchase of apartment buildings in the Medical Area to be demolished to create a new site for what was then called the Affiliated Hospitals Center, later the Brigham and Women's Hospital. One of the demands of the students who occupied University Hall was "Stop the eviction of Francis Street tenants." The fact that none had been evicted did not dissuade the SDS. Thus, student unrest spilled over into the Medical Area. The class admitted in the fall of 1969 had a significant number of Harvard students who had been radicalized by the events in April. It became their mission to reform the Harvard Medical School, starting with the Francis Street apartment buildings purchased by Harvard. I am not sure that the apartments would have been demolished had there not been the aftermath of the University Hall occupation. They remain today, however, and the new hospital was finally built without the loss of any housing. In fact, Harvard helped build new housing in the area. I mention these events because they preoccupied the Harvard University administration for many months. I had to spend a considerable amount of time meeting with students and faculty, all of which was a distraction from the major business of the dean's office, including the joint program.

In November, Richard Nixon won the Presidential election. Coincident with his taking office it became evident that the NIH budget could not increase by 15 percent a year indefinitely. With Shannon's retirement there was no longer the powerful advocate for scientific medicine that he had become. This was inevitable, just as it was inevitable that the rate of increase in the NIH budget would drop. The great optimism about scientific medicine had begun to wane. No longer was it reasonable to think that any innovative idea could persuade the NIH to provide support. All of this had its effect on fund raising, as we shall see a little later.

The Second Phase of Planning

With the discharge of the Joint Committee on Engineering and Living Systems, the second phase of planning began under the strong leadership of Irving London. The work was supervised by a Joint Faculty-Administration Committee, co-chaired by Wiesner and Ebert. This large committee was in turn divided into committees with specific missions. In some cases additional members were added. The Committee on Education in the Natural Sciences was co-chaired by Alexander Leaf and Boris Magasanik; Leon Eisenberg, Merton Kahne and Benson Snyder served as co-chairmen of a planning group in the social and behavioral sciences. The Committee on Health Care was composed of Paul Densen, Director of the Center for Community Health and Medical Care at Harvard; William Pounds, Dean of the Sloan School of Management; and Albert Seeler, Head of the Medical Department at MIT. The Committee on Administrative Structure was composed of Harvey Brooks, Paul Cusick (Comptroller of MIT), Robert Ebert, Henry Meadow, William Pounds, Walter Rosenblith and Jerome Wiesner. The latter committee made the most important recommendations.

There were urgent matters to be settled. It was necessary to define the administrative structure of the new institution. If there was to be a "school," what would be the extent of its academic authority, who would constitute its faculty, what educational programs would it be responsible for? All of this needed to be settled before a plan could be taken to the faculties of MIT and HMS for their approval and to the governing boards of the two universities for final action. That was a large order.

The summer of 1969 was a time for intensive planning. Plans were completed in the fall with a final proposal,[39] dated November 24, 1969, submitted to the MIT faculty and the HMS faculty. It was recommended that a new inter-university institution be established to be called The Harvard-MIT School of Health Sciences and Technology. It would be a school within the structure of MIT and a school in the Faculty of Medicine of Harvard. The new school would be governed by a joint governing board composed of the presidents of MIT and Harvard, members of each corporation and public members. There would be a joint administrative board appointed by the joint governing board. The Provost at MIT and the Dean of the Faculty of Medicine would alternate as chairman of the joint administrative board. It was anticipated that there would be six to eight members of the joint administrative board, including the Dean of the Harvard-MIT School of Health Sciences and Technology. Most members of the faculty of the new school would hold primary appointments in one or another of the parent universities.

Research and medical care were briefly mentioned in the proposal. Reference was made to the 150 joint research projects identified when an inventory was conducted in 1968. A purpose of the school would be to facilitate such collaboration as well as to initiate new programs. The examples of new programs given were environmental health sciences and biomaterials. Health care was referred to in general terms with the proviso that new programs should be developed in concert with the Harvard Center for Community Health and Medical Care, the Health Services of Harvard and MIT and the Sloan School of Management.

Much of the planning dealt with education. A subcommittee of the Education Committee, consisting of Blout, Siebert and Gross, proposed a far more flexible version of the combined B.S.-M.D. program discussed earlier. A five-year program was described, leading to a

B.S.-M.A., after which students could branch into a variety of doctoral programs, including an M.D. program. The program would be based at MIT, and a central part of the first five years would be human biology.

These suggestions were modified significantly when they were considered by the Committee on Administrative Structure. The recommendations of the latter committee were incorporated into the final proposal of November 24. This is what was decided:

- The Harvard-MIT School of Health Sciences and Technology would be a doctoral and postdoctoral school. It would not grant doctoral degrees, however. These would be awarded by the faculties where the final doctoral work was done.
- Undergraduates at Harvard and MIT could have an informal relationship with the joint school but would not be enrolled in it. Some courses would be open to them.
- Candidates for the M.D. degree would be chosen jointly by faculty from the Medical School and HST.
- Central to the success of the new curriculum would be the development of courses in human biology jointly taught by life scientists, physical scientists and engineers. These courses would be available to undergraduates at both universities as well as to medical students.

It is not surprising that concerns began to be expressed among members of the Harvard Medical School faculty about the magnitude of the proposed program and its impact on the Medical School. In committee discussions of the new school, it was proposed that forty to fifty students per year would enter the M.D. program. A larger group of students would be enrolled in human biology courses that would in effect cover much of what was being taught in the preclinical years at HMS. This presented several potential problems. In effect, was MIT, via the new school, starting a two-year medical school that would compete with Harvard's preclinical faculty? A distinguished member of the clinical faculty who had been active in all of the educational planning since 1966, wondered if this was the beginning of a trend that would transplant human biology from medical schools to faculties of arts and sciences, thereby causing medical schools to become two-year clinical schools. A more immediate concern of members of the clinical faculty who participated in the teaching of human biology was the strain on HMS resources if the clinical faculty had to teach at both Harvard and the new school located at MIT. This was the background for debate by the HMS faculty.

Consideration of the Proposed New Joint School of Health Sciences and Technology by the Medical Faculty

A joint program between MIT and HMS was first discussed at the September 29, 1967 meeting of the Faculty of Medicine chaired by President Pusey. At that meeting I gave a brief description of the work being done by the Joint Committee on Engineering and Living Systems. Dr. Leaf described the six-year combined B.S.-M.D. program under consideration. Dr. Blout explained that the research subcommittee had not met but talked about its agenda. Drs. Rabkin and Baumgartner spoke about the meetings of the Medical Care Subcommittee. There was no general discussion.

The first formal presentation to the Faculty of Medicine was made at the December 5, 1969, meeting, which I chaired in President Pusey's absence. I gave a general background statement describing the planning, including the role played by Irving London. I then extended a welcome to Professor Brooks from Harvard and Professors Rosenblith and Wiesner from MIT, who were kind enough to join the faculty in these discussions. Finally, I asked Dr. London to make the presentation. He began by stating that the Planning Committee recommended the establishment of a Harvard-MIT School of Health Sciences and Technology. He then went on to outline the plans for education, research and medical care. He described briefly the administrative structure of the new school, noting that it would not have departments. Most faculty would hold joint appointments in HST and a department at Harvard or MIT. An occasional person would hold an appointment only at the joint school. He emphasized that new funds would be sought to finance the enterprise, promising that it would not divert funds for existing programs at either university.

Professors Brooks, Rosenblith and Wiesner all spoke in support of the program. Dr. Wiesner stressed the need for a flexible administrative structure so that the school would not become a separate "institute." Instead it would draw together members of the two faculties. There was some general discussion in support of the proposal, but when Dr. Eisenberg moved that the faculty go on record in general support of the program, several members of the faculty said there had been too little time for debate. I therefore ruled that it would be unwise to ask for a vote. Discussion would continue at a future faculty meeting.[40]

At the next meeting of the Faculty of Medicine, held January 9, 1970, which I once again chaired in the absence of President Pusey, I began by ruling that no vote would be taken until the next meeting of the faculty so that there could be further consultations should questions arise that could not immediately be answered. There was a vigorous discussion, during which the following reservations were expressed:

- Dr. Howard Frazier worried that the departments of medicine would be overburdened if members had to assume an additional teaching load in human biology at the new school. Dr. London said that new faculty would be recruited, causing Dr. James Jandl to observe that it was hard for him to believe there was any shortage of teachers in view of the number of new appointments made at each faculty meeting (28 at this meeting).
- Dr. Eugene Kennedy wondered if a stream of students entering the clinical years from another program might further accentuate the division between the preclinical and clinical faculties. He also worried that there would be competition for the best students. These concerns were shared by Drs. Bernard Davis and David Hubel, both of whom deplored the atrophy of the preclinical departments relative to the size and strength of the clinical departments.
- Dr. Joel Alpers wondered what had motivated both MIT and Harvard other than curricular innovation. Did MIT need human biology? Had Harvard worried that MIT would start a new medical school? Was the new school really a two-year medical school?

There were also some positive reactions.

- Dr. Francis Moore said that the clinical departments had the capacity to do more clinical teaching and wondered if the proposed program " . . . might consistute a *new pathway* of entrance into an expanded clinical curriculum that would enable the school to grant a larger number of M.D. degrees."
- John Hedley-Whyte liked the idea of the new school but hoped that the emphasis might be on an undergraduate rather than doctoral curriculum so that medical education might be shortened.
- Dr. Jandl wondered if electrical engineering and physics might not be viewed as a prerequisite for the modern cardiologist or orthopedic surgeon. Perhaps the danger of a split between the preclinical and clinical disciplines was caused by a lack of relevance of the former to the latter. He strongly supported the proposal.[41]

The growing concern among some influential members of the HMS faculty could not be ignored. Answers had to be given to the reservations that had been expressed formally and informally. A more precise definition of the educational program was needed. Some estimate of the resources necessary to launch the joint effort had to be given. I asked a small *ad hoc* committee consisting of Leon Eisenberg, Don Fawcett, Alexander Leaf and Irving London to prepare a statement addressing these issues to be distributed prior to the March 13, 1970, meeting of the Faculty of Medicine. The statement with a covering memorandum from me was sent to all members of the faculty on March 4th. In my memorandum I expressed strong support for the resolution to come before the faculty on March 13th. The resolution stated that the Faculty of Medicine favored the establishment of a joint Harvard-MIT School of Health Sciences and Technology.

The prepared statement outlined in detail the courses in human biology being planned. The distinctive feature of these courses would be how they would be developed and taught. The faculty would include life scientists, including clinicians, physical scientists, engineers and mathematicians. Examples given were in anatomy, physiology, general pathology and organ system pathophysiology. The staffing pattern was estimated to be two to three anatomists, three physiologists, three pathologists, from seventeen to twenty pathophysiologists and fifteen mathematicians, physicists and engineers. There were also listed courses under development in other areas which would promote the interrelationship of the physical, engineering, social and management sciences with biology and medicine. Courses ranged from a course in physics, with the content drawn from biology and medicine, to a health services project planning laboratory.

After five years it was expected that 300–400 students would be affiliated with the school.

The approximate numbers per year were estimated to be:

1. Health sciences and technology based on engineering, physical and mathematical sciences
   Master's degree   50–70
   Ph.D.   25–30
2. Human biology-life science
   Ph.D.   25–30
3. M.D., M.D.-Ph.D., D.M.D., M.P.H.   30–40
4. Social, behavioral and management sciences
   Ph.D.   25–30

The projected operating budget after five years was approximately $5,000,000 for educational programs and $10,000,000 for research, development and health care. It was proposed to raise $50,000,000 within five years for endowment and capital costs.

The memorandum then went on to stress the need for some formal administrative organization. Courses would not preempt HMS teaching time because new resources would be provided for additional faculty. Classes would be held not only at MIT but also at Harvard College and HMS as well. There would not be competition for funds because new sources would be found. The joint school would not become a two-year medical school. It was much broader than that. Only thirty out of 150–200 students a year would be medical students. The social sciences were needed to help make technology and medicine relevant to the human condition.[42] It was hoped that the memorandum would provide members of the faculty with a better understanding of what was being proposed before a vote was taken.

At the March 13, 1970 meeting of the Faculty of Medicine, with 250 members in attendance, a vote was finally taken. After some routine business, President Pusey turned the meeting over to me for further consideration of the joint school. Dr. Paul Russell asked Professor Rosenblith, who had been invited to attend these meetings of the faculty, how the MIT faculty felt about the proposal. Rosenblith replied that the matter was to be discussed at a meeting of the faculty the following week. He fully expected a favorable outcome. The major concerns voiced were the complexity of the proposal and the magnitude of the enterprise.

- Dr. Rabkin worried about using an archaic hierarchial organization, namely, a "school" when what was needed was an informal, flexible relationship. Both Dr. John Knowles and Dr. Folkman agreed with the need for flexibility but felt that some institutional form was needed.
- Dr. Davis worried about the magnitude of the enterprise and wondered if a more modest start would be prudent. Dr. Herbert Abrams shared the concern, particularly at a time when the economy was faltering.

After further discussion, President Pusey asked if the faculty was ready to vote on the resolution, which read: "The Faculty of Medicine favors the establishment of a joint Harvard-MIT School of Health Sciences and Technology to foster the development of health-related programs of education, research and service between the institutions, provided that the necessary new resources can be obtained."

The motion was made and seconded, but before a vote could be taken, Dr. Rabkin asked to be recognized by Mr. Pusey. He moved that the Dean's resolution be amended to read a "joint Harvard-MIT program" rather than joint school. He also added at the end of the resolution " . . . and with the understanding that its primary efforts include the development of imaginative administrative arrangements to foster its aims."

The amended resolution was defeated by voice vote, following which the original resolution was passed by a large majority of "yeas" in a voice vote.[43] So ended this chapter, once a favorable vote by MIT's faculty was recorded. But another hurdle remained before it could go to the governing boards; namely, the concerns of the Harvard School of Public Health.

The Harvard School of Public Health

Relations between the Harvard School of Public Health (HSPH) and the Medical School had not always been cordial, in part because the HSPH was either ignored or made to feel like a poor relation by the wealthier medical school. Early in my tenure as dean, I made a conscious effort to improve relationships. In my view, we had important shared interests having to do with the medical care system. One of the early initiatives I undertook was to develop the Center for Community Health and Medical Care in collaboration with Dean Snyder of the HSPH. We jointly recruited Paul Densen to head the Center and Alonzo Yerby to be the official representative of the SPH at the Center. I obtained a grant from The Commonwealth Fund to launch the enterprise. When the subcommittee on medical care was formed in 1967, Dr. Yerby was invited to be a member.

But no representative of the SPH was asked to be a member of the Joint Committee on Engineering and Living Systems, perhaps because there was no one with the obvious interest of a Harvey Brooks, who represented the Faculty of Arts and Sciences. In retrospect this was probably a mistake, since it fueled the latent paranoia of the HSPH toward HMS once it became apparent that the proposed joint school might pose a threat. Irving London sought to remedy this oversight in the fall of 1969, when he asked Alonzo Yerby to discuss with the administration of HSPH the nomination of individuals to join in the planning process. But it was too late in the game. On January 5, 1970, Acting Dean Richard Daggy (Dean Snyder was on sabbatical leave) wrote to Mr. Pusey asking him to appoint two members of his faculty to join in the planning process. Discussion of the proposed School of Health Sciences and Technology at the December 1969 meeting of the Faculty of Medicine was known to the Faculty of the School of Public Health. Quite suddenly, what had started as a limited collaborative effort in bioengineering and the management sciences now appeared to be much more ambitious, even encroaching on traditional interests of the SPH, such as the environment. I was aware that Mr. Pusey was keenly interested in the welfare of the HSPH and would be sensitive to any development that potentially could damage that school. While he had been supportive of my interests in collaborating with MIT, he did not have a personal investment in the idea. His first priority would be to protect a Harvard faculty that felt itself threatened.

This was the background for a special meeting of the Faculty of the School of Public Health on April 16, 1970, called to discuss the proposed joint school. In preparation for the meeting I sent Dr. Daggy the background material for the HMS faculty meetings held in December 1969, and January and March, 1970. I also sent him the minutes of those meetings, which recorded the reservations expressed by some HMS faculty. President Pusey chaired the meeting. Others invited to join in the discussion were Brooks, Ebert, London, Meadow, Rosenblith and Wiesner.

Dr. Daggy began with a conciliatory statement, in which he said that his initial concerns had been allayed by the additional information he had been given. He said that a small committee had been appointed, chaired by Roger Revelle, to look into the proposal. It held its first meeting the week before this meeting. I made an opening statement, in which I emphasized the Medical School's need to call on disciplines not represented in its faculty if the School were to meet its obligations to society. This was my reason for wishing to work with the SPH via the Center for Community Health and Medical Care. London, Wiesner and Brooks followed with statements about the program. Wiesner said he fully understood the reasons for faculty concern at the School of Public Health. When he and I initiated discussions, we had no idea that what had started as an informal relationship would result in a proposal for a new school.

Mr. Pusey then opened the meeting to questions. Although there were expressions of support, most questions reflected an undercurrent of concern. Was the new school addressing the right problems? Would it eventually supplant the SPH? Would it compete for resources? In fact, reactions were not dissimilar to some of those expressed by the Medical School faculty. Here are some of the questions and comments:

- Dr. Jean Mayer wondered if the proposed new school was addressing the right problems. Wasn't health manpower a more important issue, not only numbers, but how to utilize auxiliary health workers more effectively? Based on conversations with staff at the Department of Health, Education and Welfare, he thought it likely that the trend will be to provide funds to increase the supply of physicians and health workers rather than support a new research-oriented school. He also pointed out that the joint sponsorship of the School of Public Health by Harvard and MIT at an earlier time was abandoned because it was too cumbersome. I pointed out that the new school would enable us to increase Medical School size economically. Dr. Wiesner said that MIT had been asked to start a medical school but had decided on the collaboration instead.

- Dr. Yerby said that in order to devise better ways to provide health care, one needed a place to test new ideas. Would the program be able to do this? Dr. London hoped that Cambridge might provide such a laboratory.

- Dr. Mott asked what kinds of individuals will come from the school in terms of manpower and fitting into the health sector of our society. Professor Brooks answered—three or four kinds. First, physicians well versed in engineering; second, persons with master's degrees who could be described as bioengineers or medical management persons; third, undergraduates at Harvard and MIT who would be exposed to some tough intellectual problems involved in the delivery of health care, not in the professional sense but as a part of general education; and finally, there would be Ph.D. specialists in bioengineering. Professor Rosenblith added that exposure of undergraduates to an interdisciplinary approach to problem-solving could provide a career incubator as well as education.

- Professor Campbell quoted from a speech made by Dr. Sanazero, Director of the National Center for Health Services Research and Development, in which he said that there was a need for greater pertinence of curriculum to the needs of health workers. He suggested that "university aggregates" would be modern successors to schools of public health. Was this what was planned for the new school? I answered no—that it would supplement and complement, but not replace. Professor Campbell hoped not but went on to say that some day the new School of Health Sciences and Technology might actually incorporate the Medical School!

- Professor Thomas Weller wondered how we would be able to recruit the necessary new faculty given the fact that from ten to thirty percent of budgeted faculty positions in the basic sciences are now vacant. I answered that initially we would not be able to find people with the necessary backgrounds. We would have to train them in what would be an evolutionary process.
- Professor James Whittenberger mentioned competition for funds and wondered how the new school would operate. Mr. Meadow answered that funds could go to either university to be used for the new school as directed by the donor.
- Dr. Reed expressed enthusiasm for the idea but worried about the role of the SPH in planning. This should go beyond courses and focus on the principles of the venture. Many of the principles seemed to be the same ones that were guiding a re-examination of the SPH review of its own plans for the future. He felt that planning should go well beyond worry about duplicating courses and consider complementing development. Dr. London replied that he would be delighted to meet with the committee at the SPH concerned with this question.[44]

The faculty meeting ended on this upbeat note but it was apparent that the SPH wanted equal partnership if it were to support the new school. A few days later, Acting Dean Daggy wrote to President Pusey asking that formal action not be taken by the Governing Boards until the SPH had made its recommendation.

On April 9, 1970, the MIT faculty passed a resolution that was worded the same as the resolution passed by the Faculty of Medicine on March 13th. On May 6 the MIT Corporation voted to authorize the Institute to proceed with plans for its participation in the joint Harvard-MIT School of Health Sciences and Technology, subject to a five-year look at the possibilities of obtaining the necessary $50,000,000 funding and subject to authorization by the Harvard Corporation of similar participation by Harvard.[45]

On May 13, 1970, the Faculty of Public Health passed the following resolution:

> The Faculty of Public Health favors the establishment of a joint Harvard-MIT School of Health Sciences and Technology between the Faculty of MIT and the Faculties of Medicine and Public Health, and other interested Harvard units or departments, on the assumption that

administrative, financial and operating arrangements will be developed which are acceptable to each of the Faculties and units. The Faculty of Public Health wishes to participate fully in the planning of the proposed School.

Finally, at a meeting of the President and Fellows of Harvard College in Cambridge, June 1, 1970:

Voted to authorize the Deans of the Faculty of Medicine and Public Health to seek to advance the suggested plan to establish jointly with the Massachusetts Institute of Technology a new School of Health Sciences and Technology in accordance with the resolution presented by the President, on behalf of the Deans concerned, to the Fellows of Harvard College at their meeting June 1, 1970.

Finances, Program and Governance The Final Phase

The votes of the two university corporations were encouraging, but seeking to advance a plan to establish a joint school subject to finding $50,000,000 was a pretty guarded mandate. Now money and turf became the hurdles to get over. How was it going to be possible to find $50,000,000 without competing with other programs? Who will decide on the boundaries of the new school so that what it offers is unique and not competitive with other programs in the two universities? How will it be governed so as to fit comfortably in two different university cultures? Early in the summer, planning for a fund-raising campaign began. On July 8, 1970, Ebert, James Killian (who had succeeded Howard Johnson as president of MIT and who had agreed to help raise money for the joint school), Revelle, Wiesner and London met to consider major prospects.[46] Dr. Killian hoped to persuade Laurence Rockefeller to chair a committee of sponsors. It was announced that Dr. Walter Koltun had agreed to serve as the principal staff member concerned with the development of resources for the new school beginning August 15, 1970.[47] A few visits to prospective donors were made during the summer, but a more formal consideration of fund raising did not occur until September. At that time some substantial disagreements became apparent.

There was skepticism that $50,000,000 (a little later increased to $60,000,000) could be raised on a noncompetitive basis. Bayley Mason, who headed the Medical School Development Office, was certain it could not be done. He worried that foundations with programs in the health field, from which HMS already received support, would ask if support for the joint school took precedence over other Medical School or School of Public Health programs. Our increased reliance on private donors as a consequence of a cutback in Federal funding caused Mason particular concern. He noted that HMS had $40,000,000 of high priority needs. HSPH had $25,000,000. The Program for Harvard Science was stalled at $20,000,000 short of its $50,000,000 goal. He said the fund-raising market does not exist for $25,000,000 worth of Harvard sponsored programs in the health field. He noted that 43% of our private monies came from foundations. He thought that if the idea of a consortium of foundations, possibly convened by The Commonwealth Fund, went forward, HMS might well be abandoned by some of our most critical donors for a three-to- five year period—Commonwealth, Ford, Rockefeller, Kellogg, Carnegie, Mellon, etc.[48]

Jack Snyder, Dean of the Faculty of Public Health, who had become a member of the steering committee since his return from sabbatical leave, had another worry. How were the funds raised to be allocated? What would be the mechanism to do this? He thought that a reasonable and fair document should be written and agreed to before $10,000,000 was raised.

I argued that we needed a case statement on which we could all agree, one that was sufficiently focused so that it did not appear to prospective donors that previous programs supported by some of them had either failed or were being taken over by the joint school. A recent draft of a document was to be used as a description of the kinds of people to be trained as health care planners and managers, economists, political scientists and public administrators concerned with public policy for health and medicine. Courses would include the application of the social and behavioral sciences to health problems and needs. It seemed to me that a program that had started as a way of bringing bioengineering into medicine and human biology had now become so global as to include about everything related to health. I thought that donors would be confused about the relationship between the programs of the proposed school and what already existed in the Medical School, the School of Public Health and the Kennedy School of Government.

I had received support from The Commonwealth Fund to start the joint HMS-HSPH Center for Community Health and Medical Care, an organization concerned with public policy and planning in the health area. I had recruited a prominent medical economist, Rashi Fein, to work in the Center. I also obtained support for Martin

Feldstein, who at that time was interested in health economics, thus helping to keep him in the Department of Economics in the Faculty of Arts and Sciences. I had received support from The Commonwealth Fund and the Ford and Rockefeller Foundations to start the Harvard Community Health Plan. I had supported the development of a joint M.D.-Master of Public Policy program with the Kennedy School. (Harvey V. Fineberg, the current Dean of the School of Public Health is a graduate of that program.) To sum up, I had invested a great deal of time and effort trying to approach problems of medical care in an interdisciplinary fashion. I had supported programs for physicians to attain competence in fields such as health policy and health services research. My plea to the steering committee was to develop a case statement that would state the unique mission of the proposed school, eliminating much of the global approach to health care.

All of this made Walter Koltun's job much more difficult. He was asked to put all fund raising on hold until

1. a statement of specific programs acceptable to Harvard and MIT had been prepared, and
2. there was agreement on guidelines for the allocation of funds.

He was asked to omit the word "school" in his case statement. In addition, he was asked to follow a set of clearance guidelines involving development offices at Harvard, MIT, HMS and HSPH. With so many restrictions he wondered if he would be able to do his job. It must have seemed to Walter Koltun that most of the restrictions were coming from Harvard, but that wasn't surprising. Harvard had more to lose than MIT if sources of funding interested in health were approached for support of the joint enterprise. There would be competition with other health related programs, most of which were at Harvard.

Whatever reservations I might have had about the global terms in which the proposed school was being described, I never had any doubts about the validity of the concept. I was committed to the idea of a joint school. I mention this because of Dean Snyder's growing disaffection with the work of the steering committee. The report of the summer study in 1970, held by Dr. Revelle's committee, had been quite positive about the potential for cooperation between HSPH and the new school,[49] but Dean Snyder did not share that optimism. He anticipated competition rather than collaboration. He found himself involved in discussions of fund raising for an enterprise that had been planned without him. He was frustrated by his inability to get satisfactory answers to questions about allocation of funds and how they would be administered.

Dr. Wiesner and I were also feeling some frustration with the difficulty in getting agreement among the various players. On January 27, 1971, we issued a progress report that spoke of the need for "establishment of a well-defined programmatic and administrative focus within each university." To accomplish this we recommended that, rather than continue with a joint general venture between two universities, we return to the original focus of an HMS-MIT joint program. We suggested that at a later time, after $10,000,000 had been raised, a joint school could be established involving other parts of Harvard in addition to the Medical School. The progress report discussed the educational programs proposed. They would span the full spectrum of higher education but would reflect the specific opportunities provided by MIT, HMS and the School of Dental Medicine. We noted the plan to admit twenty-five students chosen from Harvard, Radcliffe and MIT into a new human biology curriculum in September 1971 in preparation for the clinical years at Harvard Medical School. We discussed the projected educational budget, a research program initially focused on biomaterials and finally the need to implement a fund-raising program. In the spring of 1971 Dean Snyder wrote to President Pusey expressing his frustration with the planning process. He, too, argued that the program should be a joint HMS-MIT enterprise, although for rather different reasons.

In April of 1971 I wrote to President Pusey asking for the Harvard Corporation to designate the Faculty of Medicine as responsible for the advancement of the joint program in health sciences and technology. No action was taken by the Harvard Corporation. I can only guess that Mr. Pusey, who was to step down from the presidency in June, was of the opinion that his successor should make the decision about my request.

Meanwhile a new case statement had been developed, dated March 31, 1971. After discussing education, research and development, the following statement was made:

> Harvard and MIT will continue their current interests and programs in health care. However, the Program will provide a complementary mechanism for facilitating the application of science and technology to problems in the organization and delivery of health services. Where it is uniquely suited the Program will be engaged in the development of improved health care systems.

That was the statement that went to The Commonwealth Fund as a part of a request for a new grant. It satisfied my reservations expressed earlier.

Three notable events occurred on July 1, 1971. Derek Bok assumed the presidency of Harvard, Jerome Wiesner was made President of MIT, and Walter Rosenblith became Provost of MIT. New eras had begun at both universities, which would certainly have an impact on the joint program. Shortly after taking office, Bok stated that he would take an active interest in the development of the joint school. He did not wish to commit Harvard to fund raising in excess of $10,000,000 for the school until he could see what programs would evolve.[50] William Olney, who had been asked by President Bok to advise him on fund raising for the new program, recommended that Harvard should be as active as MIT in every aspect of the new school, including fund raising. Olney also urged that the School of Public Health be reinstated as a full partner in the enterprise. He said that the retirement of Dean Snyder offered an opportunity to appoint a new dean who would take a fresh look at the potential for collaboration between the SPH and the joint school. Olney also suggested that Harvard appoint a senior fund raiser to represent all of Harvard's interests.[51] I thought that was an excellent idea, and in my conversations with Olney I asked if Mr. Bok wanted him to assume that role, would he be willing to do so. He seemed to me to be ideal for the job given his positive thinking about Harvard's involvement. Unfortunately, President Bok had other plans for Olney.

Although President Bok wished to take an active role in planning the new school, he thought that the description of the program was too diffuse. From the beginning of his involvement he continued to ask for a more precise definition of what would and would not be included in the school's program. He disliked the generalities that so often are a part of brochures developed for the purpose of fund raising. Not only were they unconvincing, but they might have a negative impact on prospective donors.

The second half of 1971 was a time for greater optimism than the first six months had been. The two new presidents seemed intent on developing a joint program. A new, innovative educational program was ready to begin in the fall of 1971 with the admission of twenty-five candidates for the M.D. degree in a joint university program.[52] A prestigious committee of sponsors had been recruited and were scheduled to meet in the early part of the following year. There was every reason to believe that after a slow start, the $10,000,000 goal would be reached. A strong supporter of MIT had given $1,000,000 in endowment, The Commonwealth Fund had provided a new $600,000, and the NIH had approved an $863,000 grant for support of work on biomaterials.[53] An executive committee was appointed to oversee the development of the program, including fund raising.[54] The thirteen-member committee included both presidents, the Chancellor, Provost, Dean of the Graduate School of MIT, the Dean of the Medical School, the Dean of the Faculty of Arts and Sciences, and the Dean of the Division of Engineering and Applied Physics from Harvard. Irving London and Walter Koltun as Director and Assistant Director were also members. Clearly, this high level committee was in a position to make decisions. Two other members were added later in 1972. In May, Derek Bok appointed Howard Hiatt, Dean of the School of Public Health. Shortly thereafter Bok wrote to Wiesner suggesting that Hiatt be asked to join the Executive Committee. In September, Wiesner wrote to Bok saying that MIT had established a Program of Health Sciences and Technology to serve as a focus in those fields. Irving London was appointed chairman of the Program and Professor Robert Mann, chairman of its Executive Committee. Wiesner asked for the appointment of Robert Mann to the Executive Committee of the Joint Program.

At the beginning of January, 1972, in preparation for the March meeting of the Sponsors, Walter Koltun circulated a draft statement of the proposed program. Once again it was expansive in scope, stating that the collaborative effort would be directed toward "integrating the natural, social and behavioral sciences and engineering with medical education and health care." And once again I objected as I had when a proposal was being prepared for submission to The Commonwealth Fund.[55] More to the point, Derek Bok wrote to Walter Koltun saying that Harvard could not subscribe to expansion of the program into health care delivery and administration in view of its potential conflict with the School of Public Health.[56] A new statement was prepared describing the educational programs, research and development. All reference to health care was omitted.

The successes of the joint program in education and research were reasons for continued optimism over the next five years, but final institutionalization seemed endlessly delayed. Not until April of 1977 was action taken by the two university governing boards approving a permanent governance and an administrative structure.[57] There were three problem areas that caused the long delay: fund raising, program boundaries and administration. All had to do with competition and turf. I shall briefly describe how these three problem areas were ultimately resolved, but first I will comment on the successes.

Education and Research. Because of some of the constraints upon the over-all effort, it is easy to overlook the ongoing accomplishments of the joint program between 1971 and 1977. The M.D. program, initiated in 1971, was an instant success. The first class graduated in 1975, by which time 20% of the 100 students enrolled in the program were candidates for M.D.-Ph.D. degrees. From the beginning, it attracted first-rate students, as it continues to do today. New courses were developed in bioengineering by the joint program, and in the fall of 1977 a new curriculum in medical engineering and medical physics was scheduled to begin.

Joint research programs flourished. Biomaterials science was the first joint research program to begin, and in 1977 funding from the NIH amounted to $922,000. A rehabilitation engineering center was established at Children's Hospital and MIT with support of $350,000 per year from The Department of Health, Education and Welfare. Another research program supported by the NIH in the amount of $215,000 per year involved nuclear techniques in the study of metabolism and bone disease. Thus two of the three areas originally chosen for exploration when planning started in 1967 were successfully under way. But there were problems on other fronts.

Fund raising. As noted earlier, there were problems about fund raising from the start. While the stated intent was to be noncompetitive, clearly that was impossible. There were a finite number of sources, particularly in the foundation world. Major gifts from individuals usually came from persons who identified strongly with Harvard or MIT. To the extent that they were a continuing source of gifts, neither university was inclined to favor the joint program over its individual needs.

The first meeting of the Sponsoring Committee was held March 13, 1972, and twelve of the twenty members attended, including such luminaries as Charles Francis Adams, Chairman of the Board of Raytheon; Paul Cabot, former Treasurer of Harvard; Crawford Greenwalt, Chairman of the Finance Committee of duPont; John Loeb, Sr., Senior Partner of Loeb, Rhoades & Co.; James Shannon, former Director of the NIH; Charles Thomas, former Chairman of Monsanto; and Uncus Whitaker, Chairman of the Board of AMP, Inc.[58] Thus it included major benefactors of both Harvard and MIT. President Bok sent greetings, since he was unable to attend due to a recent injury. William Olney reported to him the next day that the group had heard talks about the program " . . . which were meaningful, although perhaps not exciting."[59]

With such a distinguished Sponsoring Committee, the goal of $10,000,000 seemed in easy reach. But it was not to be. Fifteen months later Walter Koltun sent a memorandum to London bemoaning the fact that the Sponsoring Committee had been of little help. At the meeting in October 1972 only seven of twenty members attended. Clearly, those with the ability to give or raise funds from others had higher priorities elsewhere. As of June 30, 1973, endowment funds received or pledged totaled $3,300,000, of which $2,190,000 had been raised during the previous year. Koltun thought it would take at least two or three years to raise $10,000,000, and he wondered if that was an acceptable timetable. He suggested that instead of joint fund raising, each university assume responsibility for raising a $3,000,000 portion of the endowment.[60]

A year and a half later, prospects weren't much better. In a memorandum to Henry Meadow dated February 19, 1975, Koltun said endowment in hand or pledged amounted to $5,000,000. He felt that in a "steady state" the program would need an endowment of $25,000,000. Therefore, he urged that the leadership of Harvard and MIT commit themselves to raising an additional $20,000,000.[61] President Bok was dubious about this goal and doubted that he would authorize it. Although he wanted to be helpful, he did not wish to give it preferred status, feeling that for Harvard the program was less important than needs such as public policy or public health.[62] Despite Walter Koltun's best efforts he was never able to obtain the full support of either Harvard or MIT in his fund-raising efforts. He did find other sources of money, such as the Palm Beach community, but he had not reached his goals by the time the program was finally approved in 1977.

Program boundaries. Repeatedly over the period from 1972 until 1977, efforts were made to define in specific terms the boundaries of the joint program. What should be included, what excluded, what controls should be exercised over the development of any new initiatives? A planning committee was appointed in early 1973 to consider this issue, among others. It was agreed, for example, that the program would not have responsibility for human biology or bioengineering at the undergraduate level at MIT. I can only assume that MIT faculty did not wish to relinquish authority over any of its undergraduate programs to an organization not completely controlled by MIT. This might not have been an issue had a joint B.S.-M.D. become a reality. Then there would have been a reason for the HST program to administer an undergraduate pathway.

Dr. London acknowledged that health planning and management were now excluded because of separate programs at MIT and HSPH. He expressed the opinion that there should be no arbitrary exclusions but accepted the judgment of the committee that the HST program should stay out of systems level projects, contributing only where it had special expertise; e.g., rehabilitation. In its report to the Executive Committee, the Planning Committee recommended that health-related activities might be classified as mutually acknowledged, collaborative and joint. The report also recommended a deans' committee where all health initiatives would be discussed. Membership would include the deans of HMS, HSPH, Harvard's FAS, MIT Division of HST, the Sloan School and MIT's School of Architecture and Planning.

As I look back on the debate about boundaries, I now believe I can identify the fundamental disagreement that caused so much trouble. It began with what I believe was a tactical error in describing the program for fund-raising purposes. The mandate for the new school was painted in such broad terms that it seemed to include almost everything related to health care. As noted earlier, this caused me concern because of its possible impact on our traditional donors. But it worried President Bok even more, for it appeared that the HST program was staking claims to areas that were traditional domains for various Harvard faculties, particularly the HSPH. He was determined to eliminate that threat by insisting that there be a precise definition of the HST program, what it would include, and what it would not include. Although Irving London was willing to make the program less global, he felt it was a mistake to be so arbitrary. He thought that the scope of the new school should be constantly re-evaluated in the light of changing conditions. For example, new opportunities in education and research being pursued independently in both universities might be more productively and economically pursued jointly. There might also be jointly sponsored supplementary activities that could enhance programs being carried out independently in each university. Although I had always objected to what I considered too global a program, I agreed with Irving London's formulation of scope. I did not believe it could ever be completely static. The resolution of this issue is described later in "The Final Solution."

Administration. There were endless meetings and memoranda about how the HST school or program should be administered and governed. But there was one underlying theme: How was it to be controlled. I suspect that a jointly governed organization will always be a source of worry to the sponsors. Will it become too autonomous? Will it invade someone else's turf? As a consequence, the temptation is to create a governance that controls the joint enterprise much more tightly than similar organizations within either university. As we shall see, the administrative structure ultimately approved by the two governing boards put in place stringent controls over new programs.

Finally, there was the question of what the HST program should be called. Irving London and I wanted it to be called a school, headed by a dean, equal in status to other schools in both universities. But there was opposition. I do not know where it came from at MIT. At Harvard, major opposition came from Dr. Hiatt, Dean of HSPH. He thought the designation "school" gave too great an emphasis to technology in medicine.

The Final Solution

I sometimes wondered if we would ever be able to institutionalize the joint program. It took a long time, but finally, there was agreement. And in April 1977 the final steps were taken. The statement approved by the Administrative Committee of the program, dated March 22, 1977, was called "Proposal for Organization and Governance of Harvard-MIT Division of Health Sciences and Technology." (Note that the proposal was for a division, not a school.)

In this document, presented to the two university governing boards for their approval, the program of the Division of HST was defined in precise terms. Two educational programs were described: (1) a curriculum developed and administered in concert with Harvard's Faculty of Medicine and the Faculty of MIT leading to the M.D. degree awarded by Harvard University; (2) a curriculum leading to masters, engineering and doctoral degrees, awarded by MIT, which would prepare engineers and scientists for careers in medical engineering and medical physics.

There were equally precise definitions of programs in research and development. They were to be concerned with important biological medical and health problems that could be addressed in an interdisciplinary manner through the collaborative efforts of biomedical scientists, physical scientists, engineers, physicians and/or public health faculty from the two participating institutions. No longer was there mention of behavioral and social scientists, health planners, etc.

The control of any new programs would be exercised by the Administrative Council (defined below) according to the following two criteria:

1. The extent to which the proposed program will provide intellectual benefits, cost savings or other advantages that cannot be achieved by either institution alone through its existing programs, or through programs already being planned and capable of being carried out within the intellectual and material resources realistically available to that institution.
2. The extent to which a new program threatens to divert funds from sources, public or private, that might otherwise be available to support existing programs or programs being planned in either institution.

I submit that those are tighter controls over new programs than are exercised over any faculty or school at Harvard and, I suspect, at MIT as well.

There were four components to the governance and administration of the Division of Health Science and Technology:

1. A governing board that would have responsibility for the formulation of educational, administrative and fiscal policies. Membership would consist of the President and one member of the Harvard Corporation and one other individual they shall select and the President and one member of the Corporation of MIT and one other individual they shall select.
2. An Administrative Council, the members of which would include the Provost of MIT, the Dean of the Harvard Faculty of Medicine, the Director of the Division of Health Science and Technology, the Dean of the Harvard Faculty of Arts and Sciences, the Dean of Engineering and Applied Physics at Harvard, the Dean of the Harvard School of Public Health, the Dean of the School of Engineering at MIT, and the Dean of the School of Science at MIT. The Administrative Council would oversee the implementation of approved programs, review plans for new educational and research programs and develop recommendations for policies and programs related to fund raising.
3. A budget committee consisting of the Provost of MIT, the Dean of the Harvard Faculty of Medicine and the Director of the Division

of Health Science and Technology. It would review and approve budgets prepared by the Director of the Division. It would also review proposals for programs, appointments in and organization of the Division of HST. When such proposals involved matters significantly affecting another Faculty or unit in either university, the dean or an appropriate representative thereof would be invited to attend.

4. A Joint Faculty Committee, the members of which would be members of the Harvard or MIT faculties with major administrative, educational or research functions in the Division. It would develop and oversee criteria for faculty appointments and other faculty matters.

Membership on the Administrative Council was designed to represent and protect the interests of all the major deans in both schools who might object to any new programs based on the two criteria mentioned earlier. The Administrative Council was also given oversight of fund raising. Thus, all the major deans in both universities were protected from competition for money or "turf." The new Division was sufficiently contained as to no longer represent a threat to anyone.

And so ended my participation in the Harvard-MIT Division of Health Science and Technology. In June 1977 I left Harvard to become President of the Milbank Memorial Fund.

Reflections on the Experience

Let me begin with a categorical statement: The Harvard-MIT Division of Health Science and Technology is a success. None of my comments to follow will in any way cast doubt on that statement. But I have learned some things along the way that may be useful to others interested in inter-university collaboration.

Collaboration between individuals or even departments in different universities present few difficulties, partly because such joint programs are usually temporary, partly because they rarely require any formal action by university governing boards. Developing formal and permanent relationships is an entirely different matter. The major reason is the non-hierarchial nature of university faculties. University presidents do not have the same powers as presidents and CEO's in the corporate world. University presidents, even with board of trustee support, cannot arrange mergers or partnership arrangements with other institutions without consulting with their faculties and deans. And university schools, divisions and departments are quick to defend their turf. That was evident in the debate about what the HST program should be called and what its boundaries would be. There was opposition to calling the joint program a school because that would have given it equivalent status with other schools in the two universities. There had to be a precise definition of boundaries, lest it compete with an established school in one or the other of the two universities. And the ultimate constraint was fund raising. It must not compete with other fund raising in either university.

I learned what kind of collaboration was possible within the boundaries of these constraints. Well defined educational programs that exploit the complementary talents in the two universities were welcome. Joint research projects with the same characteristics were equally welcome. What was not welcome was competition with existing programs in either university.

I cannot help but reflect on the different dynamics affecting the evaluation of the Harvard-MIT Division of HST and the Harvard Community Health Plan (HCHP), the planning for both of which began at the same time, with significant personal involvement on my part. Of necessity the HST program had to live within the constraints of two universities. In contrast, HCHP was established as a separate corporation—related to Harvard but independent—modeled on the relationship between Harvard and its affiliated teaching hospitals. HCHP did not have to justify its actions to any governing body other than its own board of directors. As a consequence, it was free to pursue courses of action believed to be necessary in order to grow and compete in a highly competitive marketplace. It could form new alliances with Harvard's teaching hospitals, with community hospitals, with other physician groups and other HMO's. It could negotiate as an equal partner with the Harvard Medical School in the creation of a new university department of ambulatory care and prevention. In other words, it was free to operate, to succeed or fail on its own, subject to none of the constraints experienced by the HST program. Unconstrained it has become the largest HMO in New England and one of the three most prestigious HMO's in the nation. HCHP had one other advantage. It could generate its own income, including enough to fund teaching and research.

Finally, a regret. When the Education Subcommittee began its planning, the emphasis was on a combined undergraduate-M.D. program. To begin with, the program was designed to shorten the time needed to earn the M.D. degree. Too inflexible, the critics said, so the time was lengthened. But when a program was finally put in place, it was for M.D. candidates only. I am not sure why that happened. Perhaps the resistance at Harvard College of early professionalization was a factor, for the Harvard-MIT committee felt that any joint B.S.-M.D. program should be open at both universities. Perhaps it was inertia. Perhaps it was easier to eliminate the need to develop criteria for early medical school admission. Whatever the reasons, I believe we missed a wonderful opportunity to experiment.

Notes

1. Memorandum to the files dated June 8, 1964, from David D. Rutstein re meeting with "ad hoc Committee on so-called Biomedical Engineering" at Massachusetts Institute of Technology (hereinafter referred to as MIT) on June 8, 1964.
2. Memorandum dated May 13, 1964, to selected MIT professors from Gordon S. Brown, Dean, School of Engineering, MIT re ad hoc Committee on so-called Biomedical Engineering.
3. Memorandum dated March 19, 1964, to Henry C. Meadow from Professor Murray Eden and Professor David D. Rutstein re (Progress Report) Biomedical Technological Resource.
4. Letter dated December 10, 1965, to Robert H. Ebert, Dean, Harvard Medical School, from Jerome B. Wiesner, Dean, School of Science, MIT.
5. Charge to the Joint Committee of Harvard University and the Massachusetts Institute of Technology on Engineering and Living Systems (hereinafter referred to as JCELS), dated January 23, 1967.
6. Minutes of meeting of JCELS, July 5, 1967.
7. Minutes of meeting of JCELS, May 25, 1967.
8. Minutes of meeting of JCELS, July 5, 1967.
9. Minutes of meeting of JCELS, September 19, 1967.
10. *Ibid.*
11. Minutes of meeting of JCELS, December 6, 1967.
12. *Ibid.*
13. Minutes of meeting of JCELS, January 11, 1968.
14. Minutes of meeting of JCELS, March 27, 1968.

National Academy of Engineering Contract Study Task Committees

Task Group	Harvard	MIT
Sensory Life		R. Mann
		S. Mason

National Academy of Engineering Contract Study Task committees

Task Group	Harvard	MIT
Artificial Organs	G. Austen	E. Merrill
		A. Shapiro
Skeletal Prostheses	M. Glimcher	R. Mann
		R. Alter
Organ and Cell Culture and Storage	J. Folkman	S. Miller
Biological Control Systems	E. Blout	R. Wurtman
	A. Leaf	E. Merrill
		H. Monroe
		B. Magasanik
Sub-cellular Engineering	E. Blout	P. Gross
	G. Edsall	
Neurophysiology	N. Kiang	J. Brown
	T. Wiesel	W. Peake
	J. Barlow	W. Siebert
		J. Lettvin
		W. Nauta
Physiological Monitoring	H. Bendixen	L. Smullen
	B. Lown	P. Katona
	P. Drinker	
	E. Haber	
Diagnostic Instrumentation	W. Simon	M. Rodman
	F. Lee	P. Bowditch
	B. Vallee	S. Burns
	W. Wacker	
Diagnostic Processes	O. Peterson	H. Sherman
	H. Blumgart	M. Eden
	B. Vallee	
Regionalization of Health Services (Macrosystems)	J. Hartgering	W. Pounds
	O. Peterson	J. Rockart
	P. Densen	B. Frieden
	L. Baumgartner	
	G. Rosenthal (Brandeis)	
Medical Care Microsystems	M. Rabkin	A. Drake
	O. Barnett	B. Reiffen
	D. Rutstein	H. Sherman
	C. Walter	
Bioengineering Curricula	Entire Joint Committee on Engineering and Living Systems plus list selected by Drs. Eden and Zacharias	

National Academy of Engineering Contract Study Task Committees

Task Group	Harvard	MIT
Continuing Education	H. Hiatt	H. Mickley
	D. Federman	G. Zacharias
	G. Foster	
	D. Hurwitz	
	J. Dickson (NIH)	

15. Minutes of meeting of JCELS, October 24, 1968.
16. Letter dated December 9, 1968, to Quigg Newton, President, The Commonwealth Fund, from Robert H. Ebert and Jerome B. Wiesner.
17. Minutes of meeting of Ad Hoc Subcommittee on Medical Care, May 10, 1967.
18. Minutes of meetings of JCELS, December 6, 1967, and January 25, 1968.
19. Minutes of meeting of JCELS, January 25, 1968.
20. Minutes of meeting of JCELS, December 6, 1967, including copy of undated proposal for "An Ambulatory Health Care Program."
21. Letter dated December 2, 1968, to Robert H. Ebert from Howard H. Hiatt with Proposal for the Development of an Ambulatory Care Service.
22. Minutes of meeting of JCELS, July 5, 1967.
23. Minutes of meeting of JCELS, December 6, 1967.
24. Minutes of meeting of Subcommittee on Education, January 2, 1968.
25. Minutes of meeting of JCELS, January 11, 1968.
26. Minutes of meeting of JCELS, February 6, 1968.
27. Minutes of meeting of JCELS, March 27, 1968.
28. Minutes of meeting of JCELS, May 1, 1968.
29. Minutes of meeting of Subcommittee on Education, January 27, 1969.
30. Minutes of meeting of JCELS, January 29, 1969.
31. Minutes of meeting of JCELS, July 5, 1967.
32. Minutes of meeting of JCELS, January 11, 1968.
33. Minutes of meeting of JCELS, October 24,1968.
34. Minutes of meeting of JCELS, November 15, 1968.
35. Minutes of meeting of JCELS, December 2, 1968.
36. Minutes of meeting of JCELS, February 22, 1969.
37. Memorandum dated February 25, 1969, from Robert H. Ebert to Henry C. Meadow.
38. Report of the JCELS, MIT-Harvard University, July 1, 1969.
39. "Proposed Program—Harvard-MIT Planning Committee on Health Sciences and Technology," November 24, 1969.
40. Minutes of Harvard Medical School (hereinafter referred to as HMS) Faculty Meeting, December 5, 1969.
41. Minutes of HMS Faculty Meeting, January 9, 1970.
42. Supplementary Statement, Proposed Joint Harvard University-MIT Program in Health Sciences and Technology prepared by Leon Eisenberg, Don. W. Fawcett, Alexander Leaf and Irving M. London, March 4, 1970.
43. Minutes of HMS Faculty Meeting, March 13, 1970.

44. Minutes of Harvard School of Public Health Faculty Meeting, April 16, 1970.
45. Excerpt from minutes of meeting of MIT Corporation, May 6, 1970.
46. Agenda of meeting of Steering Committee, Harvard University-MIT Planning Committee for Program in Health Sciences and Technology, July 13, 1970.
47. *Ibid.*
48. Memorandum dated October 14, 1970, to Robert H. Ebert and Henry C. Meadow from Bayley F. Mason.
49. Report to the Faculty of the Harvard School of Public Health of the Harvard School of Public Health Summer Study Conference, MIT Endicott House, July 7–10, 1970.
50. Memorandum to file dated August 23, 1971, from Henry C. Meadow.
51. Memorandum dated July 29, 1971, to Derek Bok from William Olney.
52. Press release dated September 17, 1971, from HMS and MIT.
53. Status report dated December 1, 1971; also memorandum, dated December 9, 1971, to Robert H. Ebert from Beverly Bennett.
54. Undated document (probably early 1972) entitled Harvard-MIT Program in Health Sciences and Technology.
55. Letter dated January 24, 1972, from Robert H. Ebert to Derek Bok.
56. Letter dated January 21, 1972, from Derek Bok to Walter L. Koltun.
57. Vote of President and Fellows of Harvard College, April 18, 1977.
58. Agenda, including list of attendees, of meeting of Sponsoring Committee, March 13, 1972.
59. Memorandum dated March 14, 1972, to Derek Bok from William S. Olney.
60. Memorandum dated July 30, 1973, to Irving M. London from Walter L. Koltun re Report of Fund Raising during the period July 1, 1972-June 30, 1973.
61. Memorandum dated February 19, 1975, to Henry C. Meadow from Walter L. Koltun re Plan to Raise Funds for Proposed Harvard- MIT School of Health Sciences and Technology.
62. Letter dated March 19, 1975, to Robert H. Ebert from Derek Bok.

Chapter 4

THE EARLY YEARS: 1970–1985

Irving M. London, M.D.

This account of my part in the history of HST is both institutional and personal. As an alumnus of Harvard College and Harvard Medical School, I maintained strong ties to many Harvard faculty members and followed Harvard academic activities with great interest. After graduation from medical school in 1943, I spent the next twelve years in the Department of Medicine at Columbia-Presbyterian Medical Center, except for 1944 to 1946 when I served as a medical officer in the United States Army. My service in the army was largely devoted to clinical research on the pharmacotherapy of malaria in the course of which I worked closely with Dr. James A. Shannon.

In 1955, I accepted the opportunity of helping to found a new medical school, the Albert Einstein College of Medicine, and to serve as the first chairman of its Department of Medicine. The experience in the development of this new medical school was one from which I learned a great deal in terms of the integration of the basic medical sciences with clinical medicine, the organization of clinical departments, and the responsibility for the delivery of health care in a large urban setting.

The successful establishment and growth of Albert Einstein prompted an invitation to me in 1965 from Brandeis University to advise President A.L. Sachar, and interested faculty members, on the feasibility of developing a medical school at Brandeis. Given the strengths of Brandeis in biological sciences and the prohibitive costs of developing new clinical facilities for patient care and teaching, I felt it was advisable to explore the possibility of a program to join pre-clinical sciences at Brandeis with clinical experience and teaching at one or more of the Harvard teaching hospitals. This exploration involved discussions with the General Director of the Massachusetts General Hospital, Dr. John Knowles, and Dr. Robert H. Ebert, the newly appointed chairman of the Department of Medicine of that hospital. Both of them showed a lively interest in such a possibility. It soon became clear, however, that the financial commitments that Brandeis would be required to make would seriously compromise the growth of their existing programs. Accordingly, this possibility was not pursued further.

In 1967, Dr. Ebert, newly appointed Dean of the Faculty of Medicine at Harvard, invited me to meet with the committee searching for a chairman of the Department of Medicine at the Boston City Hospital. Although the position at the Boston City Hospital was in many respects similar to the position I occupied at Albert Einstein, the conditions in Boston were much less favorable than those in New York. Nevertheless, I visited the Harvard Services at the Boston City Hospital and met with the search committee. After the meeting Dr. Ebert informed me that the committee was eager for me to accept the position at the Boston City Hospital, but I had decided not to do so. In the amicable discussion that followed, I told Dr. Ebert that the exploration of a joint program between Brandeis and Harvard Medical School had raised a question in my mind of whether a joint program between Harvard and MIT was being considered. I had heard that discussions were under way between the two universities and asked whether such a program was part of the discussion. Ebert was very pleased by my interest and he immediately suggested that we meet with Jerome Wiesner, the Provost of MIT. I was acquainted with Wiesner because both of us served on the Advisory Committee to the Director of the National Institutes of Health, James Shannon, my friend and war-time mentor. We met on a Sunday morning in February, 1968, at the Wiesners' home in Watertown when I was returning from a skiing vacation. Ebert and Wiesner told me of the previous meetings of a Joint Committee on Engineering and Living Systems with faculty members from Harvard Medical School and MIT. Much of the emphasis in those discussions appeared to be on the potential of research collaboration between engineers and physicists at MIT and clinicians at Harvard Medical School. Many examples were cited of fruitful joint research efforts. There was, however, a need for the formulation of a detailed program plan. Ebert and Wiesner asked whether I would be willing to assume the task of leading the effort to formulate a detailed program that could be presented to the faculties of MIT and Harvard Medical School. I agreed to serve as a consultant in this effort.

During the academic year 1968–69 I made several trips to Boston and Cambridge from New York City for meetings with Ebert and Wiesner and with Walter Rosenblith, Chairman of the MIT faculty. I also met with Boris Magasanik, Chairman of the MIT Biology Department, Gordon Brown, Dean of the MIT School of Engineering, and Henry Meadow, Senior Associate Dean at Harvard Medical School, as well as with Murray Eden of the MIT Electrical Engineering Department and David Rutstein, Chairman of the Department of Preventive Medicine at Harvard Medical School. I had come to know Walter Rosenblith well since we both served on the Board of Medicine of the National Academy of Sciences, the precursor of the Institute of Medicine. I was very impressed by his keen intellect, infectious optimism and generosity of spirit. Rosenblith and I held several meetings with Quigg Newton and Colin MacLeod, the President and Vice President of the Commonwealth Fund, to apprise them of the discussions that were under way between the two universities. Wiesner and Ebert appointed a subcommittee consisting of Rosenblith, Meadow, Eden, and Rutstein, with myself as a consultant, to draft a proposal to the Commonwealth Fund for a planning grant. The proposal was submitted with the indication that I would serve as a principal consultant and would have a substantial role in the planning process. The objective of the proposal was the planning and design of a program that could be presented to the faculties of Harvard Medical School and MIT for their consideration and ultimately for submission to votes of the faculties. The favorable response of the Commonwealth Fund to the proposal is described in Dr. Ebert's essay (Chapter 3). A total grant of $655,000 was made, a vote of confidence of inestimable and crucial value in launching the planning effort.

I had kept the members of the Department of Medicine and Dean Harry Gordon of Albert Einstein informed of my service as a consultant to Wiesner and Ebert during the 1968–9 academic year. They were not surprised, therefore, by my request for a sabbatical leave of one year, July 1969 to June 1970, to permit me to serve as director of the planning effort on a full-time basis. Since the Department of Medicine was in excellent condition, I felt that I could take leave for one year with equanimity, and Dean Gordon graciously concurred.

My decision to undertake the planning effort was greeted by some of my friends with cautionary warnings and puzzlement. One of them remarked that trying to get Harvard and MIT to agree on a common program was like trying to get porcupines to mate. Another friend, the wife of a department head at MIT, said that she could not understand why I would take on the myriad problems in one institution, let alone in two. Despite these dispiriting comments, I was encouraged by the enthusiastic attitudes of several of the faculty members whom I had come to know in both universities. At the very start of the planning effort I was approached by George Benedek, Professor of Physics at MIT, who was eager to develop a basic introductory course in physics in which the illustrative examples of physical principles could be derived from biology and medicine. To assist George Benedek in the initial phases of this work, we enlisted the help of Philip Aisen, a distinguished physician and a physicist at Albert Einstein who also found this project an interesting educational challenge. I was confident that we would find many other faculty members in the two universities who would have similar adventurous spirits. To help organize the planning office, I was fortunate in receiving an application from Virginia Safford, a secretary with long experience in the Harvard system and a person with very good judgment and a very pleasant personality. I was similarly fortunate in having the enthusiastic support of H. Frederick Bowman who served as administrative officer of the Joint Committee on Engineering and Living Systems (JCELS) and who was exceptionally knowledgeable and experienced with the administrations of MIT and HMS.

The Spirit of the Times

It is important to remember that the years 1968, 1969, and 1970 were years of student and faculty turmoil in many universities in the United States and abroad. Protests against the Vietnam War, the assassinations of Martin Luther King, Jr., and Robert F. Kennedy, the riotous Democratic National Convention in Chicago in 1968, the Civil Rights movement and the demand for greater minority representation and affirmative action for selection of faculty members and students in universities—all of these elements made for a spirit of change. There was a strong desire on the part of many academics to be engaged in activities beneficial to society. This was especially true among engineers and physicists who had been in defense work and now wanted to be engaged in solving societal and medical problems.

At the same time there was a growing interest on the part of some leaders in academic medicine in establishing an organization that would be called The National Academy of Medicine. In response to such interest, The National Academy of Sciences appointed a Board on Medicine to consider whether a National Academy of Medicine should be developed within the framework of The National Academy of Sciences or whether it should be an independent and unaffiliated organization. James Shannon, Walter Rosenblith and I served on the Board on Medicine. I chaired the committee that was charged with recommending the preferred institutional form. There was much heated debate within our committee on the relative merits of complete independence compared to affiliation with The National Academy of Sciences, but one principle was universally accepted: health and medicine require representation of other professions and disciplines such as the biological, chemical and physical sciences, engineering, law and the social and behavioral sciences. This view prevailed, and when the Institute of Medicine was created as a constituent organization within The National Academy of Sciences, it was stipulated that at least twenty-five percent of the membership would come from professions and disciplines other than medicine.

Themes and Influences on Planning

In approaching the planning effort, I was influenced by my earlier experience as a student at Harvard College and Harvard Medical School and as a faculty member at the Columbia College of Physicians and Surgeons and at the Albert Einstein College of Medicine. These influences were reflected in certain principal themes that, I hoped, would guide our planning.

The first of these themes was the integration of medical education into university education. The Flexner revolution in medical education in the early twentieth century had succeeded in establishing university standards for medical faculties; but medical schools, closely associated with pre-existing hospitals, were very often geographically and intellectually distant from their parent universities. It seemed preferable to view medical education as a continuum beginning at the undergraduate college level and extending through the medical school curriculum to postgraduate education and training. In this continuum, one could seek to bring to bear on education for medicine the full range of sciences basic to medicine. These would include biology, chemistry, mathematics, physics and engineering, and, since medicine is a major service in society, medical education and research should also comprehend the social and behavioral sciences. Such a range of sciences can best be found in a university rather than in a medical school alone.

A second theme held that students of medicine are candidates for a doctoral degree and should be treated as graduate students who participate very actively in their own education. This approach favors learning in interactive seminars and by the solving of challenging problems. All students should be encouraged to engage in research and to present a written thesis as a qualification for the M.D. degree. Since many students might choose to pursue a Masters or Ph.D. program in addition to the M.D. curriculum, administrative flexibility should be encouraged to accommodate the diverse interests and needs of the individual students.

The third theme was related to research. There were numerous examples of successful research collaborations between individual faculty members at Harvard Medical School and MIT. Joining the two universities in a common program devoted to health and medicine could provide an infrastructure for mounting multi-disciplinary research activities on a scale suitable to the dimensions of the problems to be solved. MIT's experience with interdepartmental research laboratories had shown the advantages of such large-scale undertakings. The prospect of addressing major health problems by developing inter-university multi-disciplinary research programs was an attractive challenge.

Health care policy and management constituted the fourth theme. It was evident in 1969 that the health care system in the United States was seriously flawed. One could hope to create educational and research programs in health care policy and management that would represent very valuable contributions to American society by taking advantage of the strengths of the two universities in economics, management and political science as well as in medicine and in public health.

Finally, in creating a joint program of two universities, each with its own history, traditions and culture, the original focus on collaborative research might not survive the centrifugal forces of large, diffuse institutions. For the joint program to thrive and achieve permanence, one would need the cohesive influence of faculty and students engaged in successful educational programs.

The Planning Committee co-chaired by Robert H. Ebert and Jerome B. Wiesner met in plenary session on July 2, 1969. Forty-seven faculty members of Harvard Medical School, Harvard University, Harvard teaching hospitals and the various schools of MIT were present. I outlined the scope of the planning effort and announced the names of the faculty members who agreed to lead in various elements of the plan:

I. *Education* would comprehend: A.) Medical education with two principal curricular streams: the natural sciences chaired by Alexander Leaf and Boris Magasanik and the behavioral and social sciences chaired by Leon Eisenberg, Merton Kahne, Elliot Mishler and Benson Snyder; B.) Bioengineering, chaired by William Siebert; and C.) Programs to be considered such as an M.D./Ph.D program or a medical scientist training program, and a program in managerial sciences and administrative medicine.

II. *The Research and Development Committee* chaired by Judah Folkman and Murray Eden would consider a proposal for a major research effort in bio-materials science. Consideration would also be given to the development of an information exchange program within the Harvard-MIT community for the benefit of faculty members and students.

III. *The Committee on Health Care* was to be chaired by Paul Densen and William Pounds.

IV. *The Committee on Administrative Structure* was composed of Harvey Brooks, Robert H. Ebert, Henry C. Meadow, William F. Pounds, Walter A. Rosenblith, Jerome B. Wiesner, and myself.

These committees were asked to meet during the summer and to report at a second plenary session to be held in September. The Committee on the Behavioral and Social Sciences was to hold a summer study at Endicott House to consider the role of these sciences in medical education.

Administrative Structure

The Committee on Administrative Structure got off to a very fast start and held its first meeting on July 11, 1969 at the Woods Hole Oceanographic Institution. At this first meeting, Brooks, Ebert, Pounds, Rosenblith, Wiesner and I were present.

The task of the committee was to design the administrative structure best suited to implementation of proposed HST programs in education, research and development, and health care. The characteristics to be achieved in the design of the administrative structure were: 1) It should provide for effective utilization of existing personnel and resources of both universities; 2) it should facilitate the creation of necessary new facilities and the appointment of new personnel as may be required; 3) it should provide attractive career opportunities for faculty members whose primary commitment is to the success of the institution's program; 4) it should afford new opportunities for students at various levels of university education and especially in areas at the interfaces between medicine, the biomedical sciences, the other natural sciences, engineering, and the social and behavioral sciences; 5) it should have physical facilities that would provide loci for the community of faculty members and students engaged in the joint programs and promote their productive interaction; and 6) its viability and stability should be assured by financial support that provides endowment for faculty positions, adequate aid for students, and funds for the creation of needed physical facilities. This financial support should be new and should not divert funds from existing programs of Harvard and MIT. The ratio of resources to services in the new institution should be higher than in the universities generally so that some funds of the new institution may be available to support appropriate activities in the universities. The institution should have a clearly visible identity which will enhance its chances of obtaining the requisite financial support.

Dr. Wiesner suggested the following administrative structure: a Joint Governing Board with one third of the members coming from the Harvard Corporation, one third from the members of the MIT Corporation, and one third being independent members. Reporting to the Joint Governing Board would be the Joint Administrative Council consisting of the Deans of Harvard Medical School, the Division of Engineering and Applied Physics, The Faculty of Arts and Sciences and the JFK School of Government at Harvard, and the Provost and the Deans of Engineering, Science, and Management of MIT and the Dean or Director of the School of HST. The Dean or Director of the HST would report to the University Presidents, the Dean of HMS and the Provost of MIT.

There was general agreement that this structure would be appropriate to the needs and objectives of the institution.

A second major proposal related to faculty appointments. Faculty members whose primary commitment is to the program of the School of HST could have joint appointments in the School of HST and in another school of either Harvard or MIT or appointments in the School of HST alone. Faculty members whose primary commitment was to another school of either university but who spent part of their time in the program of the School of HST could hold joint appointments. Joint appointments would be made in conformity with the procedures of the appropriate departments or schools of the universities, and the procedures of the appointments and promotions in the School of HST would be established by the Joint Governing Board in consultation with the Joint Administrative Council. Tenure appointments and promotion to tenure rank in the School of HST would be recommended by *ad hoc* committees composed of faculty members of Harvard and MIT.

The Committee on Administrative Structure met again on July 18, 1969 at Woods Hole and on July 29, 1969 at MIT. The principal matters considered at these meetings were: a) the similarities and differences that exist in salary structure and fringe benefits and rules concerning tenure for faculty members at Harvard University, Harvard Medical School and MIT; b) the mechanisms that would be most appropriate for raising funds, applying for grants and disbursing funds from public and private sources; and c) the differences between MIT and Harvard in terms of the number of years a faculty member spends before achieving tenure, and the average age of the faculty members on achieving tenure in each university.

On August 12, 1969 the committee considered the mechanisms for the admission of students to the School of HST. It was proposed that undergraduates at Harvard and MIT would be apprised of the opportunities afforded by the School of HST in career guidance, curriculum planning, tutorial instruction, and particularly in courses and seminars on subjects relating to health and medicine. During the undergraduate years students could take advantage of the resources and facilities of the School of HST, but they would not be formally enrolled in the School.

Admission of M.D. Candidates: A Joint Admissions Committee composed of faculty members of Harvard Medical School and of the School of HST would be responsible for the admission of students who would be afforded a program in Human Biology in the school of HST and clinical education leading to the M.D. degree at HMS. Forty to fifty students per year were envisaged in such a program. Students would be eligible to apply not only from Harvard and MIT but from other colleges and universities. There was a further suggestion that it might be desirable to admit a group of students into the school of HST who, after completion of the program in Human Biology, would be eligible for admission into the clinical years of a medical school either at Harvard or elsewhere.

Admission of Ph.D. Candidates: A joint committee composed of faculty members of the appropriate department of Harvard or MIT and of the School of HST would be responsible for admission of candidates for the Ph.D. degree. The Ph.D. degree would be granted by Harvard or MIT upon the satisfactory completion of the requirements established by the department or school of the university concerned.

The principal decisions of the Committee on Administrative Structure were summarized in a memorandum by Henry Meadow and Walter Rosenblith: These were: 1) To establish a school of Health Sciences and Technology; 2) At MIT this school should have the status equal to that of other MIT schools; 3) At Harvard this school should be within the framework of the Faculty of Medicine along with the Medical School and the Dental School; 4) A joint Governing Board should consist of the Presidents of Harvard and MIT, two members from each corporation, two to four members from areas of interest outside of Harvard and MIT, and the Chairman of the Joint Administrative Board; 5) The Joint Administrative Board consisting of eight to twelve members would be appointed by the Joint Governing Board; half the members would be nominated by the Provost of MIT and half by the Dean of the Faculty of Medicine; the Dean or Director of the School of HST would also be a member of the Joint Administrative Board; 6) A Joint Policy and Planning Committee appointed by the Dean or Director of HST who would serve as chairman with the advice and consent of the Joint Administrative Board; 7) The Joint Administrative Board should be a successor to the Joint Committee on Engineering and Living Systems; and 8) Steps should be taken to provide a formal means of representation from junior faculty members and students.

A striking feature of the work of the Committee on Administrative Structure was the ability of the committee to establish, in a very short time, the principal organizational guidelines for the new Harvard-MIT Program. The members of the Committee, particularly Jerome Wiesner, Robert Ebert, Walter Rosenblith, Henry Meadow, Harvey Brooks, and William Pounds, possessed wisdom, experience, enthusiasm, good will, and administrative authority such that they could define the basic structure with confidence and optimism. I can attest to the fact that working with the members of this committee was an exhilarating experience.

The second Plenary Session was held on September 16, 1969. Eighty-five faculty members of HMS and MIT assembled in the Little Theater of the Kresge Auditorium at MIT. The attendance by leading members of both faculties reflected their interest in the development of the Harvard-MIT Program. Dr. Alexander Leaf reported on the deliberations of the committee concerned with the medical curriculum. He discussed the change in the curriculum at HMS with the adoption of a semester system that could coincide with the semester system at MIT. The suggestion was made that this new curriculum would benefit if new approaches were interlaced in some areas by having MIT faculty members teaching in this curriculum, for example, by using a systems analysis approach to human organ physiology.

Paul Gross, reporting for Elkan Blout, William Siebert and himself, stated the main conclusion of their subcommittee was that to have a national impact, a large-scale effort was needed. It was especially important to help develop clinicians who are much better scientists than are now being produced. Accordingly, a specific recommendation was made that a human biology sequence should be provided at MIT, making use of HMS faculty to prepare students to be well qualified for the clinical years at HMS.

William Siebert presented a possible scheme leading to the clinical years in greater detail. A human biology sequence with intensive scientific content was a principal feature of this scheme. He proposed a five- to six-year program leading to a B.S. or M.S. degree in Health Sciences and Technology which would encompass the basic MIT requirements in mathematics and in the sciences and then would include one and one half years devoted to the medical sciences. With electives and thesis, the total time required for the M.S. degree would be five to six years. The student would then be prepared for the clinical years of an M.D. curriculum or the pursuit of the Ph.D. degree in a biological science or in health policy or management or in medical engineering or medical physics.

Professor George Benedek presented the work that he and Philip Aisen had been doing for the course in which physical principles would be taught with illustrations from Biology and Medicine. Professor Leon Eisenberg summarized the report of the Committee on the Social and Behavioral Sciences with emphasis on the teaching of the Human Sciences and their relation to medical education. I presented a brief report on the overture from Dr. Theodore Cooper, the Director of the National Heart Institute, who was interested in our development of a research program in biomaterials, and I reported that a committee was at work to ascertain the type of response that should be made to this overture. In health care there was agreement that a major effort for the HST program seemed appropriate but planning had not yet begun. Finally, with regard to the administrative structure, Dr. Jerome Wiesner reported on the deliberations of the Committee on Administrative Structure.

Dr. Wiesner stated that the initial contacts leading to the formation of the JCELS were made because faculty members wished to facilitate collaborative research as well as academic programs. He expected that the joint effort would result in new research programs in biomedicine and bioengineering. With regard to academic structure, he stated that the Harvard-MIT School of Health Sciences and Technology would have a Joint Government Board consisting of members of the Harvard and MIT corporations as well as independent members, and a Joint Administrative Council consisting of Deans of the principal schools related to the sciences and technology of health and medicine. With respect to funding, he indicated that 40 to 100 million dollars would be sought and that shortly an advisory council composed of senior faculty of Harvard and MIT would be established to succeed the Joint Committee on Engineering and Living Systems. With regard to faculty appointments, there would be joint appointments between the new school and other departments of both universities with easy access for present faculty to collaborate with the joint institution. Physical facilities would be built initially at MIT.

I was very pleased by the recommendation that a program in Human Biology should be developed. It would be available to advanced undergraduate students. Such a program would include anatomy, physiology, genetics, anthropology, and ecology and could serve as an introduction to the pre-clinical sciences of medical school or dental school. This program could be available for graduate students in biomedical engineering and for graduate students in health policy and management who would profit from a knowledge of human biology. This proposal could also serve the broader purpose of integration of medical education into university education and could help to bring to bear on education for medicine the full range of science basic to medicine.

The work of the Committee on Administrative Structure in the summer and fall of 1969 provided ample evidence of the enthusiasm and harmonious spirit of the leadership of MIT and Harvard Medical School in promoting the development of the School of Health Sciences and Technology. Despite this strong support, I was convinced that it would be necessary to develop grass roots support in the faculties of the two universities. Accordingly, I arranged to meet with all of the departments in Harvard Medical School and the relevant departments at MIT. There were literally scores of meetings in which I attempted to describe in as much detail as possible the plans that were being formulated by the planning committee. These meetings were essential in generating faculty support or, at the very least, in minimizing resistance. I was somewhat disappointed to find that some friends of long standing on the faculties were not only not supportive but were actually resistant to the plans that were being proposed. On the other hand, very strong support was voiced by faculty members who found the proposed programs very much to their liking and realized that the Harvard-MIT school would enhance their opportunities and would not jeopardize their activities.

In the course of meeting with the various departments, I explored the possibility of enlisting the services of faculty members for the various courses which were being planned for our medical sciences curriculum. One experience deserves particular mention as an illustration of some of the problems that were encountered. When I met with the Department of Neurobiology at Harvard Medical School, the Chairman welcomed me but made it clear that I would have no help from his department in the development of a course in the neurosciences. When I met with the Head of the Department of Psychology at MIT, I was told that I could not count on help from any member of his department, especially not from the eminent neuro-anatomist Walle Nauta. Since an introductory course in the neuro-sciences was an essential part of our planned curriculum, I was faced with the problem of seeking help elsewhere. After weeks of fruitless searching, I received a call from Dr. Nauta who asked to meet with me. He informed me that he had learned that I had been told that he was unavailable for teaching but the contrary was true. He asked whether I would accept him as a faculty member to head the course in the neuro-sciences. Needless to say, I accepted his offer with alacrity and joy. And, indeed, Dr. Nauta developed a great course in the neuro-sciences for our students.

The numerous meetings held with departments, department heads, and individual faculty members served to promote a much better understanding of the developing plans and at the same time provided the planning committee with a sense of the hopes and fears or anxieties of faculty members who might be most directly involved in the activities of the new school. In order to provide further opportunity for faculty discussion of the developing plans, Dr. Ebert decided to have a presentation of the planning effort and program in the nature of a progress report at a meeting of the Harvard Medical School faculty in December, 1969. In his chapter he describes the reactions, both positive and negative, to the presentations. It was clear that much more work was needed to present a more fully developed plan. Accordingly, a formal proposal was drafted by a small subcommittee consisting of Leon Eisenberg, Don Fawcett, Alexander Leaf and myself. Its principal features are presented below:

The Proposal for a Joint Harvard-MIT Program in Health Sciences and Technology, dated February 26, 1970, presented to the Faculties of Harvard Medical School, MIT, and the Harvard School of Public Health, may be summarized as follows:

In 1968, the Joint Committee on Engineering and Living Systems reached the following general conclusions:

Harvard University and the Massachusetts Institute of Technology have both an obligation as well as an opportunity to advance the welfare of mankind by the joint application of their complementary resources to the life and health sciences in education, in research, in development, and in health care.

A new inter-institutional framework should be established to provide identity, coherence, and structure for the joint enterprise, a framework in which engineers, social scientists, physical scientists, physicians and biologists may contribute as equal partners.

Major new resources must be secured to provide facilities as well as support for the programs of the new institution.

On the recommendation of the Joint Committee, Presidents Johnson and Pusey requested the financial support of the Commonwealth Fund to facilitate the detailed planning of the programs and an administrative structure for their implementation. The support requested was granted in the spring of 1969.

The detailed planning effort is being carried out with the aid of a joint Faculty-Administration Committee whose members are Dr. Robert H. Ebert, Dr. Jerome B. Wiesner, co-chairmen. Senior faculty members and administrators of Harvard Medial School, the School of Public Health, the faculty of Arts and Sciences Division of Engineering and Applied Physics, and MIT Schools of Science, Engineering, and Management constitute the membership of the Committee.

The remarkable progress achieved in recent years in the biological and medical sciences has raised the expectations of our society for good health care, but despite the commitment of a growing proportion of our national resources to health needs, there is an increasing gap between these expectations and the capacity of our health care system to meet these needs. To meet the challenge of planning, building, and operating health care systems which are commensurate with our economic and intellectual resources, education and medical institutions, government agencies, and industry must orient themselves toward the creation and productive utilization of a broad spectrum of the new and emerging health professions. The full potential that may derive from joining the strengths of the two universities can be realized most successfully by the development of joint education programs. To provide for the effective coupling of the two universities in programs which can be integrated harmoniously into the activities of both universities, the Planning Committee recommends the establishment of a Harvard-MIT School of Health Sciences and Technology.

Education for the health professions should be viewed as a continuum, beginning in the pre-baccalaureate years and extending through the years of pre-doctoral education into the post-doctoral years of fellowship, internship and residency, or other professional training.

To promote the productive interaction of the biological and medical sciences with the physical and engineering sciences and with the social and behavioral sciences, and to facilitate the development of coherent curricular programs that provide continuity in the educational process, education for the health professions should be effectively integrated into general university education.

The School of Health Sciences and Technology would offer graduate education leading to a wide range of career opportunities in the health sciences based upon significant interactions of biology and medicine with the other natural sciences and engineering, and with the social, behavioral, and management sciences. Programs leading to Masters and Doctoral degrees would be sponsored jointly by the School and by the appropriate university departments that grant these degrees. These programs would be under the control of joint faculty committees whose members would be drawn from the faculty of the School and from the appropriate departments at Harvard and MIT. These committees would be responsible for the screening, preliminary qualification, and final examination of candidates for advanced degrees. Programs under the sole control of the faculty of the School would not be precluded; such programs would be desirable when faculty competence would be a subject area existing solely in the School. The following programs are envisaged:

1.) *Programs at the interfaces of human biology and engineering and the physical and mathematical sciences.*
2.) *Programs in human biology as an integral part of higher education in the life sciences.*
3.) *Programs in the social, behavioral, and management sciences as these relate to health and medicine.*
4.) *Programs that would provide suitable preparation for the pursuit of a degree in Public Health.*
5.) *Programs which would qualify the student to enter the clinical years of medical school or dental school. Some students could be admitted to the School of Health Sciences and Harvard Medical School with a commitment to proceed to the MD Degree at Harvard on the completion of satisfactory preparation in human biology.*

Selected undergraduate students at Harvard College and MIT would be offered the opportunity to enter in their sophomore or junior year programs which could lead to combined bachelor's and graduate degrees. These programs would be jointly supervised by a department offering the bachelor's degree and by the School of Health Sciences and Technology. The student would have the opportunity to select a sequence of subjects, seminars, laboratories, and tutorial sessions best suited to fulfill his educational goals. As an undergraduate, the student would be formally enrolled as a candidate for the bachelor's degree at MIT or Harvard College.

Courses under development or that are being planned are offered as illustrative examples in biophysics, biophysical chemistry, biomedical engineering, biomechanics, health services project planning, human genetics, child development with particular emphasis on cognitive processes, and computer modeling applied to population genetics, epidemiology, and social medicine. Courses in human biology to be developed include human anatomy, physiology, and pathophysiology, and will be developed in concert by life scientists, physicians, and physical scientists, engineers, and applied mathematicians. These courses in human biology will provide pre-clinical preparation for the clinical years of an MD curriculum. Post-doctoral programs that are envisaged include:

1.) Medical scientist programs for the development of medical scientists with a strong science base, whether this base be in the biological sciences or in the other natural sciences closely related to biology and medicine, or in the social and behavioral sciences as these relate to health and medicine.

2.) Programs for physicians and other health professionals seeking careers in management and administration.

3.) A program in biology and medicine for qualified engineers and other physical scientists interested in pursuing careers in bioengineering and at the interface between biology and the physical sciences.

In research, it would be the purpose of the School to facilitate the numerous joint research efforts involving faculty members and students of both universities, to provide a forum for the exchange of information, to select areas of investigation deserving of particular emphasis and chosen to take advantage of the strengths afforded by the two universities, and to find settings especially suited to multidisciplinary fields or areas of studies. Examples of the kinds of research that might be undertaken include a program in environmental health sciences and a program in biomaterials science.

Development as a concept refers to the deliberate applications of research findings to important health needs. Such development may encompass the design and production of prototype instruments for diagnosis and treatment, prosthetic devices such as sensory devices for the blind and the deaf, artificial organs, automated laboratories, model emergency rooms and operating rooms that effectively utilize the advantages afforded by modern science and technology. In health care, the application of managerial science and engineering technology to health services should enhance the quality and availability of health care and the efficiency of the delivery system. To be effective, education, research, and demonstration programs in health care should have one or more operational bases. It will be desirable to integrate such programs into the activities of the School and into the activities of the Harvard teaching hospitals, the MIT and Harvard Health Services, the Center for Community Health, the School of

Public Health, and the Sloan School of Management. Studies will be undertaken to determine the possibility of development of comprehensive health care programs in Cambridge and in Boston.

The characteristics to be achieved in the design of the administrative structure of the new institution are as follows:

1.) *It should provide for effective and joint utilization of existing faculty and resources of Harvard University and MIT.*
2.) *It should facilitate the creation of necessary new facilities and the addition of new faculty.*
3.) *It should be able to provide career opportunities equivalent to those of more traditional departments for faculty members who choose to make their primary professional commitment to the purposes and success of the new School.*
4.) *It should afford new opportunities for students at various levels of education and especially at interfaces between medicine, the biochemical sciences, the other natural sciences, engineering, and the social and behavioral sciences.*
5.) *It should have physical facilities that will provide foci for the activities of faculty members and students engaged in the joint programs and will promote their productive interaction.*

To achieve the goals of the programs and the desired characteristics of the administrative structure, the committee on Administrative Structure reached the unanimous conclusion that a new inter-university institution to be called the Harvard-MIT School of Health Sciences and Technology should be established. This School would be a school in the Faculty of Medicine at Harvard and a school within the structure of MIT. The School would be governed by a Joint Governing Board composed of the Presidents of Harvard and MIT, members of each corporation, and representatives of the public. In order to enhance the interaction of faculty members of different disciplines and in order to avoid the development of units that would parallel existing departments in the two universities, the School will not have a departmental structure.

Most faculty members in the School will hold joint appointments, with primary appointment in an existing department of either university and a secondary appointment in the School. Some faculty members whose primary commitment and responsibilities are in the School would also hold joint appointments insofar as possible with their primary appointment in the School. In exceptional cases, ap-

pointment in the School alone would occur for unusual individuals whose scientific disciplines do not conform to the existing departments of either university.

The viability and stability of the School should be assured by financial support which provides endowment for faculty positions, adequate aid for students, and funds for the creation of needed physical facilities. This financial support should be new and should not divert funds from existing programs of Harvard and MIT.

To implement the objectives of the programs, it will be necessary to develop a variety of new facilities at Harvard College, MIT, Harvard Medical School, and its teaching hospitals.

The meetings of the Harvard Faculty of Medicine and the School of Public Health to consider and vote on the proposal of a Harvard-MIT School of Health Sciences and Technology are well described in Dr. Ebert's chapter in this book. I should like to add some personal observations.

The meetings of the Medical School faculty reflected strong support for the basic principle of bringing to medical education, research and health care the strengths of the biological, chemical, and physical sciences and engineering, as well as the strengths of the social, behavioral, and management sciences. There was enthusiasm for undertaking a new and promising adventure. But there was also some concern over the impact of the proposal, especially if it should be very successful, on the various existing programs. The very favorable vote of the Medical School faculty was in a large measure a vote of confidence in Dean Ebert, who expressed his strong support of the proposal. At the meeting of the MIT faculty shortly after the favorable vote of the Medical School faculty, the proposal was approved without dissent. Again, I believe, the enthusiastic support of Jerome Wiesner, Walter Rosenblith, and Howard Johnson was critical in achieving this unanimity.

As for the School of Public Health, its faculty had mixed emotions. It was concerned with questions of territoriality at the same time that it perceived possibilities of enhanced opportunity through joint efforts with faculty members of MIT, the Medical School, and other Harvard faculties. The vote of the Harvard Corporation on June 1, 1970, authorizing Deans of the Faculty of Medicine and Public Health to seek to implement the plan for a Harvard-MIT School of Health Sciences and Technology was viewed as "a mandate to the Faculty of Public Health to give the most careful consideration to the problems and promise of the proposed new school and its potential effects on the objectives, operations, financing, and teaching and research programs of the Harvard School of Public Health."

To respond to this mandate, a committee at the HSPH was appointed with Professor Roger Revelle as Chairman. I was asked to participate in a summer study of HSPH and its relation to the proposed Harvard-MIT School. I happily accepted the invitation and agreed to have the study financed with our planning funds. The conference, held at Endicott House from July 7–10, 1970, was planned to consider ways in which teaching and research in HSPH could be coordinated with the Harvard-MIT School of HST with special emphasis on environmental health, the roles of social, behavioral, and management sciences as related to health and medical sciences, the health of disadvantaged populations, human population problems, and basic public health sciences such as biostatistics and epidemiology. The actual conference, however, dealt largely with a critique of HSPH educational policy and little consideration was given to coordination with the proposed School of HST.

The Revelle Committee had planned a second four-day conference scheduled for September 8–11, 1970, but it was postponed, according to Dean John Snyder of HSPH "because the fund raising procedures of MIT during July and August raised very difficult problems both for the Harvard Medical School and the Harvard School of Public Health." I was present at a meeting of Dean Snyder and James R. Killian, President Emeritus of MIT, to discuss fund raising for the Harvard-MIT Program. At this meeting, Dean Snyder was much more concerned with determining the allocation of funds to HSPH than with participating in the raising of funds. This attitude was very disappointing to Dr. Killian, who was quite prepared to devote much of his own time and effort to HST fund raising.

Dr. Ebert and Dr. Wiesner came to the conclusion that the original concept of a Harvard Faculty of Medicine-MIT Joint Program should be reinstated. As they wrote in a Progress Report dated January 27, 1971:

> progress toward the development of joint programs and the joint School would be facilitated by the establishment of a well-defined programmatic and administrative focus within each university. A sharp focus is preferred to a more general joint venture amoung all of MIT and several Schools of Harvard . . . As the joint Program evolves and when an estimated $10 Million of necessary new resources are ob-

tained, a joint School of Health Sciences and Technology will be established . . . Faculty members and students from all branches of both universities will, as now, be welcome to participate fully in the joint Program.

The favorable votes of the Harvard and MIT Corporations in June 1970 endorsing the establishment of a Harvard-MIT School of Health Sciences and Technology represented successful completion of my task as director of the planning effort. My sabbatical leave from Albert Einstein was near its end, and I was expected to return to my position as Chairman of the Department of Medicine. Wiesner and Ebert, however, urged me to accept the directorship of HST with appointment as Professor of Medicine at Harvard and Professor of Biology at MIT (the latter appointment had been in effect since July 1, 1969). They were concerned that the plans that had been adopted after so much effort might not be successfully implemented if I were to leave. I was faced with a difficult choice. I had strong bonds to my friends and colleagues at Albert Einstein with whom I had worked so happily for fifteen years. I had also forged new bonds of friendship and shared commitment to the goals of HST with many Harvard and MIT faculty members. Whereas I was confident that the Department of Medicine at Albert Einstein was very firmly established and would continue to prosper without me, I was sensitive to the argument that implementation of the HST program would be jeopardized were I to leave. After soul-searching discussions with my wife and our sons, I decided to accept the Directorship of HST.

The Scope of HST

Given the multiple institutions at Harvard and MIT with strong interests in health and medicine, what is the proper function of HST? Should it restrict its agenda to activities that are not being pursued in either university or should it seek to create synergistic collaborations that are more productive than one university can achieve on its own? These questions came to the fore early in the history of HST.

In 1972, Derek C. Bok became President of Harvard University, Jerome B. Wiesner became President of MIT, and Walter A. Rosenblith became the Provost of MIT. Their warm and amicable relations created a very favorable atmosphere for inter-university programs. Nevertheless, President Bok requested that Health Policy and Management be excluded from the scope of HST because of the territorial claim of HSPH. I understood the reason for President Bok's decision, but I felt nevertheless that it was unfortunate. I had envisaged an inter-university effort which would seek to marshal some of the strengths of both universities in economics, political science, and management as well as the strengths of HSPH and HMS in public health and medicine. I thought that HST could try to catalyze the development of outstanding programs of education and research in health policy and health services administration and management that are very much needed in this important sector of our society. It seemed regrettable that programs commensurate with the extraordinary strengths of the two universities in the relevant fields have not been developed.

A possible role for HST in health care had been attractive to faculty members interested in the development of model systems of medical care that could be replicated. There were promising discussions with Dr. James Hartgering, the Commissioner of Health in Cambridge, who was enthusiastic about the possible use of Cambridge and Cambridge City Hospital as sites for such study and model development. But Dr. Hartgering soon found that powerful political forces in Cambridge were opposed to such possible developments, and he felt obliged to discontinue the discussion. A role for HST in health care would have to be deferred as we concentrated our attention on the principal foci of education and research.

Defining the Educational Programs

The Planning Committee had recommended the development of a program in human biology that would be appropriate for undergraduates of Harvard College and MIT. There was much to recommend such a program, but far too little had been done to explore or develop the interest of key faculty members at Harvard College and at MIT. When I met with the Head of the Department of Biology at Harvard, his reaction to the proposal of a program in human biology was to declare that he saw no difference between human biology and snake biology and that he would certainly be opposed to any program such as was being recommended. At MIT there was concern that a program in human biology would probably become the preferred path to Medical School and would result in diversion of many of the best undergraduate students from choosing the Biology Department for their major course of study. It became clear that considerable time and effort would be required to formulate and develop a program in human biology for undergraduates that would be acceptable to both the Harvard Faculty of Arts and Sciences and the MIT faculty. Accordingly, the decision was made to defer the development of such a program to some future time that would be more propitious. We chose to begin with a focus on the Biomedical Sciences Curriculum leading to the M.D. degree at Harvard Medical School.

In an effort to foster the influence of the physical and engineering sciences on medical education, we sought to introduce principles of physics and engineering science by associating physical scientists and engineers with the various courses in the pre-clinical curriculum. These efforts met with mixed results. In functional anatomy, and in cardiovascular, pulmonary, and renal pathophysiology, the introduction of physical principles enhanced and illuminated the course contents. In other courses, however, success was achieved with an emphasis on the molecular and biochemical basis of clinical medicine rather than on the application of physical principles.

The recruitment of a faculty of very high quality was a most important part of the initiation of the educational program. With the cooperation of various department heads, principally at Harvard Medical School, we were able to attract faculty members who were not only very well qualified, but who were also very much interested in the programmatic objectives of HST. A critical core group was assembled rather rapidly. This group included David Hamilton and Farish Jenkins in Anatomy, Harvey Goldman in Pathology, Walter Abelmann and Roger Mark in Cardiovascular Pathophysiology, Daniel Shannon in Respiratory Pathophysiology, Martin Carey in Gastroenterology, Cecil Coggins and Alexander Leaf in Renal Pathophysiology, William S. Beck in Hematology, Dwight Robinson in Musculoskeletal Pathophysiology, W. Hallowell Churchill in Hematology and Introduction to Clinical Medicine, Walle Nauta in Introduction to Neuroscience and Paul Gallop in Biochemisty. It is remarkable that so many of this original group of faculty members have remained in leadership positions in the educational program. They have shown not only exceptional qualities as educators, but they have had a sustained dedication to the goals of HST.

Admission to the Biomedical Sciences M.D. Program

The decision to admit a first class of twenty-five students in the fall of 1971 was made early that year. This permitted very little time to publicize the program and admission to it. Accordingly, it was decided to offer admission to students who were accepted or on the waiting list for admission to Harvard Medical School. The selection of twenty-five students from this pool of 280 students was made by Dr. Herrman L. Blumgart, Chairman of the HMS Admissions Committee, and by me. Dr. Blumgart was Professor Emeritus of Medicine and former Chairman of the Department of Medicine at the Beth Israel Hospital. He was a good friend of mine, ever since my own student days at Harvard Medical School when I worked in his research laboratory. I was delighted to be associated with him again. Given the outstanding qualifications of applicants to Harvard Medical School, it was not difficult to select a class of twenty-five excellent students who were also willing to be pioneers in this experiment in medical education.

In subsequent years, an HST Admissions Committee operated as a subcommittee of the HMS Admissions Committee. It was agreed that the decisions of the HST Admissions Committee would require ratification by the HMS Admissions Committee. In practice, however, the decisions of the HST Committee were rarely overruled by the HMS Committee. The ready acceptance of the judgments of the HST Admissions Committee was based not only on the qualifications of the HST Committee members but also on the excellence of the students selected for admission to HST.

There were several policy issues to be decided. Should admission be restricted to students from Harvard College and MIT? If medical education is viewed as a continuum beginning in the undergraduate years, should students be encouraged or permitted to enroll as candidates for the M.D. degree while still undergraduates and candidates for a Bachelor's degree? If the curriculum is oriented toward students with a strong interest in the natural sciences or engineering, which sciences should be favored—mathematics, physics, and engineering; or molecular biology, genetics, and biochemistry? This is a debate that has continued to the present. A bimodal distribution has existed with the physical sciences as one mode and the biological sciences as the other. In many respects, this bimodal distribution is advantageous because it promotes interaction between the two groups which is stimulating and informative.

If one were to seek a single mode, defined by advanced mathematics, physics, and engineering, one would not only risk turning away superb candidates from the biological sciences, but one would face the dilemma of teaching the medical sciences with subject matter that remains to be formulated in terms that can take advantage of the students' strengths in the mathematical and physical sciences. The bimodal distribution has provided a creative tension which has proved to be quite productive.

A few students have been admitted as candidates for the M.D. degree while still undergraduates working for a Bachelor's degree. On the whole, however, students have chosen to apply for entrance after graduation from college. Nearly half of the successful applicants come from Harvard and MIT and the other half from distinguished colleges and universities elsewhere.

The Admissions Committee has been fortunate in having outstanding chairmen. Herman Eisen, William S. Beck, and Daniel Shannon have led committees composed of faculty members drawn from the two universities in the medical sciences, in the biological sciences, and in the physical sciences and engineering. The committee has also included HST students as regular voting members.

From the very beginning, the HST program has attracted superb students who are eager to accept the dual challenge of becoming excellent physicians and excellent scientists. We encouraged the development of combined degree programs. The flexibility of the HST curriculum made it possible to develop individualized M.D.-Ph.D. programs at a time when there was no formal M.D.-Ph.D. program at Harvard Medical School. Following the lead of HST, a formal NIH funded M.D.-Ph.D. program was established at Harvard Medical School with HST students occupying approximately half of the positions in the program.

A special feature of the HST Biomedical Sciences curriculum has been the thesis requirement. As candidates for a Doctoral degree, HST students are expected to present a thesis based on original work and independent study. If the student is a candidate for the Ph.D., the Ph.D. thesis serves to meet this requirement. If the student is a candidate for the M.D. degree only, then the thesis is required. This thesis work has been the basis for the achievement of graduation with honors by a substantial proportion of HST students.

One of the very first educational initiatives of HST was the development of a course and textbook, *Physics with Illustrative Examples from Medicine and Biology,* by George B. Benedek and Felix M.H. Villars. First offered as a course for MIT students in 1970, its success prompted the publication of the first edition of the textbook in 1973. A second edition in three volumes, *Mechanics, Electricity and Magnetism, and Statistical Physics,* published in 2000, has been widely acclaimed and is a valuable resource for medical scientists and biophysicists.

Other HST initiatives worth noting were the presentation of a course in Medical Ethics by Sissela Bok and by Charles Fried of Harvard Law School and a course in Economics of Health Care by Allen Detsky, an HST graduate with both an M.D. and Ph.D. in Economics.

Development of the Medical Engineering and Medical Physics Program

While the faculty of the School of Engineering at MIT and the Division of Applied Science at Harvard had been engaged in bioengineering teaching and research for over a quarter of a century, it was not until 1971 that a formal graduate program in Biomedical Engineering was developed under the auspices of the Dean of the Graduate School. The creation of the HST program in 1970 fostered the growth and development of this interdepartmental program through its support of students, curriculum development, and clinical associations. The interdepartmental program attempted to provide interdisciplinary training in the natural sciences and engineering to an extent not possible in the doctoral programs in the various departments. Participation was small and the program suffered from the lack of formal structure, particularly with respect to providing a strong foundation in the biomedical sciences and appropriate exposure to clinical medicine.

In response to these deficiencies, a group of faculty members from Harvard and MIT joined forces in 1975 to develop a new graduate program within HST which would prepare students for a new profession of Medical Engineering and Medical Physics (MEMP). This program is based on a new concept: students, well qualified in physics or engineering, are also educated in the basic biomedical sciences and have hands-on direct experience in a clinical care setting under medical supervision. The purpose is to confront the budding medical engineer or physicist with real-life clinical problems so that he or she can formulate the questions of clinical care from the vantage point of the principles of engineering or of physics and can interact or collaborate with physicians or surgeons on an equal basis.

After two years of planning by a committee led by Ernest Cravalho and Fred Bowman, the program was approved in 1977 by the MIT and Harvard faculties. To assure a high quality of candidates selected for admission, the successful applicant must be accepted by a department at MIT or at Harvard, and then by HST. The degree of M.S. is awarded on recommendation of the department, and the Ph.D. is awarded on the recommendation of HST. The key components of the program are advanced study in engineering or physics, pre-clinical studies in the biomedical sciences, extensive clinical experience, and thesis research of an original nature.

The program has proved very successful, as judged by the quality of the students and by the positions which graduates of the program have held since its inception. The graduates are very much in demand for leadership positions in other academic institutions, in industry, and in major health care centers. The details of the program are presented in Professor Roger Mark's chapter in this book (Chapter 9). I should like to add one comment.

Despite the obvious success of this program, a committee charged with a review of the HST program in 1984 made the suggestion that the MEMP program be terminated and that a few places be made available in the Biomedical Sciences curriculum to accommodate students from the MIT Interdepartmental Program in bioengineering that had become dormant with the advent of MEMP. This suggestion was made principally for financial reasons and could not be justified based on the performance of the students or the excellence of the educational program. Fortunately, this suggestion, which would have been a grievous mistake, was not followed, thanks to the vigorous and reasoned opposition of MEMP students and HST faculty. The leadership of Ernest Cravalho, Roger Mark, and Fred Bowman was an essential element in the success of this program.

Governance of HST

After five years as a Program, there was general agreement that HST should be institutionalized. To prepare for such institutionalization, a constitution and rules of procedures for appointments and promotions of faculty were required. Two years of drafting with repeated revisions were carried out by the Administrative Committee, principally led by Walter Rosenblith, Henry Meadow, Eleanor Shore (serving as special assistant to President Derek Bok), Ernest Cravalho, and myself. President Bok was very helpful in providing a critical review of each revision. The final document, dated March, 1977, is summarized below.

The experience of seven years as a Program demonstrated that Harvard and MIT can join successfully and productively in common efforts in the health sciences and technology. From the beginning and increasingly as the Program has developed, it has been recognized that an appropriate, stable institutional structure is essential to the full achievement of the Program's objectives.

To secure the most successful utilization of the intellectual and physical resources of Harvard and MIT in medicine and health, joint programs of education and research have been established. The stability necessary for the optimal development of these and other joint programs requires an administrative structure which should:

1.) be an integral part of the two universities;
2.) provide a framework for interdisciplinary, educational, and research efforts, and for the development of new professions, such as medical engineering and medical physics;
3.) facilitate the appointment of necessary new faculty members and the development of necessary new facilities;
4.) provide attractive career opportunities for those faculty members whose primary commitment is to the achievement of the programs directives;
5.) provide visibility for the commitment of the two universities to this joint enterprise and thus enhance the chances of obtaining the requisite financial support.

The rather ambiguous term "Division" was chosen as the name for this administrative academic structure instead of the original term "School" which had been proposed in the resolution adopted by both university corporations in 1970. This decision was said to be due to the different meanings of the term "School" at Harvard and MIT. It was clear, however, that there was some resistance to conferring the status and title of school on an academic structure that might impinge on the territory of one or more existing schools. Accordingly, in 1977, the Harvard-MIT Division of Health Sciences and Technology was established by vote of the Corporations of MIT and Harvard University.

The purpose of the Division is to provide a means of collaboration between Harvard and MIT that makes available educational and research opportunities that could not be exploited as effectively by either institution through its own efforts. Conversely, the Division should not be administered in a manner that results in an unreasonable duplication of effort or an undue competition for funds with either of the two participating institutions.

The educational programs will include:

1.) A curriculum leading to the MD Degree awarded by Harvard University.
2.) A curriculum leading to Masters and Doctoral degrees in Medical Engineering and Medical Physics.

Programs in research and development will be concerned with important biological, medical, and health problems, which can be addressed in an interdisciplinary manner through the collaborative efforts of biomedical scientists, physical scientists, engineers, physicians, and/or public health faculty from the participating institutions. To ensure that these objectives are achieved, every proposal for a new educational program or a new research or development program must be submitted to the Administrative Council for review. All new educational programs and every major new research program must also be submitted to the Governing Board, with final approval requiring the agreement of both Presidents.

The organization and administration of the Division are as follows:

Governance:

1.) Governing Board. Responsibility for the formulation of educational, administrative, and fiscal policies will be vested in a Governing Board. Membership will consist of the President and one member of the Harvard Corporation and one other individual they shall select, and the President and one member of the Corporation of MIT and one other individual they shall select. The Governing Board will authorize major programs of instruction and research, subject to the specific consent of the Presidents of Harvard and MIT.
2.) Appoint a committee to visit the Division of HST.
3.) Review and approve the annual budget of the Division of HST together with policies and programs related to fund raising and forward such budgets to the governing bodies of their respective institutions for final approval.

A second major body is the Administrative Council. Membership will include the Provost of MIT, the Dean of the Harvard Faculty of Medicine, the Director of the HST Division, the Dean of the Harvard Faculty of Arts and Sciences, the Dean of Engineering and Applied Physics at Harvard, the Dean of the Harvard School of Public Health, the Dean of the School of Engineering at MIT, and the Dean of the School of Science at MIT.

The Administrative Council will:

1.) Oversee the implementation of approved programs in the participating faculties and schools.
2.) Review the plans for new educational and research programs of the Division of HST and discuss plans for new educational and research programs in other schools or faculties of the two universities relevant to the activities of the Division of HST.
3.) Develop recommendations for policies and programs related to fund raising on behalf of the Division of HST for submission to the Governing Board.

The Budget Committee consisting of the Provost of MIT, the Dean of the Harvard Faculty of Medicine, and the Director of the Division of HST will:

1.) Review and approve budgets prepared by the Division of HST prior to submission to the Governing Board.
2.) Review proposals for programs, appointments, and organization of the Division of HST. Where such proposals involve matters that affect another faculty or unit in either university, the dean or appropriate representative thereof should be invited to attend.

Joint Faculty Committee:

The development and conduct of HST programs are the principal responsibilities of the Joint Faculty Committee. Membership will consist of those members of the faculties of the two universities having major educational, research, and administrative functions within or in relation to the HST Division. Members will be appointed by the Director of the Division of HST with the advice of the Administrative Council. The Joint Faculty Committee will determine criteria for appointment of the faculty of the Division of HST, establish requirements for new faculty and staff positions whose primary responsibility is to HST and initiate requests for appointments to meet these needs, request and receive reports from faculty committees established to implement the academic programs of the HST Division, and maintain liaison with related activities of Harvard and MIT through service on appropriate committees in either institution. The rules and procedures for appointment to tenure and for term appointments are specified in detail and in a manner that conforms essentially to the rules and practices of the two universities.

It will be the policy of the HST Division to develop and conduct its programs primarily with faculty who are appointed to positions in either or both Harvard and MIT. However, it is recognized that it may be necessary to appoint a small number of faculty members whose primary responsibility will be to the Division of HST.

The carefully drafted constitution was adhered to by President Wiesner, Provost Rosenblith, and President Bok, but with the retirement of Rosenblith in 1981, the Administrative Council lapsed into inactivity as a result of sparse and sporadic attendance by the Provost and various deans. As for the Joint Faculty Committee members, those who were appointed to represent their departments or school but who had no stake in the success of the HST Division attended Joint Faculty Committee meetings only occasionally. Accordingly, these meetings were essentially devoted to reports of standing committees such as the Curriculum, Admissions, Research Program, and Finance Committees. The Joint Faculty Council meetings were useful for informational purposes, but they did not provide a suitable forum for discussions of policy.

During the first ten years of HST's existence, we derived great benefit from a committee that met weekly for a period of at least two hours. Its members were Provost Walter Rosenblith; Senior Associate Dean of the Faculty of Medicine, Henry Meadow; Assistant Dean of the Faculty of Medicine, Robert Blacklow; Special Assistant to President Bok, Eleanor Shore; Associate Director for Medical Engineering and Medical Physics, Ernest Cravalho; Assistant Director for Resources, Walter Koltun; Assistant Director for Research and Development, Irving Berstein; Senior Academic Administrator, Fred Bowman; and I. This committee was very effective. The administrative problems that arose in the joining of the two universities in a common effort were resolved speedily and amicably. This was, in effect, an excellent executive committee.

In joining the two universities in common educational and research programs, the Harvard-MIT Division was anchored at Harvard in a well-organized Faculty of Medicine. At MIT, however, despite very intensive educational and research activities related to health and medicine, no similar academic focus existed.

There was need for an appropriate administrative structure within MIT for programs in health-related activities beyond the defined scope of the Harvard-MIT Division. To help meet these needs, President Wiesner and Provost Rosenblith proposed the creation of a College of Health Sciences, Technology, and Management. This new college could provide an administrative home for the Harvard-MIT Division and, like the division, it would be multi-disciplinary and without internal departmental structure. Since health and medical problems are complex and difficult to study, let alone to solve along uni-disciplinary lines, the concept of a multi-disciplinary academic institution whose faculty members hold joint appointments whenever possible in the existing departments was an integral part of the proposal of the Harvard-MIT Division as well as of the new College of Health Sciences, Technology, and Management. With the enthusiastic and effective leadership of the Chairman of the Corporation, Howard W. Johnson, and President Wiesner, and with the successful achievements of the Harvard-MIT Program as a basis, the MIT administration raised $26,000,000 in support from Uncas and Helen Whitaker, the Pew Memorial Trust, and the Kresge Foundation. These funds made it possible to establish the Whitaker College of Health Sciences, Technology, and Management in 1978, to provide for the construction of physical facilities to house the new college, and to provide essential administrative and laboratory facilities for the Harvard-MIT Division. To promote the harmonious development of both Whitaker College and the Harvard-MIT Division, I was asked to assume the Directorship of Whitaker College while at the same time continuing to serve as Director of the HST Division.

In initiating the activities of Whitaker College, I was aided by two very able Associate Directors, Ernest Cravalho, Professor of Mechanical Engineering, who had played a major role in the development of the Medical Engineering and Medical Physics Program of HST, and Christopher T. Walsh, Professor of Chemistry and Biology. We undertook several developments simultaneously: planning and design of the physical facilities for the Whitaker College Building, recruitment of new faculty members by search committees in the human neurosciences and the basic biology of cardiovascular disease, and the development of a training program in health policy and management. The faculty searches resulted in the recruitment of outstanding scientists, Ronald McKay, Robert Rosenberg, and Monty Krieger. With the support of the Kaiser Family Foundation, the Program in Health Policy and Management was developed under the leadership of Edward Roberts of the Sloan School, Harvey Sapolsky of the Department of Political Science, and Peter Temin of the Department of Economics.

In 1980, there was a major change in the MIT Administration.

President Wiesner and Provost Rosenblith retired and were succeeded by Paul Gray and Francis Low, respectively. When construction of the Whitaker College building was completed, the MIT Administration chose to convert Whitaker College into a home for the newly-named Department of Brain and Cognitive Sciences, formerly the Psychology Department. Professor Emilio Bizzi, head of the Department of Brain and Cognitive Sciences, was named Director of Whitaker College, and the programmatic association between Whitaker College and the Harvard-MIT Division was interrupted. The funded training program in Health Policy and Management was permitted to lapse, despite the obvious need for well-qualified professionals to deal with the flawed health care system in the United States. As for the newly appointed faculty, Ronald McKay left MIT for the NIH and Robert Rosenberg and Monty Krieger were integrated into the MIT Biology Department. The original concept of a college of Health Sciences, Technology, and Management was not realized at that time but remained, in the view of many, a goal to be attained.

Research

A principal objective of HST has been the promotion of multidisciplinary collaboration between the faculties and students of MIT and Harvard Medical School in research on major health problems. Programs developed by HST have ranged from fundamental scientific research to applied research and development. The HST Division seeks to bring together teams of physicians, scientists and engineers to work on scales appropriate to the dimensions of the problems under study. Emphasis is placed on the development of programs that take advantage of the strengths afforded by the two universities and that have a high potential for productive and valuable results. Our experience has helped us to develop a strategy for fostering collaborative research. An announcement is made of a meeting open to all who are interested in pursuing research on a given subject. At the meeting, we seek to identify one or more leaders. With the help of such leaders, a schedule of exploratory seminars and information exchange meetings is established. The principal questions to be addressed are formulated, and then there follows a period for the development of research grant proposals that can form a coherent program. In general, this process takes about eighteen months from the initial announcement to the time when a research grant proposal can be submitted to an appropriate funding agency such as the NIH.

This procedure was developed with the leadership of Dr. Irving Berstein, who was Assistant Director for Research Program Development. A Ph.D. in chemistry, he had been a successful CEO of a small biotech company. He promoted and facilitated the interactions between scientists of different disciplines, and he helped to create a climate in which physicians, engineers, and scientists could work together productively as equals.

During the first thirteen years of the existence of HST, major multidisciplinary research programs were established. These included the Program in Biomaterials Science, ably administered by Robert W. Mann; the Harvard-MIT Rehabilitation Engineering Center led by William Berenberg and Robert W. Mann; the Optimization of Dose Distribution in Cancer Radiation Therapy directed by Martin Levine and Bengt E. Bjarngard; the Harvard-MIT Biomedical Center for Clinical Instrumentation directed by Roger Mark; the Harvard-MIT Research Program in Short-Lived Radio-Pharmaceuticals directed by S. James Adelstein and Gordon Brownell; the Center for Health Effects of Fossil Fuels Utilization directed by Gerald Wogan and William Thilley; the Research Program in Hyperthermia Treatment of Tumors, initially supervised by Padmakar P. Lele and subsequently directed by H. Frederick Bowman, Terrence Herman, and Norman Coleman; and Thromboresistant Materials directed by Edwin Salzman and Robert D. Rosenberg. During the period of 1971–1984, eighty new research programs were launched. These programs were supported at the level of approximately $51,000,000. As of 1984, there were 115 research faculty and senior research staff associated with HST research programs, approximately equally divided between MIT and Harvard faculty members. These large-scale inter-university research programs have required excellent administrative staff support. We were fortunate in having the administration and management of these programs in the hands of Fred Bowman and Keiko Oh.

Resource Development

When the HST Program was first established in 1970, there was a great sense of optimism that it would be quite easy to raise $10,000,000 of endowment. Dr. Walter Koltun, an alumnus of MIT and a Ph.D. in biochemistry, was appointed as Assistant Director for Resources. He was an experienced fund raiser who was confident that this goal could be achieved relatively quickly. To help launch the fund drive, a distinguished sponsoring committee of friends of Harvard and MIT, mainly alumni of these universities, was appointed. Several members of this committee were quite wealthy and were considered very good prospective donors for the joint program. As it turned out, however, very little help was derived from this sponsoring committee. The joint effort of Dr. James Killian, representing MIT, and Dr. George Thorn, representing both Harvard Medical School and MIT, was far more effective in raising funds for the HST Program.

Dr. Koltun had been led to believe that he would be helped in fund raising by the Development Offices of the two universities. In practice, however, he was not made a member of either Development Office, and he was asked to clear prospects for fund raising with both offices to be certain that he would not be approaching individuals or foundations that were already targeted by either university. This clearance procedure was required of HST, but the system was not made reciprocal; the Development Offices did not clear any of their prospects with Dr. Koltun. His task was, therefore, quite difficult. Nevertheless, he succeeded in developing fruitful relations with potential donors who had no previous association with either university. By 1984, more than $10,000,000 of endowment had been successfully raised.

Some Reflections on the Founding and Development of HST

The joining of two great universities in common programs of education and research affords obvious advantages. The mobilization of complementary resources can achieve substantial synergy and can lead to greatly enhanced opportunities for faculty members and students. By seeking to bring to bear on medical education and research the full range of the sciences basic to medicine, one can hope to produce physician-scientists and medical engineers and physicists who continue to grow intellectually throughout their professional lives, who advance the scientific and technologic base of medicine, and who are dedicated to humane professional service in our society. I believe that this major goal of HST has served us well and should continue to guide us in the future.

If the scope of the joint effort is restricted to one that neither institution can undertake alone, the potential for mounting major inter-university collaborative programs may be severely and unnecessarily limited. In defining the scope of HST, it would be preferable, I believe, to consider whether a joint effort would achieve a better result than would independent effort by each institution.

The constitution and by-laws that were designed for HST were meant to provide a stable administrative structure. This worked well when the leaders of the two universities supported the administrative structure that was defined in the constitution. But when leaders were less supportive, they could simply ignore the basic provisions of the constitution. One might ask, therefore, how one can achieve institutional stability with preservation of the rights presumably guaranteed by the constitution. Stability can be achieved by mounting programs of education and research that are of unassailable excellence. Stability is also promoted by the ability to generate the financial resources required to endow faculty and student activities and to create essential physical facilities. A substantial endowment is a powerful stabilizing force.

I have often been asked to comment on the causative influences in the success of HST. There are several principal elements. First, the leaders of the two universities, Jerome B. Wiesner, Robert H. Ebert, Walter A. Rosenblith, Howard W. Johnson, and Derek C. Bok, provided creative administration, guidance, and support. A second element has been the quality of the faculty members committed to the HST programs. They have been outstanding scholars with strong dedication to the achievement of excellence in education and research. A third element has been the superb student body seeking a deeper understanding of the science of medicine. Our students have recognized the importance of promoting the progressive penetration of the medical sciences by the sciences basic to medicine. They have excelled not only in the medical sciences but also in clinical medicine and surgery and in the associated specialty fields. A fourth element has been adherence to the principle that a doctoral degree, whether in medicine or in medical engineering and medical physics, should reflect original and independent research. Research as an integral part of the curriculum is a principal characteristic of HST.

Finally, on a personal note, I feel honored and privileged to have been able to participate in the founding and development of HST as an institution bridging these two great universities.

Chapter 5

THE MIDDLE YEARS (1985–1990)

A Memoir

Richard J. Kitz, M.D.

In the fall of 1968, while still at the Karolinska Institute in Stockholm on sabbatical leave from the College of Physicians and Surgeons of Columbia University, my interest in moving to Boston was first kindled. The lure was a position offered as Anesthetist-in-Chief at the Massachusetts General Hospital, Henry Isaiah Dorr Professor of Research and Teaching in Anesthetics and Anaesthesia at Harvard Medical School, also principal investigator of the Harvard Anesthesia Research Center. The key individuals in the recruitment process were Drs. Gerald Austen, Surgeon-in-Chief at MGH; John Knowles, General Director of MGH; Robert Ebert, Dean of HMS and one of the two grand architects of HST. After the usual *pas de deux,* I assumed the position in September of 1969. The Harvard Anesthesia Research Center was supported by a five- year grant from the Institutes of General Medical Sciences of almost a million dollars direct cost to fund all anesthesia related research among the Harvard teaching hospitals. One of the projects was to establish a Bioengineering Unit to support engineering and technology requirements of the investigators for commercial equipment or unique devices to further their mission. Fifty thousand dollars annual support for this purpose was committed.

With these center grant funds, a biotechnology instrumentation and support group was established, first under the direction of Dr. Joseph Cywinski, later under the supervision of Drs. Ronald Newbower and Jeffrey Cooper. Relationships with MIT and the Harvard Division of Applied Sciences were developed, technology support services organized, and appropriate instructional courses implemented.

These inter-institutional activities were facilitated because of a relatively unique situation. In the mid-sixties, Dr. James Shannon, Director of the NIH, had approached the administrations of MIT and MGH to establish still another new medical school in Boston with NIH supporting the venture initially with a commitment of $50,000,000. Shannon and others were convinced that the practice of medicine was then highly empiric, more of an art than a science and hardly evidence-based. The purpose of the new school would be to educate as medical students those who had previously been graduates of programs in the physical sciences such as engineering, chemistry, mathematics, and physics. It was assumed that such students would be more rigorous in their medical practices thereby requiring quantitative evidence to support diagnoses and therapies. After vigorous debate among the respective faculties and medical staffs, this revolutionary project was rejected.

However, the Harvard-MIT-MGH committees that sifted through the principal issues were astonished to find a large number of inter-institutional research and educational projects often unknown to the respective administrations. Because these were more extensive than realized and were fulfilling relatively unique pedagogic and research needs at both institutions, it was recommended that Harvard Medical School and MIT create a structure that would formally accommodate these inter-institutional activities. Professor Irving London, Chairman of the Department of Medicine at Albert Einstein College of Medicine in New York, was asked to design and recommend an appropriate entity into the two universities. Consequently, the Harvard-MIT Program in Health Sciences and Technology (HST) was formally established in 1970 with Professor London as its first Director.

On a sunny Sunday afternoon in the Fall of 1970 I had a chance encounter with Dr. London while attending a performance at Harvard's Loeb Repertory Theatre in Cambridge. We had known each other in New York City and had a good friend in common, Dr. Emmanuel M. Papper, who had been my chief of anesthesiology at the Columbia Presbyterian Medical Center. During intermission in the course of our conversations, Dr. London readily sensed my long-held interests in technology and asked that I consider membership on the Joint Faculty Committee of HST. This group of senior faculty from MIT and Harvard Medical School continues today and serves as a counseling and advisory group to the HST administration. We have monthly meetings and enjoy periodic *ex cathedra* retreats.

Through these interactions I became an advisor to students who were considering medical careers and various educational, research, and training opportunities. The operating room and critical care environments of the Anesthesia Department at the MGH were special magnets for HST students because these care- taking and research activities are dependent on sophisticated technology.

In the mid-seventies, HST established one of the more rigorous doctoral programs at MIT. The Medical Engineering/ Medical Physics Program (MEMP), described in detail in Chapters 9 and 11, was designed to equip outstanding engineers and physical scientists to address important health-related problems. The program features intense course work in the medical and clinical sciences at HMS in addition to departmental based graduate study in the physical sciences at MIT and Harvard. Dr. Ernest Cravalho, Professor of Mechanical Engineering, together with Dr. Fred Bowman, the principal architects of MEMP, asked that I join the admissions committee on which I subsequently served for many years.

It was in 1980 that I first met Dr. Roger Mark. Roger, a dynamic leader with a medical degree from Harvard and an engineering degree from MIT, was given the mission to form a bioengineering center incorporating appropriate research groups from Harvard, its teaching hospitals and the departments at MIT. Because of our Bioengineering Unit at MGH, we were asked to participate. I attended the initial series of organizational meetings and then asked Ronald Newbower and Jeffrey Cooper, Directors of our Bioengineering Unit, to participate. It was clear that Roger Mark was a special person indeed, a leader with professional and personal characteristics that enabled him to work at the interface between two major institutions, represented by scientists of varying backgrounds and interests.

In the spring of 1985 I had a call from the Office of the Dean of the Medical School, Dr. Daniel Tosteson, to arrange an appointment between us. When we met a week later he asked whether I had an opportunity to meet with the special committee appointed by the presidents of Harvard University and MIT to examine the current status and future of the Harvard-MIT Division of Health Sciences and Technology. The committee was chaired by the ex-president of MIT,

Professor Howard Johnson. Because I had been in Europe at the time of the committee's meetings, I had not had an opportunity to meet with them. Dean Tosteson briefly reviewed some of the recommendations of the Johnson Committee report. In particular we discussed the desirability of increasing the size of the M.D. program and phasing out the MEMP program. The Dean indicated that the director, Professor Irving London, would be stepping down at age 65 and that the Johnson Committee recommended a co-directorship. MIT and HMS would each have their own representatives who would work closely with each other to direct the affairs of HST. He then asked me to consider my being the HMS representative. I told him that indeed I was interested depending on the nature of the charge, and of equal importance, the identity of the other co-director. Incompatibility in just about any aspect of vision, management and style would lead to failure. In addition, I pointed out that I had had no experience with a co-directorship and that the one proposed involved two culturally and operationally different institutions separated by the Charles River. Dean Tosteson believed that the MIT administration was uncomfortable with a single director who must be a physician if he/she were to be responsible for the M.D. program. The Dean pointed out that for HMS, MIT is the only venue for these kinds of educational and research programs. That is to say, there was almost no alternative. If the Harvard-MIT Division were to go forward, then it had to be with the MIT requirement for the co-director format.

I mentioned to Dean Tosteson that I was not a disinterested person when it came to HST. I was very much in support of the HST vision and if I assumed the position he suggested, then he would be appointing someone who would be a vigorous advocate of HST. He asked why I felt so strongly and I suggested to him this probably derived from the understanding that my specialty, anesthesiology, is dependent in its care of patients on the trilogy of biochemical pharmacology, pathophysiology, and technology. HST employs these same disciplines, in part, to achieve its mission.

Dean Tosteson thanked me for my interest and candor and requested that I meet with Dr. James Adelstein, Executive Dean for Academic Programs, to review the Johnson Committee report and discuss potential candidates for the MIT co-directorship. Dean Adelstein sent along a copy of the report in anticipation of our meeting a week later. After thorough discussion he and I concluded that some of the recommendations were warranted and that others would be difficult to implement. In addition, the venture had not yet been considered by the Harvard University and MIT central administrations. We then reviewed the CVs of two candidates for the MIT co-directorship. One of them, Dr. Roger Mark, was superbly qualified, having earned his M.D. degree at Harvard Medical School and his Ph.D. in electrical engineering at MIT. Of course I remembered Roger as having organized the Bioengineering Center application to the NIH. Alas, he resided in Dover, Massachusetts, which is also my home. Jim then suggested that Roger and I meet to consider how some of the recommendations might best be implemented and why others should not. In the course of these discussions we would learn whether or not we could work together as a team, sharing a common vision and management style.

Although I'm not necessarily a believer in instant rapport, sitting down with Roger Mark proved to be just that. Not only did we live less than a mile apart, but we basically had the same philosophy: that HST was too good to disappear or be modified in major, detrimental ways. We agreed that we needed to make certain that we identified the issues that led to the current concern about HST programs and the need to design remedial initiatives rather than to implement a major restructuring. Our individual ideas coalesced into a unified plan.

We discussed the dangers inherent in a co-directorship and quickly concluded that the partnership would work only if Roger and I were identified by our administrations, faculty and students, as a single entity. To do this would require that I know almost as much about MIT as did Roger, and he in turn, know as much about HMS as did I. To implement this arrangement, we agreed to have lunch together twice a week to educate each other and develop strategies and plans which could be supported vigorously by both of us. We reported these agreements to our respective leaders: for me, Jim Adelstein, Executive Dean for Academic Programs, and for Roger, Vice Provost at MIT, Ken Smith. We were told of an impending meeting with the Presidents of the Institute and the University and to include Provost John Deutch, Dean Daniel Tosteson, Vice Provost Ken Smith, Executive Dean for Academic Programs Jim Adelstein and selected members of the respective Visiting Committees. We would be invited to meet with this group at a luncheon to discuss our plans for HST.

Roger and I then made an appointment to see Professor Irving London. Conversations with Dr. London are always fascinating and informative and ours proved little different. In his matter-of- fact, unhurried and incisive style he reviewed the beginnings of HST, its current status and his concerns. We took notes, told him we would seek his counsel privately from time to time but asked him to join an HST Administrative Committee that we would form and continue his membership on the Joint Faculty Committee (JFC). He agreed.

One of the principal recommendations of the Johnson Committee was to phase out the Medical Engineering Medical Physics Program and expand the M.D. component by transferring some of the MEMP positions and explicitly reserving them for candidates for both M.D. and Ph.D. degrees, the latter in engineering. The MEMP program had had its teething problems but was now maturing as one of the best and most rigorous doctoral programs at MIT. The Johnson Committee had failed to interview MEMP students who were very upset with that omission. The student body nominated two senior students, Deborah Burstein and Martha Gray, to argue this case. They met with Provost John Deutch and vigorously articulated cogent reasons why the MEMP program should continue. Likewise they presented their arguments to a special meeting of the JFC which was convened on November 19, 1984. After vigorous debate, the JFC unanimously endorsed a resolution to delay termination of the MEMP program pending implementation of specific strategies designed to address the issues cited by the Johnson Committee. This recommendation was forwarded by letter to the Provost and the Dean. Later, Roger and I brought the Joint Faculty Committee Resolution to the luncheon meeting with our institutional presidents and gained their tacit support.

During these first weeks, Dr. Mark and I met with Vice Provost Smith and Executive Dean Adelstein to constitute ourselves as the HST Executive Group. We were given the privilege of convening the Executive Group each month to coordinate our HST initiatives. It soon became clear that this was a most effective strategy as it provided us with timely counsel and advice that virtually precluded wrong decisions on our part. In addition this procedure gave us confidence and material support for those initiatives that were endorsed. If the period 1985–1990 is judged to have been important for HST, then much of the credit must be assigned to the wisdom and support of the Executive Group's leadership.

The meeting with Presidents E. Paul Gray of MIT and Derek Bok of Harvard took place in the MacLaurin room at MIT. After the usual introductions, Dean Adelstein reviewed my credentials and Vice Provost Smith, those of Roger Mark. We were asked about our plans for addressing the issues raised by the Johnson Committee, our own visions and proposed initiatives for HST. We reviewed our concerns about the recommendations to phase out the MEMP program and reported on the consternation of the MEMP student body and the Joint Faculty Committee. We discussed our plans to enhance the Joint Faculty Committee involvement in HST activities and the importance of the Executive Group in implementing our plans. As a general strategy, we hoped to institutionalize HST at both MIT and HMS by increasing the number of core faculty, raising program endowment and securing endowed chairs. We then requested that a Visiting Committee for HST be convened with Dr. Richard Johns of Johns Hopkins as chairperson. Further, we asked that the Edward Hood Taplin chair be activated so that an appropriate HST professor could be established on the MGH campus.

General discussion yielded the following: the decision to eliminate the MEMP program would be deferred pending further study and possible recommendation of remedial actions by the co-directors. The enhanced roles for the Joint Faculty Committee and the Executive Group were supported. A request to increase the number of core faculty was denied but joint fund raising on behalf of HST would be implemented. The HST Visiting Committee was re-titled "Advisory Committee" and was authorized to meet every other year to review issues identified by the co-directors and to report to the Provost and Dean. In general, we were directed to formulate strategies, seek endorsements, and implement plans to address the concerns identified by the Johnson Committee. These directives and our new initiatives would be implemented by the Executive Group and reported annually to the Provost and Dean.

It was clear that the presidents were in support of the concept of HST but were not on the verge of committing substantial resources for an entity at a crossroads state, under new and untried leadership. Consequently, Dr. Mark and I committed our joint mission to reinvigorating and institutionalizing HST. Later, the HMS commitment was underwritten by incorporating the HMS M.D. student body as one of the five medical student societies in the New Pathway to medical education. In addition, HMS would commit the Robert Ebert Chair in Molecular Medicine to the co-director of HST.[1]

Although Roger and I parallel processed a number of issues, we assigned highest priority to establishing monthly meetings under the aegis of the Executive Group and designing a strategy to save the MEMP Program. Because Vice Provost Ken Smith had selected Roger, and Executive Dean for Academic Programs Jim Adelstein likewise had selected me, our two superiors had almost as much dependent on the outcomes as did the co-directors themselves. We formulated the agendas and scribed the minutes of our two-hour monthly meetings. Our proposals were always thoughtfully and objectively considered, and we were the beneficiary of sage counsel that not only improved our initiatives but aborted those that were considered ill conceived for whatever reason. Perhaps even more important, the initiatives that were endorsed enjoyed the support of two most important and influential institutional executives. The meetings themselves were always conducted on Friday afternoons in Ken Smith's office, though once a year the co-directors convened a meeting in a local restaurant as special thanks to our patrons.

To fulfill the dictates of our presidents, the Executive Group reported annually to the Dean and the Provost. One meeting was held in the hospital room of Provost John Deutch. He had been hospitalized to repair a leg fractured when crossing Massachusetts Avenue and struck by an MIT graduate student riding a bicycle. These meetings were always highly enjoyable, providing an opportunity for the co-directors to report on the state of HST, to review initiatives of the past year and proposals for the future. Roger and I recognized what a special privilege we had in working with the leadership of both our institutions.

Because of this hierarchical, consultative relationship we had quiet assurance in reporting our proposals and strategies to HST's student body, administrative leadership and Joint Faculty. Our management philosophy could probably best be termed "A Guided Democracy." The threat of HST's retrenchment was thwarted and the Program, now a Division, began to thrive once more. For the co-directors, this was a period of enthusiasm and energy as we thoroughly enjoyed working in harmony, processing our agendas in parallel. As described in detail in Chapter 9, MEMP was streamlined somewhat, but preserved and stabilized.

To decrease the vulnerability of HST to vicissitudes of changes in institutional leadership, the co-directors sought to extend the base of support locally by broadening and enhancing the mission of the JFC. In addition, the HST Advisory Committee represented not only a traditional method of working issues and plans but served to educate its members about HST and thereby extended its influence.

Members of the Joint Faculty Committee were carefully selected from those with a strong HST bias and represented appropriate disciplines and departments at HST and HMS. Instead of a group to which the co-directors reported initiatives and actions, this became a prime consultative committee that energized the various programs proposed by HST leadership. By soliciting joint faculty input and factoring their advice into the various proposals, the basis of support for these initiatives was broadened and deepened. The Joint Faculty Committee was convened monthly during lunch at the MIT Faculty Club.

The HST Advisory Committee was triumphant from the beginning. Dr. Richard Johns, Massey Professor and Director, Department of Biomedical Engineering at Johns Hopkins University, agreed to head the committee which planned to meet in Cambridge/Boston every other year. With the advice and consent of Jim Adelstein and Ken Smith, committee members were selected, based not only on their national and international reputations in areas of importance to HST, but also because of the institutions they represented across the country. By reviewing the missions and programs of HST, they better understood and in turn supported the Division and its vision. In that way, the HST Division became better known across the country, not only enhancing its image but increasing the number of graduate school applicants.

Roger Mark and Fred Bowman were the dual engines behind the organization of the two-day meeting of the committee. The standard meeting format always included a pre-meeting dinner organized by the chairman to review charges and agenda with committee members. The next day began with a report by the co-directors, following which the members were divided into groups to review or discuss specific agenda items with students, core faculty, course directors, etc. This would include tours of laboratories as might be required by specific agenda items. On the second day, the co-directors were invited to have breakfast with the committee to answer questions that had arisen during the committee's deliberations. The chairman would cite the general conclusions of the committee at that point and ask the co-directors if they had comments. The committee then resumed its meeting in executive session and reported their conclusions to the Dean, Executive Dean, Provost, and Vice Provost.

Within a month, a formal report was sent to the Provost and the Dean. The report of the Advisory Committee was generally one of enthusiasm for HST and an endorsement of most of the initiatives proposed by the co-directors. With this kind of broadened support from within the institutions by the Joint Faculty and beyond our schools by the Advisory Committee, HST began once more to prosper within the limits prescribed.

This was also the period when Dean Tosteson completely reorganized the medical student body, dividing it into five separate societies in a manner similar to that in vogue at Oxford and Cambridge. The purpose of this New Pathway to Medical Education, as it was titled, was to enhance the educational experience by enabling groups of students to work more closely together and more intensively with faculty.[2] HST in a very real sense was the first of these societies. It enjoyed its own section of the HMS Admissions Committee and had its own curriculum, a core faculty, and administrative and laboratory space in the Whitaker building on the MIT campus. In 1985, culminating three years of intense study by faculty, students, and administration, the New Pathway was launched at HMS and adopted by the other four societies. I was appointed Master of the HST Society composed of our medical students and associated faculty. HST selected those attributes of the New Pathway appropriate to its mission. Dean Tosteson secured funding to totally redesign one of the buildings on the quadrangle at HMS then dedicated as the Medical Education Center, housing quarters for the five societies around a large atrium. HST was awarded prime space in the Medical Education Center with dedicated student areas, computer carrels, laboratories, and meeting rooms. These were replicated in the other society areas.

HST's medical students were joined by MEMP students during the first two years for a marvelous, inter-institutional educational experience. Because a research thesis was required for graduation and the student body selected with academic careers a likelihood, student research efforts flourished broadly. Few HST students completed their programs in the minimum of four years while a third earned advanced science degrees. Of the 150 M.D.-Ph.D. students at the Harvard Medical School at any one time, over half are HST students. We benefitted greatly by having available laboratories at Harvard University and MIT in Cambridge, the Medical School and its hospital affiliates in Boston. No richer research and educational opportunities exist anywhere.

One of our more frustrating ambitions for HST was the attempt to increase the number of core faculty. Both institutions were unwilling to increase the numbers, mostly because they perceived HST as a division between two institutions and not enjoying the usual departmental prerogatives. Operationally, this meant that HST would always be cast as a non-equal to the traditional departments. Without the usual perquisites that attend departmental status, it is not possible to commit adequate resources to the faculty thereby to ensure perpetual growth and development for HST. The institutions believed that it was best that HST have a small core faculty and to recruit other faculty from the traditional departments depending upon HST's programmatic needs. But without the leverage of departmental status and resources, the co-directors were too often placed in a position that was in conflict with departmental needs. Annually, we importuned the institution's leaders and annually were denied!

There was sympathy for HST's position among several key faculty members, and we considered the possibility of asking our administrators to transfer these professorships to HST's core faculty. Indeed, Dr. Nelson Kiang transferred his professorship to HST, while Drs. Richard Wurtman and Robert Langer accepted joint appointments. Important cooperative programs were launched. Thus, NIH awarded a major training grant to HST entitled "A Training Program for Speech and Hearing Sciences" with Professor Kiang as its Director. The MIT Clinical Research Center was transferred to HST in 1987. Dr. Richard Wurtman served as its director, and Dr. Robert Rubin was recruited later as associate director with a primary HST endowed chair.

At about that time, the MIT Medical Department was being reorganized and one of our HST course directors, Dr. Arnold Weinberg, was appointed its director. The Medical Service was located in the Whitaker College Building, shared with HST and others. A natural collaboration ensued with students selecting electives on the Medical Service and faculty involved in their instruction also meriting HST appointments.

New courses were designed with MIT basic scientists assigned as co-directors with many clinical course heads to make certain that fundamental science was incorporated in all courses. This was highly successful and made for an enduring synergy. It had always been an HST tradition to evaluate all courses periodically. Principally through the efforts of Dr. Walter Abelmann, course evaluations were increased in frequency and rigor. This, at least in partial measure, accounts for the excellence of HST course offerings.

If the term biomedical engineering is interpreted broadly, then many MIT faculty and departments are involved in biomedical research. Initially, there was no coordination of these efforts to provide students and faculty with guidance, support and review. Dr. Mark founded an HST "Graduate Committee" termed the Biomedical Engineering/Physical Sciences Committee. It was to be the common touchstone group for all biomedical research at MIT. Each of the traditional departments that offer biomedical research and educational opportunities was represented on the committee. It was not an easily workable committee. Thus, its efforts were only partially successful. Full cooperation of the traditional departments was never achieved. It was clear to the co-directors and many others that the imaging sciences were, and would continue to be, a major opportunity for research and teaching, surely with almost immediate societal payoff. Nonetheless it was difficult to promulgate the idea because the imaging sciences cut across the traditional departmental lines which, at MIT, made progress difficult and sometimes acrimonious. Fortunately, the idea was too good to die. It was ultimately endorsed, and a search for faculty began in 1994. Significant endowment for this initiative was gifted in 1999.

In 1994, the Edward Hood Taplin Chair in Medical Engineering was awarded to Dr. Ernest Cravalho, Professor of Mechanical Engineering, a long-time HST faculty member. The MGH agreed to house the Taplin professor and ceded many of its diverse biomedical engineering activities to the new hospital department. Our hopes were that the Taplin chair would be responsible for all MIT/HST students on the MGH campus, research between the institutions would be enhanced, technology would be represented at the policy making tables, and clinical service improved. Unfortunately, none of these goals were achieved. After three years, the experiment was declared a failure, and Dr. Cravalho's position at the MGH was dissolved. The idea was certainly a good one; perhaps the times and the personnel were inappropriate.

After five years working with Dr. Mark as co-director of HST, and in my seventh decade, I began to consider the increasingly short time I had to continue my commitment to HST and the large department at the MGH. HST was now stable and thriving, its existence no longer threatened.

At the MGH, the faculty and resident staff were increasingly concerned that too much of my time was being devoted to off-campus activities. Indeed that was true in large measure and especially so when Dean Daniel Tosteson established the medical students societies, HST being one. A new series of time commitments were required and it became quite apparent that I needed to make a decision: should I step down from the full-time responsibilities of being a chairman of anaesthesia to part-time status so that I could give increasing amounts of time and energy to HST? It was clear to me that younger leadership was now appropriate for the HST co-director and that I should return full time to the MGH and to plan the transition to my successor.

In the fall of 1990, I asked Dean Tosteson to relieve me of my responsibilities as co-director of HST and Master of the HST Society the next summer. He reluctantly agreed and committed the Robert Ebert chair to my successor as co-director. After a world-wide search Dr. Michael Rosenblatt was selected to be the first Ebert professor and my successor as co-director of HST.

Conclusion

There is a general consensus that the period 1985–1990 in the history of HST was successful and perhaps some would argue most successful. Why is that so and why did it happen? HST not only survived an interregnum of some turmoil and uncertainty but was suffused with new energy, purpose and destination: the Division thrived again under conjoint leadership.

And why did this occur? Reasons that are cited include: the superb faculty, a legacy from Dr. Irving London; the quality of the student body; the support of the Executive Group; and the endorsements of the Advisory Committee. As this is a personal story, I exercise my prerogative of respectfully demurring with those judgements though agreeing that they and others played important roles. Unequivocally, the harmonious relationships between the co-directors, their common goals and perfectly complementary styles led to a singular entity that was indeed greater by far than their individual contributions. I consider those five years the halcyon period of the thirty I have spent at Harvard and its hospitals. I thank Deans Tosteson and Adelstein for making this possible and especially Roger Mark for making it so.

Notes

1. D.D. Federman, H. Goldman, D.A. Goodenough and M.B. Ramos, "Academic Societies," in D.C. Tosteson, S.J. Adelstein and S.T. Carver, eds., *New Pathways to Medical Education. Learning to Learn at Harvard Medical School* (Cambridge, MA: Harvard University Press, 1994), pp. 167–172.
2. Ibid.

Chapter 6

HST: 1992–1995

Michael Rosenblatt, M.D.

On March 1, 1992, I had the privilege of succeeding Dr. Richard Kitz of the Massachusetts General Hospital as the "Harvard" Co-Director of HST. Selected by a search committee composed of faculty and administration from Harvard Medical School (including its affiliated hospitals) and MIT, the recruitment was conducted collaboratively by the Dean of the Harvard Medical School, Daniel C. Tosteson; the Chairman of the Department of Medicine at Beth Israel Hospital, Dr. Robert M. Glickman; and the Provost of MIT, Mark Wrighton. Harvard Medical School assigned a newly endowed chair, the Robert H. Ebert Professorship in Molecular Medicine, to the Co-Director position, and Beth Israel Hospital established a new Division of Bone and Mineral Metabolism within the Department of Medicine. The efforts of the new Co-Director were to be divided evenly between HST and Beth Israel Hospital. Perhaps predictably, both roles soon became "full-time."

I discovered in 1992 that the HST was an organization with an outstanding record of past achievement. Previous leadership, including Dr. Irving London, Dr. Richard Kitz and Dr. Walter Abelmann, contributed greatly to the excellence and evolution of HST. Nevertheless, although there remained great promise and opportunity in its interdisciplinary mission at the interface of medicine and engineering, and its status as a joint venture of Harvard and MIT, HST faced a number of issues in the path to continued success. On the MIT campus, HST is a "Division" of the Institute, formally established by the MIT Corporation. A small number of primary faculty hold appointments in the Division, but a much larger number hold primary appointments in other departments and participate in the educational and research programs of HST as "affiliated faculty." This arrangement has been both a strength and a weakness. It gives HST the ability to reach broadly across the diversity of the MIT faculty and deeply within certain of its departments, especially those involved in biomedical engineering. Fortunately, in the MIT culture, conventional department groupings do not act as barriers. Consequently, HST enjoys loyal and dedicated effort from an eclectic group of MIT faculty which sustains its programmatic objectives. On the other hand, the lack of "departmental" status is a liability. Prior to 1992, even new "primary" HST faculty appointments had to be made in conjunction with a conventional department at MIT. Although the responsibility for professional development of HST primary faculty was shared between HST and the department, the promotion and tenure process was based in the conventional department. While the arrangement served to "certify" HST faculty within the context of the MIT academic structure, it also created a certain tension for faculty and often placed an unrealistic set of obligations on them which originate from the need to serve two "departments." Furthermore, the small number of "core" faculty alone could not carry out the broad Divisional mandate and populate its numerous committees and infrastructure.

On the Boston side of the Charles River, a different set of issues was evident. HST is constituted as one of the five Academic Societies at Harvard Medical School.[1] HST, therefore, is configured as a major educational organ of the medical school, maintaining the curriculum and generating innovations in medical education. As an Academic Society, HST also supports the non-curricular aspects of student academic life and provides an infrastructure of advising, career counseling, and enrichment programs to meet student needs. The Dean and other leaders of Harvard Medical School and its affiliated hospitals recognize HST to be an exemplary Academic Society. In many respects, HST served as the model for the Academic Societies at HMS. It has its own curriculum and has constructed a number of mechanisms to fulfill previously "centralized" functions in support of the students. For instance, HST has its own set of student advisors who meet regularly as a board. HST also conducts its own curriculum retreats, course assessment, and convenes its own Admissions Committee.

Despite its accomplishments and visibility as an Academic Society, HST nevertheless was in some respects separate from the rest of HMS. Its programmatic differentiation, although highly successful, seemed to detach HST from the mainstream of medical education at HMS, where exciting and major medical educational reform was taking place. Primary faculty appointments in HST at HMS were not possible in 1992; they were simply viewed as not necessary. HST was strictly an educational organization and the tradition of devoting time to teaching was strong amongst HMS faculty. Hence, there was no real problem enlisting faculty (even the most senior and distinguished) from the HMS departments to HST's educational initiatives. Although there seemed to be no real need for primary faculty from HMS, nevertheless, there were a small number of faculty who identified more strongly with HST than with their "home" department. These faculty sought mechanisms to strengthen and formalize their affiliation with HST. For these reasons, some HMS department chairpersons wanted to explore joint recruitment and appointment with HST.

It was in this setting that a new team of Co-Directors assumed leadership of HST. Dr. Roger Mark had already served as Co-Director from MIT for seven years. He and I worked together on all aspects of HST administration, policy, and new initiatives. We avoided dividing the labor along MIT and Harvard lines. Nevertheless, although we both concerned ourselves with issues on both campuses, we each tended to represent HST on our respective home campuses. Therefore, for purposes of this chapter, I will focus mainly on events related to the M.D. program from 1992–1995.

In these efforts to improve the program, innovate in medical and graduate education, and enhance student advising and other supports for the student community, we were joined by Joseph Bonventre, M.D., Ph.D. We had the good fortune to succeed in recruiting Dr. Bonventre to the position of Associate Director and Associate Master of HST. Dr. Bonventre was, in many respects, the ideal person to assume this role. He is a graduate of the program, holds M.D. and Ph.D. degrees, and is a highly successful physician-scientist whose research is at the interface of medicine and modern biology and biophysics. Combined with his exceptional interpersonal skills, he is a role model for HST students. As Associate Master, he serves on the HMS Council of Masters. In addition, he is a member of the Renal Unit at the Massachusetts General Hospital and (at the time of this writing) is Associate Professor of Medicine at HMS.[2]

My first year was spent meeting and learning about the people who comprise HST, becoming informed about and evaluating the HST educational programs (M.D., Ph.D., combined M.D.-Ph.D., Medical Engineering and Medical Physics, Speech and Hearing Sciences Programs), and examining HST's role at HMS and its interface with the four other Academic Societies. After one year of surveying the "waterfront," several new opportunities were identified.

It is clear that the HST M.D. curriculum and the New Pathway curriculum (which is followed by the other four Academic Societies)[1] can benefit mutually from increased communication and the sharing of ideas. In a very real sense, two educational experiments of national significance were being conducted in parallel at HMS, in a nearly ideal environment which includes some of the very best medical students in the country and outstanding faculty. The educational missions of the two curricula (HST and New Pathway) are different: HST has as its mission to train physician-scientists who will one day be leaders in biomedical research; the New Pathway has a broader and more diverse mandate, which includes the training of primary care physicians, specialists, and leaders in health policy, as well as physician-scientists. Both programs share the same commitment to broadly educating physicians who will be excellent and who will be in the top tier in their fields.

In order to stimulate educational innovation, the Dean convened the Council of Masters which met with him weekly. In this forum, the heads of the Academic Societies met together to discuss issues facing the medical education program and to plan curricular change. In short order, an effective bridge was built between HST and the other four Academic Societies. Informational traffic increased dramatically in both directions to the benefit of all. In HST, the sense of ownership by the faculty for the organization and its programs continued to be a "role model" for the Academic Societies. HST provided the New Pathway with a new example of how to organize the student research experience as a formal course. In addition, HST has led the medical school in developing computer-based approaches to medical education.

The New Pathway successfully demonstrated the importance and value of having students learn about ethics during their time in medical school. Now, HST has begun an effort to incorporate ethics into the curriculum at three critical junctures. These positions in the curriculum were selected because of the belief that they represent times at which the students would be receptive to learning about ethics: at the beginning of the laboratory experience, when they learn about ethics in the conduct of scientific research; at the beginning of the clinical experience, when they learn about ethical issues in the patient-doctor relationship; and in a clinical research elective, when they learn about the ethics of conducting experiments with human subjects. In addition, aspects of the pedagogic philosophy of the New Pathway are being incorporated into the HST curriculum. There is now more emphasis on problem-based learning, the tutorial format, students taking responsibility for active learning, and developing the habit of life-long learning and self-study using primary sources.

As the Masters exchanged information amongst themselves and decided to collaborate and work together to take charge of all aspects of both curricula, a mechanism for "dividing the labor" was instituted. The concept of "stewardship" arose. Each Master assumed responsibility for a large segment of the curriculum as it appears vertically through all the years of the curriculum. Within the area of stewardship, each Master works with faculties and department chairpersons to improve and refine the representation of that discipline within the curriculum. The Master also is responsible for providing the impetus for curricular innovation and the infrastructure for experiments in education. As Master of the HST Society, I assumed stewardship of "medicine." Other Masters became stewards of neurology and psychiatry, obstetrics and gynecology, and pediatrics, primary care and the patient-doctor courses, etc. Also, added to the HST area of stewardship was biostatistics and epidemiology, social medicine and health care policy, the student advising system at HMS, and the HST pre-clinical curriculum.

An important outgrowth of the "stewardship" concept was the opportunity for HST to develop a full four-year curriculum in addition to the basic medical sciences of years I and II. As steward for medicine, we began to work in collaboration with the hospitals to design new clerkships in core medicine and the medical subspecialties. The most important of these efforts is ongoing at the time of this writing. We are engaged in a cooperative effort to design a new Core Medicine Clerkship I, co-sponsored by HST, which will emphasize pathophysiology and technology. The objective is to build bridges from the clinical experience back to years I and II. The concept has met with great enthusiasm by all Core Medicine I clerkship directors from the four hospitals which offer the course. HST is now in the process of developing a faculty syllabus which will focus on approximately ten major diseases which students encounter during the Core Medicine I clerkship. For each of these diseases, a chapter will be written by experts oriented toward the basic pathophysiology of the disease and the scientific basis of technology applied in that area of medicine. Cost-benefit analysis and the limitations of the technology will also be explored. In this manner, we hope to provide the attending physicians with a level of comfort sufficiently high to enable them to introduce these topics into attending rounds. We also plan to identify HST-affiliated faculty to serve as clinical mentors of the students at the hospital sites. Since HST has been in existence long enough to have alumni who are now on the HMS faculty, it is our hope that some of the mentors can be selected from amongst our alumni.

Major opportunities for HST have arisen in the area of clinical research. In the early 1990s, the MIT administration was examining the role of and potential for the MIT Clinical Research Center (CRC) which is under the direction of Dr. Richard J. Wurtman. The MIT CRC is the only NIH-funded CRC not located in a hospital. Since its emphasis is on clinical research, but it is nested in a university that has no medical school or hospitals, the CRC encounters greater than usual difficulties in forming close ties to other MIT departments. Therefore, the MIT administration asked HST to assume departmental oversight for the CRC in an effort to better integrate the CRC into the MIT academic community and to foster interdepartmental collaborations.

Fortunately, within a short period of time, an opportunity arose for HST to broaden the mandate of the MIT CRC from clinical research exclusively to inclusion of a training mission. Dr. Robert H. Rubin, who serves as Chief of the Transplantation Infectious Disease Unit at the Massachusetts General Hospital, was recruited to join HST's primary faculty and establish a new Clinical Investigator Training Program. When Dr. Rubin joined the HST core faculty, he became the first incumbent of a newly endowed professorship, The Osborne Associate Professorship in Health Sciences and Technology. Dr. Rubin attracted major support from Pfizer, a multi-national pharmaceutical company, for development of the new program. In collaboration with the CRC at Beth Israel Hospital, and under the auspices of HST, he and Dr. Alan C. Moses of Beth Israel launched one of the largest training programs in clinical investigation in the nation.[2] The program has ten two-year positions, for a total of twenty trainees at any time. One-half of the positions are allocated to Beth Israel Hospital and the other half to the MIT CRC. In its first few years, the Clinical Investigators Training Program has attracted highly accomplished individuals with advanced subspecialty training from a number of medical disciplines. Some of the work done by the trainees has already achieved national recognition, especially in the area of functional imaging of the central nervous system.

An important by-product of the program has been the design of a one-month elective clerkship in clinical research which will be open to all HMS students. The HST leadership realized that there are many students enrolled in HST and HMS who are interested in laboratory research. After they are exposed to clinical medicine, many of them become very enthusiastic about the practice of medicine and some of those seek mechanisms for combining their research interest with clinical medicine. At the time of devising this new clerkship in clinical research, there was no formal offering in this area at HMS.

In the area of student advising, the HST model of a highly active group of advisors who meet regularly as a board is in the process of being emulated by the other Academic Societies under HST guidance. Specific areas have been targeted for improvement, including internship advising, career counseling, and a special advisory program for M.D.-Ph.D. candidates. In the latter case, a new primer was written by Dr. Barry Sleckman, an HST M.D./Ph.D. alumnus. In the area of career guidance, HST held two symposia on careers outside academic medicine. In particular, opportunities in the biotechnology sector were showcased.

One of the new courses developed under HST auspices is a tutorial-based approach to advanced medicine. Dr. Steven E. Weinberger of Beth Israel Hospital designed a course for fourth-year medical students which relies on problem-based learning and case-method teaching to emphasize the basic pathophysiology and scientific underpinnings of medicine. The course has been extremely popular—more students apply than can be accommodated.

The review process for HST courses was revised and enhanced to evaluate not only individual courses but to assess each semester and each year of the HST curriculum as a grouping of courses in order to examine course integration, avoid duplication and omissions, and configure courses optimally for educating physician-scientists. In June 1995, Dr. Frederick J. Schoen of the Brigham and Women's Hospital chaired the Curricular Review Committee. The Committee conducted an extensive one-year long review of the HST curriculum. They recommended the establishment of new courses, a decrease in time allocated to some existing courses, and utilization of new pedagogic techniques. Pursuit of the recommendations promises to change dramatically the HST M.D. curriculum for the next decade.

A major change in the administrative status of HST was obtained by the Co-Directors. At MIT, the Division was granted all the rights and privileges of a department, including the ability to appoint faculty based exclusively in the HST Division. At HMS, the privilege of making primary HST faculty appointments also was granted. As a result, the HST primary faculty was expanded. As mentioned earlier, Dr. Robert H. Rubin was appointed the first HMS incumbent of the Osborne Chair. Elazer R. Edelman, M.D., Ph.D., an HST alumnus (Class of '83), was appointed to the Cabot Associate Professorship at MIT. In addition, Dr. Lee Gehrke was promoted to tenure at Harvard Medical School as the Lawrence J. Henderson Associate Professor of Health Sciences and Technology. Funds were raised for the J. W. Kieckhefer Chair as well. Martha Gray Ph.D., also an HST alumna (MEMP '86), became its first incumbent. The expansion of the "core" faculty and addition of several faculty in the early stages of promising careers has enhanced the vitality of the HST Division.

A major new initiative for HST is under way at the time of this writing: to establish a functional imaging center at MIT. Two senior endowed professorships will be dedicated to this effort. The new facility will be housed in the Francis Bitter Magnet Laboratory at MIT. Based on the virtual explosion of knowledge in this area and the opportunity to form links between the new imaging technologies and modern biology, this area was deemed worthy of a major investment of resources by HST and MIT. It is anticipated that collaborative ties will develop with many of the departments at MIT, such as Chemistry, Biology, and the Clinical Research Center. It is also hoped that links will develop with the new "Mind, Brain, Behavior" initiative based at Harvard, which involves several Harvard faculties. The Functional Imaging Center will be not only a research center but also a major training and educational center.

The era we are currently entering creates numerous challenges for HST. Firstly, Dr. Roger Mark announced his intention to leave the Co-Directorship of HST after nearly a decade of exceptional service. It will be difficult to replace his talents and dedication to HST. The appointment of a new Co-Director and the new directions chosen by him or her will be of vital importance to the future of HST. In addition, we are entering an era in which technology is sometimes misunderstood or even under attack in the "managed care" environment. The attractiveness of specialized medicine compared to general medicine has declined, and many research-oriented HST students feel insecure about the future. However, the interface between academia and industry is growing and creating new research opportunities for HST and its graduates. These arenas will be highly active in the next few years and will challenge HST leadership, faculty, and students to produce the best program they can to prepare HST graduates for careers as physician-scientists and leaders in biomedical research.

Notes

1. D.D. Federman, H. Goldman, D.A. Goodenough and M.B. Ramos, "Academic Societies," in D.C. Tosteson, S.J. Adelstein and S.T. Carver, eds., *New Pathways to Medical Education. Learning to Learn at Harvard Medical School* (Cambridge, MA: Harvard University Press, 1994), pp. 167–172.
2. A.C. Moses, "A Model for Training Clinical Investigators," in Proceedings of the 1996 Fall Symposium of the Association of Professors of Medicine, *Biomedical Research in Academic Departments of Internal Medicine: Challenges and Solutions*, 1997.

Chapter 7

FUND RAISING FOR THE HST PROGRAM 1969–1993

Walter L. Koltun, Ph.D.

In 1969, during the planning phase of the HST Program, the Commonwealth Fund made a grant of $600,000 to the two universities for the detailed planning of educational programs in Health Sciences and Technology and for the design of an administrative structure for their implementation. During the following year many issues were explored in depth, including the fiscal requirements to establish a joint enterprise on a permanent basis. The need for and the desire to engage in a major collaborative effort were strengthened by this process, and a major fund-raising program was initiated to meet the cost of the proposed undertaking.

When the two universities agreed to establish the joint Program in 1970, they also agreed on certain fund-raising goals and operating procedures. The major ones were:

1. The Program would have its own fund-raising office and funds would be raised jointly by both schools together, rather than separately. In the fall of 1970, Dr. Walter L. Koltun was appointed Assistant Director for Resources to coordinate efforts. His office was to provide staff support for the senior officers of both universities in concert with the respective development offices as well as support for the Program Resources Committee (see 3 below), and for

the Sponsoring Committee (see 4 below). Therefore, the chief role of the Program's Assistant Director for Resources was to support the fund-raising efforts of others. Only secondarily was he to raise funds himself.

2. An endowment goal of $10,000,000 was established as the minimum necessary to underwrite the Program and to support a major fraction of the needed core senior faculty. This was to be raised within five years. Simultaneously, operating funds also were to be raised. In 1970–71, Uncas A. Whitaker, a member of the M.I.T. Corporation, contributed $1,000,000 to the Institute for the Program and helped launch the fund-raising effort.

3. The senior officers of both universities and the Director of the Program were primarily responsible for raising the funds. It was expected that the usual on-going fund-raising efforts of both institutions also would raise funds for the Program's purposes. The responsibility for raising the needed funds was to be shared, therefore, among Harvard, M.I.T., and the Program itself. The primary focus for fund raising at Harvard was to be the Medical School. An internal development committee, the Program Resources Committee, was established in 1971–72 and given oversight responsibility for raising the necessary funds and for implementing the joint fund-raising concept. It was to provide the focal point for decision making with respect to fund raising, including the development of strategy, clearance of prospects, and solicitation of prospects.

4. A National Sponsoring Committee, composed primarily of distinguished business and community leaders, was established in 1971–72 to help achieve the financial goals. By their personal stature and experience, and through their endorsement, the members of the Committee were to give the Program increased national visibility and national impact. The Committee was to provide leadership and advice and leads to promising sources of funding, both individual and corporate. Individual members were to participate in fund raising as circumstances would permit. The Committee was to meet periodically to assess progress in the development of resources.

5. Funds were to be raised from new sources; i.e., from donors who either had never given to Harvard and M.I.T. before or from previous donors who, while maintaining their prior support, would give additional funds earmarked for the HST Program. Donors could give endowment funds to either Harvard or M.I.T. for purposes of the Program or to the joint Program itself. In the latter

case, the funds were split between the two universities and invested separately by each institution. This was necessary as the Program was not a separate corporate entity. Similarly, operational funds could be given to either Harvard, M.I.T. or the Program. In the early years, income and expenses were divided equally, and therefore it did not matter to whom the gifts were made.

6. All HST prospects were to be cleared by both Harvard and M.I.T. before any fund-raising action could be taken.

By June 30, 1972 the fund-raising structure was in place and operating. In 1971–72, $1,982,000 was raised, including $1,120,000 for endowment, $600,000 for operations, and $262,000 for HST teaching laboratories. The total funds raised the following year, 1972–73, were $1,302,000, including $1,208,000 for endowment and $94,000 for operations. By June 30, 1973 it was clear that, although the fundraising apparatus was functioning as planned, the optimistic fundraising goals would not be met. Only $3,330,000 of the $10,000,000 endowment goal had been raised.

An analysis of the fourteen proposals requesting $6,945,000 submitted as of June 30, 1973 and the grants received showed that for both endowment and operating funds the yield was $1,900,000 or 27%. This was approximately the same yield as for all proposals Harvard and M.I.T. had submitted to private sources. It had been hoped and expected that the joint Program would be more attractive to donors since it involved the union of two major universities in the area of health. Unfortunately, the conditions under which fund raising for the HST Program had to operate, namely from new sources and clearances by both institutions, restricted the number of first-class major prospects. While recognized as an essential requirement to avoid conflicts, the clearance procedure resulted in the elimination of many promising prospects. Each university was unwilling either to release its major donors for an HST approach or to agree to a joint approach to many major prospects, be they individuals, foundations, or companies.

To some extent, fund raising reflected the hesitancy and uncertainty, and the amorphous and slow decision making which the joint Program experienced broadly. This resulted in a long time scale for decisions and actions. It became clear that unless there were changes in the restrictive ground rules under which HST fund raising operated, and the institutions or specific individuals were willing to take responsibility for raising the additional $6,700,000 of endowment, the promise and full potential of the Program would not be realized.

This was the situation in the summer of 1973 when James R. Killian, Jr. of M.I.T. and George W. Thorn of the Harvard Medical School agreed to take responsibility for raising the additional $6,700,000 needed to reach the $10,000,000 goal. It was largely through their efforts, along with those of Walter Koltun, that over the following four years $5,765,000 was raised—$4,347,000 for endowment and $1,418,000 for operations and facilities. By June 1977, the endowment totalled $7,680,000, and while this was still $2,320,000 short of the desired $10,000,000, it represented major progress.

The failure to reach the $10,000,000 goal clearly reflected the lack of sufficient major prospects. The development offices of both universities continued to resist clearing their major donors for HST, and in a number of cases each preferred to approach major prospects individually for other purposes rather than jointly for HST. These issues were discussed at the Program Resource Committee meetings. However, as the efforts of Killian, Thorn and Koltun bore fruit, the Committee felt less urgency and became less active. The Committee met five times in 1971, four in 1972, three in 1973, two in 1974, once in 1975; it held its last meeting in May 1976.

Nevertheless, in spite of all the difficulties, significant funds were raised, enough to give the universities confidence that the remainder would be forthcoming soon. Early in 1977, they voted to establish a permanent joint enterprise, the Harvard-M.I.T. Division of Health Sciences and Technology. It is unfortunate that this act marked the beginning of the end of the direct involvement of Drs. Killian and Thorn in HST fund raising. Thus, at a time of expanded academic opportunities and increasing financial needs, the new Division of Health Sciences and Technology found itself without a fund-raising organization except for Dr. Koltun's office. The Sponsoring Committee and the Program Resource Committee had ceased to operate, and the withdrawal of Drs. Killian and Thorn left a fund-raising leadership vacuum. The Division was left to do its own fund raising and Dr. Koltun turned his attention to Palm Beach and to small foundations as potential sources of funds.

One of the promises made to the faculties of both institutions was that every attempt would be made to raise funds for the Program from new sources. This was taken seriously by all involved. Palm Beach has perhaps the greatest concentration of personal wealth of any community in the United States. Moreover, there is a tradition of philanthropy that interacts strongly with social activities. Accordingly, commencing in 1972 and for the following two years, Walter

Koltun explored Palm Beach in depth. He quietly cultivated Palm Beach as a new source of prospects, learned the culture, came to know the press, and brought the HST Division to the attention of numerous key people. Significant amounts of money began to come to HST in 1975 and continued to do so. Overall, more than $1,000,000 was raised from Palm Beach sources.

Believing that foundations with listed assets of $10,000,000 or less, so-called "small foundations," might be good sources of funds and would be readily cleared for HST solicitations, Dr. Koltun launched a systematic review in the spring of 1977. Over the succeeding years more than 200 foundations, primarily in New England, New York, and other selected areas, were explored. While only a small fraction, less than 10%, resulted in grants, over the years significant amounts of money were raised from foundations making grants in the range of $2,000–20,000. Moreover, a few of these "small" foundations made grants in the tens and hundreds of thousands of dollars.

From 1970–71, when the HST Program was established, to 1992–93, excluding research funds, a total of $20,669,000 was raised for academic purposes. This was roughly equally divided between endowment, $10,850,000, and operations, $9,819,000.

Whereas in the first seven years, both universities engaged in joint fund raising, this changed in 1986–87 when, following the appointment of HST co-directors to replace Dr. Irving London, HMS took financial responsibility for the biomedical sciences program which was centered at HMS, and M.I.T. took similar responsibility for the medical engineering and medical physics programs which were centered at the Institute. Thus, fund raising can be divided into two periods: 1970–1978, joint fund raising pre-Division establishment period, and 1978–1993, HST fund raising, post-Division period. In the first seven years, when both universities engaged in joint fund raising, an average of approximately $1,600,000 per year was raised. In the last fifteen years, with the Division doing its own fund raising, approximately $630,000 per year was raised. Most of these funds were for student aid; i.e., scholarships, fellowships, and research assistantships. These figures do not include the $99,600,000 raised to support the HST Division's research activities. Taken together, $120,000,000 was raised between 1971 and 1993 for the Division's activities. It is interesting to note that the original endowment goal of $10,000,000 was not reached until 1991–92, twenty-one years after the initiation of the Program.

Chapter 8

THE HST EXPERIENCE

Walter H. Abelmann, M.D.

In compiling the history of the HST Program, the central role played by key individuals, both in the planning and in the implementation of the program, became very evident. A new inter-institutional, interdisciplinary enterprise, which could not rely on replication of an existing program, had to depend upon individual creativity on the one hand, and a favorable, receptive, institutional and general climate on the other. Many of the most important determining factors that made this program possible are not easily derived from the existing archival material, but are known to many of the individuals who played significant roles in the planning and implementation of the program. Therefore, it was decided to supplement the historiography as presented by contributors to this volume and existing records with an oral history as reflected in taped interviews of additional key individuals.[1] These interviews were carried out by the editor of this volume between 1993 and 1995; almost all took place in the interviewee's office or laboratory, and they were generally limited to one and a half hours or less. The individuals interviewed were selected on the basis of their significant involvement with the program over time.[2] The interviewee was given the opportunity to add comments off the record and was provided a copy of the transcription, providing an opportunity for corrections. Although the interviews were conducted generally as free conversations, an attempt was made to cover certain relevant topics, such as circumstances surrounding their initial engagement in the program, expectations, comparisons of involvement in this versus other programs, interaction with students, effects upon research and research collaborations, views of the program as it evolved, disappointments and critique.

The individuals interviewed differed widely with regard to the nature of their involvement; the timing of their participation; the balance among their teaching, mentoring and research activities; and the extent of their planning and administrative responsibilities. Although perceptions varied, the interviews reveal a remarkable degree of overlap, if not communality. This chapter is based largely upon these comments, which not only constitute an important aspect of the Harvard-MIT Division of Health Sciences and Technology, but may be of significance for the planning and operation of any inter-university and interdisciplinary academic enterprise.

At the Massachusetts Institute of Technology, the Professors of Physics or Engineering who became early participants in the program did so from a base of earlier interest in biological and biomedical sciences and their perception that there were major questions and unsolved problems in the biomedical sciences, as well as in medicine, to which the methods of physics and engineering could be profitably applied. In the HST Program, they saw opportunities to extend their expertise and contributions through collaboration with biomedical scientists both in teaching and in research. The quantitative sciences offered opportunities for elucidation of physiologic as well as pathophysiologic processes. The physical basis of a number of diseases remained to be worked out; engineering sciences offered potential for rehabilitation by replacement of functions lost.

Members of the Faculty of Medicine of the Harvard Medical School, on the other hand, were attracted to the program because it offered an opportunity for close contact with highly selected students with documented interest in knowledge and investigative pursuits, in small groups, with the opportunity to attract some of these students to their research laboratories. The large size of the Harvard Medical School's faculty resulted in many faculty members having little involvement in teaching beyond occasional didactic lectures, and hence little close contact with students. The HST Program appeared to offer such opportunities. For some, the program also provided an opportunity for career building and enhanced the chance for tenure. Although the expectations for student contact, personal rewards from teaching and attraction of students to the laboratory were generally fulfilled, the impact upon career development and potential tenure status was often disappointing. Contributions to the HST Program, while greatly appreciated by the HST leadership, were not necessarily esteemed by the faculty member's home department. Although it is difficult to document that any one career was disadvantaged by commitment to HST, this was often the perception.

Students

If there was one topic on which all interviewees agreed and waxed enthusiastically, it was the caliber of students. Their intelligence, curiosity, motivation, enthusiasm and responsiveness were recognized as the most important and attractive aspects of the entire HST Program. The students were praised not only for their outstanding intellectual abilities, but also for their individualism, their creativity, and the broad spectrum of their interests, both curricular and extracurricular. Interviewees stressed how exciting it was to know students as individuals. Thus, teaching in HST courses was highly valued as a scintillating and rewarding experience. A few quotations are appropriate:

"The secret weapon of the HST Program was the quality of its students."

"They are interested in a rigorous approach."

"I much prefer dealing with [HST Students] because they have a real appreciation of the importance of being able to trace a clinical problem, to see how it relates to pathophysiology."

The students in class also elicited comments and praise. Their fruitful interactions were appreciated. The course on Functional Anatomy was given full credit for its major role in this process (see below). While these qualities of the student body sufficed to attract many members of the faculty to teaching in this program, another important motivation was the opportunity to attract some of these students to their research laboratories, whether it be for the mandatory M.D. thesis project, for a full year of research or for Ph.D. dissertation research.

When asked to compare HST students with students in the regular Harvard Medical School Class, faculty considered HST Students a superior group, comparing favorably with the best students in the HMS class.

"The overall opinions of most all the clinical teachers, who have been around for a long time and have been teaching generations of students, are that the HST students are a lot better than the HMS students."

"HST students are no brighter, but much more motivated toward science aspects of the curriculum."

"Unlike many HMS students, HST students did not object to the 'socratic' method of teaching favored by a number of members of the faculty. The result was a divergence of the cultures of the two groups."

The strong motivation for an academic career is also reflected in the significant number of students who, often without compensation and usually at their own initiative, taught courses or seminars in the HST Program on such topics as immunology, biochemistry (metabolic pathways), pharmacology (review), health policy, and medical economics.[3] Such offerings were facilitated by the flexibility of the HST curriculum.

In the early years of the program, HST students were concerned whether their heavily science-oriented pre-clinical curriculum would equip them as well for the clinical years as the more clinically oriented courses offered in the regular HMS program. Thus, most students also studied handouts or notes from the regular courses. In time, it became evident to the HST student body that they did well on national board examinations and held their own quite well when joining members of the regular class in the clinical clerkships, and this concern subsided.

The reactions of the regular HMS classes to the early HST classes are of interest, partly fueling the above concerns. HST students were "considered the robots, the MIT kids, the nerds, the outsiders. In the first years, they were not allowed to participate in the second year show. Even in lectures, some HMS faculty members would denigrate HST students."

The Admission Process

The consistently high quality of the students in the program must be attributed to the combined effect of recruitment of applicants and the process of selection. In the first years of the Program, Harvard College and MIT provided most of the competitive applicants. Harvard

College's system of House Premedical Advisors, as well as MIT's Premedical Advisory Council, facilitated efforts to reach the undergraduate body of these two institutions. It took time for the description of the program in the application forms to the Harvard Medical School, as well as the efforts of the Director of the Program, to reach a wider array of colleges and undergraduate premedical advisors. The leadership, as well as members of the Admissions Committee, regularly contacted colleges throughout the United States. Eventually a separate pamphlet describing the program was included in the Harvard Medical School's application packet. Special efforts were made to reach minority groups. As a result of these efforts, the applicant pool consistently exceeded the places available (twenty-five in early years, thirty in later years) at least ten-fold. The Admissions Committee has been considered one of the most important committees of the program, generally comprising ten members of the faculty—drawn from both Harvard and MIT—and an equal number of students. Each applicant was given a numerical rating by each member of the committee. Approximately 100–150 applicants were selected for interviews by members of the Admissions Committee. Although the criteria for selection varied somewhat according to the composition of the committee, consistent emphasis was placed upon overall intellectual ability and evidence of creative scholarship in addition to the usual premedical requirements plus advanced mathematics and physics courses. Interviews afforded opportunities to verify sincere interest and ability in intellectual and scientific pursuits and also allowed an evaluation of suitability for human interaction and a caring profession.

It was almost a requirement that candidates had motivation and creative involvement, demonstrated in hands-on laboratory or, occasionally, library research. Meritorious applicants generally evidenced strength and advanced standing in either biological/chemical or quantitative mathematical/physics/engineering fields, although a surprising number of applicants manifested strength in both areas. A significant number of applicants had advanced degrees, primarily Ph.D., in a broad array of fields. Whereas applicants with Ph.D. degrees in physics or engineering fields might be considered ideal candidates, many of them presented special problems. Some applicants had turned to medicine because they were disillusioned with their field and were looking for human interaction in a profession which would allow them to contribute directly to human well-being. Some of these individuals thus turned their back to basic sciences and did not meet the program's expectation that they would work at the interface of biomedicine and quantitative sciences.

Special efforts were made to exert affirmative action and to assure diversity of the class. In the twenty years from 1975 to 1995, a total of 561 students were admitted to the HST-MD Program. One hundred and seven, or 19.1% of admissions were women, and twenty-one or 3.7% were African-Americans. Four or 0.7% were Hispanic.

Faculty

Recruitment of faculty (Appendix D) for the HST courses has been a challenge. Although the potential pool of candidates at the two universities is very large, and many members of the faculty of the Harvard Medical School have few teaching obligations, once the criteria for membership in the HST faculty are defined, the pool of potential candidates becomes limited. Prerequisites include creative scholarship, demonstrated interest and ability in teaching, and ability as well as freedom to make a significant commitment. With regard to faculty drawn from the Medical School, the emphasis was upon physician-scientists who would teach at the forefront of their field, as well as act as role models. From the onset of the program, it was expected that core faculty of each course would attend all lectures and exercises, be prepared to advise students and consider participation in relevant committees.

Inasmuch as the HST Program, even after achieving Division status in 1977, was allocated only very few full-time faculty positions, much of the core faculty had to be drawn from either MIT or Harvard. Although a few tenured professors who could dispose of their own time, especially at MIT, were attracted to the Program, seeing an opportunity to reach for new horizons, most candidates had to obtain the permission of their department chairman to make commitments to HST, usually involving release from major departmental teaching obligations.

Although many of the younger members of the faculty, especially those who elected to teach in major courses such as pathology or neurosciences, did obtain permission from their respective departments, they continued to worry about the effect of the time commitment on their research activities, upon which promotion and advancement in the field depended.

"Young faculty take risks, because [the HST Program] does not have a clear-cut tenure track," was a criticism frequently heard. The concerns, however, were often balanced by the attraction of close contact with a highly motivated, excellent group of students, and the opportunity to recruit some of them to the laboratory. There was also the expectation that collaborative research might result. In order to facilitate departmental cooperation, the HST Program offered some pecuniary compensation for faculty time, to be used at the department's discretion. Some departments passed this on as an extra stipend to its members, constituting an additional motivational factor. At MIT, some faculty members "who had devoted their intellectual energies to solving military problems, were beginning to feel that they wanted to use their energies in more constructive, socially appropriate directions." A different spirit was abroad in the land.

Once involved in the Program, most individuals became enthusiastic and loyal members of the enterprise, willing to work on committees and in educational workshops as well as serve as advisors to students, in addition to their formal teaching obligations. However, there remained a risk for younger faculty: with less commitment to their own departments, some encountered difficulty in promotion, especially to tenure. This became known and acted as a deterrent to acceptance of major teaching commitments. In the words of a course head of over twenty years' standing: "the only way you really could get [top people] to come on board to take on a major teaching assignment, is to have them leaned on by the chairman of the department."

Although most members of the faculty with major administrative or oversight involvement hold the view that the full-time HST core faculty is much too small and should be expanded, "it should never get to the point that there is only one body of faculty who belong to that group and teach in HST. The interchange between people from different departments and schools is very good;" or, "HST benefits the rest of the school all the time by offering new ideas, offering comparisons, offering a little competition, offering variation in approaches, which is extremely valuable." Another route of faculty recruitment was via research projects sponsored by HST (See Appendix F). Investigators in collaborative projects became known to the director of the program, and then could be recruited to course faculty and also become student research mentors. Thus, there were important bridges between research and education.

Many members of the faculty interviewed gave testimony to the professional fulfillment derived from their involvement in HST. "The attitude always was to treat you like a university, that you are the professor in charge [of the course] and it is up to you to build the course and take the credit or blame;" or, "It was smart to get faculty involved in all aspects of the program, to identify with the program. [Thus HST] became like a college." The following was another cogent view of a faculty member participating in the program:

> I think the fact that HST is a separate and smaller component of the medical school, with a different set of goals and a different means of approaching them, and hence gathers students and faculties together making a joint effort to try to accomplish these goals, and that the numbers of students and faculty are small enough that they can know each other and know what they all are doing, establishes a feeling of community which is very good, and very rewarding for both and it's fun belonging to a group and having contact with the students. I mentioned the other day that if HST didn't exist, you would have to invent it.

The Curriculum

From the beginning of the HST Program, its formal curriculum (Appendix C) was the centerpiece of its educational enterprise. The Curriculum Committee was comprised of both faculty and students and had the responsibility of defining and planning courses, recruiting faculty, and evaluating courses. The HST curriculum was conceived as comprising its own pre-clinical courses as well as its own Introduction to the Clinic (the course covering history taking and physical diagnosis) but afterwards to funnel its students into the regular clinical curriculum at the Harvard Medical School and its affiliated hospitals.

The early design of the curriculum was based upon several principles which still inform the creation of additional courses and curricular offerings today. A critical requirement for the program's courses was their incorporation into the offerings of both universities, reflecting the strengths of both cultures, and their accessibility to qualified graduate and even undergraduate students of MIT and Harvard's Faculty of Arts and Sciences, Medical School, and School of Public Health. In keeping with these principles, courses were taught in a semester or half-semester format—in contrast to the block system generally in use at the Harvard Medical School—and were adapted as much as possible to the academic calendar of both universities. The month of January was to be devoted to short, intensive and largely elective courses. As much as possible, each course was to include faculty members drawn from both universities.

Each course head was given full responsibility for designing his or her course and was encouraged to give most of the didactic presentations personally. Larger courses were designed to have a core faculty of two or three, who were expected to attend all sections of the course and be available for questions and discussions. Rigorous scientific content was expected of courses, and stress on quantitative aspects of the subject was encouraged. Class size being generally limited to less than fifty (from twenty-five to thirty HST M.D. candidates, up to ten MEMP students, and a few graduate students). Student/faculty interaction was possible and encouraged, even in didactic sessions, as was teaching in the form of seminars and discussion groups. Problem sets, a standard part of the MIT culture, were introduced in most courses. In the pathophysiology courses, the case method was used from the beginning of the program; its use was increased in time. The development and use of computer-based educational programs and self-learning was encouraged. Provision for student teaching assistants was made for larger courses, encouraging the development of teaching skills as well as providing financial support for qualified students who acted as teaching assistants.

In order to accentuate the affiliation of the program with both universities and increase accessibility to students from other departments, an effort was made to teach an approximately equal number of courses at each site, HMS and MIT. To be of maximum value for graduate students, courses were generally designed to be self-sufficient with minimal prerequisites. This required inclusion of the normal structure and function in the pathology and pathophysiology courses. Thus, the pathology course was designed to include normal histology, and the pathophysiology courses comprised normal as well as abnormal function of the individual organ systems. An effort was made to minimize specific course requirements while adhering, in general, to the curricular requirements of the Harvard Medical School, the degree awarding faculty. Thus, in keeping with general graduate school policies, no individual courses were required as such. However, no student chose to omit anatomy, pathology or microbiology. It was possible, however, for students to study individual subjects independently; e.g., biochemistry, the musculoskeletal system or the reproductive system.

These features of the curriculum provided a flexibility most valuable for a group of students of whom many were actively involved in research projects, permitting reduction of the course load, extension of the four-year traditional M.D. curriculum to five years or more, or combining it with a Ph.D. program.

From the beginning of the Program, the Curriculum Committee encouraged course heads to consider the use of audio-visual methods, as well as interactive computer programs to supplement traditional pedagogical methods. To this end, inventories of available materials were made. It became quite evident, however, that what was available was mostly unsuitable for the HST curriculum. As a result, several course directors proposed to develop new teaching materials, and the Program made additional stipends available to permit students to participate if not lead in the application of computer technology to teaching. A close collaboration with the Decision Systems Group in the Department of Radiology at the Brigham and Women's Hospital, under the direction of Robert A. Greenes, M.D., Ph.D., was most helpful in this regard. For several pathophysiology courses, interactive computer teaching sequences relying heavily upon the case method as well as review quizzes, were developed.[4] Experience showed, however, that these projects required prolonged and intensive efforts, usually over several months, followed by field testing, revisions and updating. When high quality and relevance were finally reached, student acceptance was high.

In courses which included a good deal of visual material, traditional loose-leaf notebooks of color photographs were found most helpful, especially when—as in Renal Pathophysiology—a picture of a healthy or diseased organ could be followed by a page of questions. The incorporation of the case method proved especially popular and effective. Answers were provided later in such books. One student devoted his obligatory M.D. thesis to the transfer of such a notebook into an interactive computer program, which was offered to students as an alternative method of study.[5] The evaluation found that, while the results of later examinations did not differ, students who used the computer program devoted less time to study.

Personal involvement in research was made obligatory and culminated in the M.D. thesis. The thesis was to reflect scholarly work based upon laboratory research, clinical investigation or, under special circumstances, critical analysis of a significant problem. A minimum of three months' work was envisaged, plus one month of writing. A thesis proposal was to be submitted by autumn of the year prior to expected graduation, and the thesis was due in early February. Theses were read by two reviewers. If the student requested consideration for honors and if the readers agreed, a formal thesis defense would follow. In the case of M.D./Ph.D. students, the Ph.D. dissertation fulfilled this requirement but could not be counted for honors. Ph.D. candidates were encouraged, however, to submit meritorious material not included in the doctoral dissertation as an M.D. thesis competing for honors. The thesis requirement was fully accepted by the student body, research being incorporated as an important part of the educational process. Most students actually spent considerably more time in research than required, often devoting an extra year to it. However, a few students, who had entered holding a Ph.D. degree already, protested this requirement—to no avail.

Beginning in 1987, special funds were made available for research assistantships, in the form of tuition support, which acted as a welcome incentive. Another effective incentive for taking an additional year is Harvard Medical School's rule that four years' tuition is the maximum due for an M.D. degree, so that additional years are essentially tuition-free.

Notwithstanding—or perhaps because of—the wide-ranging opportunities to join a laboratory for the research experience, the process of choice was often most difficult for the student. Compendia of faculty research interests and activities, designation of faculty coordinators/advisors for key areas of research, and the personal student advisory system all played a role in helping students with this choice. Yet, mismatches remained a problem for a small number of students. These were mostly related to the research supervisor's misunderstanding or other personal qualities, to laboratories too large to offer close supervision or to projects chosen poorly. Early recognition of such mismatches permitted successful switching of laboratories.

It is of interest to consider the topics chosen by students for their thesis research. In general, over the years, there has been a balance of students who entered the program with majors in physical or engineering sciences on the one hand and biological sciences on the other. Yet, thesis topics in biological fields have consistently dominated bioengineering topics. (See Figures 1 and 2, as well as Appendix E.) This clearly reflects a recognition of the increasing role of molecular biology and genetics in biomedicine. This expressed student interest actually preceded the introduction of comprehensive courses in molecular biology and genetics into the HST curriculum.

From the beginning days of the Program, the need for evaluation was recognized, and the Curriculum Committee accepted responsibility for this. In addition to discussing individual courses, as well as

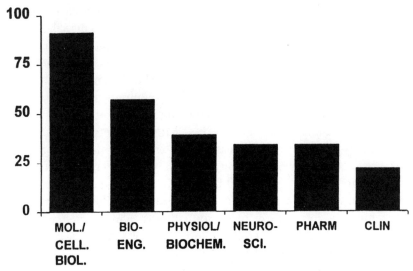

Figure 1.   Distribution of MD Theses by Field (N=277) 1978–94

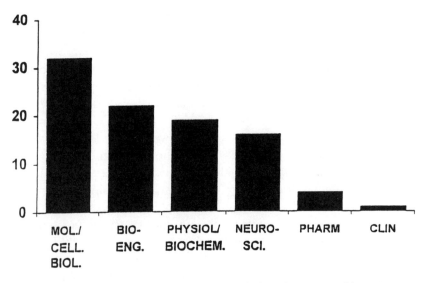

Figure 2.   MD/PhD Graduates Distribution of PhD Theses By Field (N=94) 1978–94

their inter-relationships, at regular meetings of the Committee, sub-committees were appointed to review individual courses in depth. The subcommittees included not only members of the Curriculum Committee but also members of the Harvard and MIT faculties who were not involved in HST as well as additional students. The meetings were open. Separate subcommittees would review each course at least every three years, more frequently if there had been a change in course leadership or problems were evident. Detailed recommendations were made to the Curriculum Committee and the course leadership. In addition, the Curriculum Committee, and at times separate committees, considered the curriculum in general and specific areas such as neurosciences, as well as interfaces between courses. Annual Curriculum Retreats, attended by both faculty and students, also were used to discuss aspects of the curriculum in depth, to gain broader perspectives, and to launch innovations.[6]

Courses

Whereas the traditional medical curriculum offers basic science courses (e.g., anatomy, physiology, pathology, biochemistry, pharmacology) followed by systemic pathophysiology courses, the HST curriculum's pathophysiology courses (Appendices B and C) were to start with the basic sciences relevant to each system, followed by pathophysiology and some applied clinical material or exercises.

One of the greatest challenges of the curriculum was the stated goal to stress quantitative aspects of biological and medical problems. Several members of the MIT faculty were recruited to help achieve this goal, and an effort was made to assign at least one member of the MIT faculty to each course. Two MIT professors had considerable background in applying the quantitative and analytical methods of physics to the understanding and solving of biomedical problems, having taught undergraduate courses in physics with illustrative examples drawn from medicine and biology.[7] They found, however, that "the relevance of the quantitative approach had to be reinforced consistently, whereas the relevance of molecular biology and genetics was obvious." Students whose background was stronger in biology than in physics often were strongly motivated toward acquiring the desired quantitative skills to pursue the interface between quantitative sciences and biomedicine, whereas the students with strong backgrounds in physics and engineering were more interested in filling gaps in their background in molecular biology and genetics.

The first semester included two major courses, Functional Anatomy and Human Pathology, as well as Quantitative Physiology and Immunology. The course in Functional Anatomy was to become not only central to the curriculum, but also one of the most important, formative experiences of HST students. Designed "to provide a thorough grounding in the structure of the human body and certain of its functions,"[8] it retained full dissection of the human body in groups of four, included embryology, biomechanics and some molecular biology, and did not hesitate to use comparative anatomy where applicable. This course provided students close contact with each other as well as with faculty and acted as an invaluable focus for socialization and formation of a class. In this as well as all courses, the small size of the class and the mix of the students (i.e., their diversity) were considered key assets. In the words of one course head: "Small groups allow for Socratic discussion."

MEMP and other graduate students were appreciated as "clear assets, bringing a different perspective and a different goal for their careers." To stress quantitative aspects of science, several lectures by members of the MIT faculty and the Division of Applied Sciences of Harvard's Faculty of Arts and Sciences were incorporated into the anatomy course. These lectures dealt with topics such as the branching patterns of anatomic structures but were quickly recognized as being at some distance removed from the reality of anatomy. Furthermore, these lecturers did not come to the laboratory where most student/faculty interaction took place. Later, a professor of biomechanics in the Department of Orthopedics was more successful: he presented prosections as well as lectures and addressed structure/function inter-relationships in joints, including clinical implications! The Director of the course in Functional Anatomy recalled that

Our course is different [from standard courses in anatomy] because in our lectures, we very seldom, if ever, simply describe the material. Take the limbs for example: we really don't go much through a recitation of what's in the limbs. Rather we would take the approach of how you can understand—from the point of view of development as well as phylogeny—why the limbs are structured the way they are, and then, more importantly, how they work. So students come out of our course, for example, with a very advanced appreciation of the extremities, in particular the functioning of the human hand and human gait. The best of our lectures are those that you could find nowhere in a book, they have been made up by the individual. So that is functional human anatomy. It's an emphasis on function, and we try to get our students to think that way in the laboratory.

Another important aspect of this first semester course, with a time commitment of twenty-one hours per week, is what has been called socialization of the class.

By our personal interactions and by our direct care of the students, and by being just who we are, we model each class, we give it a class spirit, and I think there is some merit. This course provides such a large amount of student interaction with faculty who are diverse and great teachers that I think it sets a very distinctive tone for the whole program. In recent years, enrollment, in addition to 30 HST M.D. candidates, has comprised 6–8 MEMP students, as well as graduate students from the Departments of Anthropology, Organismic and Evolutionary Biology at Harvard, from the Harvard School of Public Health, and also an occasional undergraduate student. The quality of the non-M.D. candidates is reflected in their performance: As a group, they almost always are in the upper half of the class, and sometimes lead the class.

The Human Pathology course constituted a radical departure from traditional medical school curricula in that it also was taught in the first semester and included microscopic anatomy, no separate histology course being offered. Thus the abnormal could be juxtaposed with the normal structure as well as function. The simultaneity with the anatomy course made it possible for the head of the pathology course to make diagnostic rounds of the cadavers, view all organs, take samples for histopathology and then review the sections with the students. The pathology course introduced case presentations and state-of-the-art seminars with outside discussors. This course also experimented with the introduction of lectures by physical scientists on quantitative topics, such as dimensional analysis and statistical applications as well as radiation physics. Even experienced enthusiastic teachers, however, were not able to conquer the students' perception that such topics were at best marginal to the course. Nonetheless, a few students appreciated these thoughtful and often original contributions and were stimulated by them. An example is the mathematical treatment of the evolutionary strategies for increasing the surface area for transport across membranes.

In time it was recognized that the initial decision to incorporate physiology into the individual pathophysiology courses left a number of topics in general physiology either uncovered or touched upon in several courses albeit only superficially. Therefore, in 1978, Professor F. M. H. Villars of the Physics Department at MIT agreed to offer a course entitled "Quantitative Physiology," dedicated to the study of integrated performance of diverse organ systems and their adaptation to external stress and organ dysfunction. Emphasis was placed upon respiratory and cardiovascular transport systems and the associated feedback controls, as well as the electrophysiologic basis of neural control and communication. Quantitative systems modeling was employed, and new concepts were developed. This course truly was a collaborative effort of the HMS and MIT faculty in a quantitative curricular offering, true to the goals of HST. Although this course was well received by a significant number of students, it raised considerable concern and criticism in others. One might well have expected that students with strong backgrounds in quantitative sciences would especially appreciate this course, and students whose strengths were in the biological sciences would have difficulties and might object. While this was so in many instances, the course also evoked different reactions. Some students seized this opportunity to review physics and calculus. These students also availed themselves of an elective informal seminar in calculus given by Dr. Alan Natapoff of the Aeronautics and Astronautics Department in the fall semester. Nonetheless, the course was discontinued in 1988 and some of the material was incorporated in the respective individual pathophysiology courses.

The course "Introduction to the Clinic," which comprised instruction in history taking, physical examination and differential diagnosis, was given in the fourth semester. In order to optimize integration of clinical data with the general scientific and pathophysiologic approach of the preceding semesters, this course was taught to HST students as a group primarily at one hospital (Brigham & Women's Hospital). In the selection of preceptors from medicine, surgery and pediatrics (Children's Hospital), preference was given to clinician-scientists.

The Educational Role of HST Courses for Non-HST Students

To the extent that space permits, and at the discretion of course heads, individual HST courses are open to qualified undergraduate and graduate students registered at either Harvard University or MIT as well as qualified students at other educational institutes in the greater Boston area. Although in most HST courses the great majority of students are matriculated in one of the HST educational programs, a significant number of non-HST students take one or more HST courses. Most HST courses are listed in the MIT *Bulletin* and many are also included in the *Course Catalog* of the Harvard Faculty of Arts and Sciences as well as in the separate HST *Course Catalog*.

In the majority of cases, non-HST students take courses relevant to their area of research or career planning. In recent years, an average of forty-one non-HST students took HST courses for credit, not counting formal and informal auditors. These were mostly MIT students. However, certain courses regularly attract students from Harvard College, the Harvard Graduate School of Arts and Sciences, and the Harvard School of Public Health. Among these courses, "Functional Anatomy" may be mentioned as being attended regularly by students in physical anthropology. Access to HST courses is important to many graduate students because pre-clinical courses in the regular HMS program are not taught on a regular semester schedule but in concentrated blocks.

Thus, the HST program has had a significant impact upon the educational offerings in the two institutions. Non-HST students, in turn, made significant contributions to individual HST courses—especially the pathophysiology courses—by increasing the diversity of backgrounds and points of view.

The Advisory System

From the beginning of the HST Program, it was recognized that, notwithstanding the small class size and accessibility of faculty, each student should have a personal faculty advisor and that this new program would be served best by having a small group of advisors thoroughly familiar with the goals and features of the program. Accordingly, the initial Board of Advisors consisted of a small group of senior members of the HST Faculty, each taking on about six members of each entering class. Students were obligated to meet with their advisors at least twice a year when study plans had to be discussed and study cards signed. They were encouraged to meet more often. The chairman of the Board of Advisors would review the progress of advisees with each advisor at least twice a year. Later, as the number of students increased, not only by increasing class size, but also by an increasing number of students who took a fifth year as well as M.D./Ph.D. students, the Board of Advisors was increased, and formal meetings were held at least twice a year. This rather formal system was considerably more rigid than the advisory system extant at HMS for the main student body. In the 1990s, the HST Advisory System became the model for a revised HMS system.

In the first clinical year, students were encouraged to seek out an internship advisor in their area of interest although internship plans were also reviewed and finalized with the primary HST advisors and the Chairman of the Board of Advisors. In the early 1990s, the drafting of the Dean's Letter was assigned to the Masters and Associate Masters of the Academic Societies, one of which is the HST Society. This assured that the student's academic status and plans were tightly supervised within the leadership of HST.

Among the most challenging responsibilities of the HST Advisors, in addition to supervising the selection of courses, was the guiding of selection of research laboratories, research supervisors, and research projects. In time, oversight of the latter selection process was assigned to one individual for the entire program, who received the thesis proposal at an early date, and then the M.D. thesis in early February of the senior year. He was free to select consultants for evaluation of the proposal and later solicited two readers for each thesis. The selection of research projects and laboratories, although in good part informed by the students' contacts with course faculty and guest lecturers, was also facilitated by lists of research interests of the faculty—initially in notebooks, later on the computer. This system, which was rather faculty intensive, should be given some credit for the success of our students. The accumulated experience with investigators and laboratories was most valuable in giving students advice and in guiding them to laboratories with special interest in and concern for students.

The great value of the informal advisory system provided by the HST offices, at both MIT and HMS, must also be acknowledged. From the admission of the first class in 1971, Ms. Virginia Safford, Administrative Assistant to the Director, and Dr. Irving London, in his MIT office, were ever ready to inform and advise students on curricular, administrative and personal matters. After her untimely death in 1985, Ms. Safford was succeeded by Ms. Almena Palombo, and later by Ms. Gloria McAvenia. In 1978, a second office of the HST Program was opened at HMS, where similar functions, with emphasis upon curricular matters, were carried out by Ms. Carol Cogliani, and after 1990 by Ms. Patricia Cunningham. The support to students—as well as faculty—provided by these ladies cannot be overestimated; it is widely reflected in comments by interviewees as well as alumni.

Views of M.D. Graduates Culled from Alumni Surveys

The following quotations were obtained from alumni beyond their post-graduate training.[9]

"We were encouraged to reason, not memorize."

"I enjoyed the closer contact with professors and was given a perspective on physiology which I could not have gotten in the regular program. Also, the supportive attitude toward basic research was a major plus."

"I believe my experience as an undergraduate at MIT had the most influence on my ultimate decision to pursue a career in basic research. Nevertheless, the quantitative approach of HST was considerably more stimulating than the conventional medical curriculum."

"The thesis requirement was probably more influential in exposing me to 'hands-on' research."

"I think that the benefits of HST include a small group of people who are bright and interested in basic science research, flexible scheduling of courses and research activities, and close interaction among students and faculty."

"Unquestionably, this has been the greatest and most enduring education benefit I received. Creating testable hypotheses, testing them, measuring outcomes are an indispensable habit of mind for anything I've done since."

"Not so much for the content as for the environment and diverse, extremely interesting students and teachers, as well as small classes."

"I enjoyed the small size of classes. I found the quantitative approach interesting but of little clinical relevance in the long run. Would choose again."

"Small class size and individual attention make a huge difference."

"Because of my engineering background, I think the HST curriculum suited me better, also I liked the small classes."

"I chose an academic position with research opportunities because of the exposure to medical scientists and their teachings and role model as part of the basic science curriculum."

Alumni also submitted a number of suggestions:

"I would have liked more emphasis on Epidemiology and Biostatistics as well as an emphasis on Public Health/Preventive Medicine."

"One area that HST did not overly address is that of the realities of funding and politics in academic medicine."

"More guidance on the process of research grant writing, limitations on the academic physician."

"Provide a better understanding of the network of science and scientific community and strategies needed to maintain funding."

Research

From its inception, a principal objective of HST has been the facilitation and sponsorship of interdisciplinary, inter-university research. It has been the goal of HST to develop productive, collaborative research relationships by bringing together multidisciplinary teams of physicians, engineers and scientists from the Harvard Medical School, its affiliated teaching hospitals and MIT to focus on major medical and health problems and to work on a scale suitable to the dimensions of the problems. Emphasis was to be given to areas of investigation with a high potential for valuable results that take advantage of the strengths afforded by the two universities and the provision of settings especially suited for multidisciplinary, large-scale studies. The need for rapid and efficient application of research findings by a systematic engineering approach was recognized. Development was seen to encompass the design and production of prototypes such as instruments for diagnosis and treatment, sensory devices for the handicapped, prostheses, artificial organs, automated laboratories and model health care facilities.

To quote from the original proposal for a joint Harvard-MIT Program in Health Sciences and Technology, of February 26, 1970:[10]

Research

An inventory conducted in 1968 revealed that there were very numerous joint research efforts involving faculty members and students of Harvard Medical School, MIT and the Division of Engineering and Applied Physics at Harvard. It would be the purpose of the School to facilitate such research, to provide a forum for the exchange of information, to select areas of investigation deserving of particular emphasis and chosen to take advantage of the strengths afforded by the two universities, and to provide settings especially suited to multidisciplinary or large scale studies.

Examples of the kinds of research that might be undertaken may be cited:

1. A program in environmental health sciences that would involve numerous disciplines such as the earth sciences, various branches of engineering, biology, genetics, human pathophysiology, urban planning, economics and others.

2. A program in biomaterials science that would focus on the interaction of biological surfaces, and membranes with chemical synthetic surfaces and would involve the study of the chemical constitution and physiologic behavior of biological membranes and the biological consequences of interaction of body tissues and fluids with synthetic surfaces.

Development

Development as a concept refers to the deliberate application of research findings to important health needs. Such development may encompass the design and production of prototypes such as instruments for diagnosis and treatment, prosthetic devices such as sensory devices for the blind and deaf or the "Boston Arm", artificial organs, automated laboratories, and model emergency rooms or operating rooms that utilize effectively the advantages afforded by modern science and technology.

Health Care

These programs should take advantage of the wide range of knowledge and competencies of faculty members and students in both universities and of their commitment to address the urgent medical and social problems related to health care. The application of engineering and management technology to health services should enhance the quality and availability of health care and the efficiency of the delivery system.

To be effective, education, research and demonstration programs in health care should have one or more operational bases. Accordingly, it will be desirable to integrate such programs into the activities of the School and into the activities of the Harvard teaching hospitals, the MIT and Harvard Health Services, the Center for Community Health, the School of Public Health and the Sloan School of Management.

Studies will be undertaken with a view to the development of comprehensive health care programs in Cambridge and in Boston. These studies will include the design of institutional forms that will be best suited to reflect the interest and needs of the communities to be served and that will provide appropriate settings for the joint efforts of public and private health agencies and of faculty members and students.

With reference to the last paragraphs quoted from the original proposal, opposition developed within Harvard University—primarily on the part of the Harvard School of Public Health—against the program including the study of quality, availability and effectiveness of health care among its goals. Development of a program in human biology also encountered disinterest, if not opposition, in the Department of Biology at Harvard's Faculty of Arts and Sciences, as well as in the Department of Biology at MIT.

In short order, major collaborative, interdisciplinary and inter-institutional programs were launched. Early examples were the program in biomaterial science, the rehabilitation engineering center, metabolism and bone disease, optimalization of dose distribution in cancer radiation therapy, nuclear medicine, energy and health, and the Center for Health Effects of Fossil Fuel Utilization. A full listing of research projects is provided in Appendix F.

The magnitude of efforts needed to bring together scientists from the different departments of the two universities around significant, timely and supportable projects was recognized and resulted, in 1972, in the appointment of an Assistant Director for Research Program Development. The first incumbent of this position, Dr. Irving A. Berstein, held a Ph.D. in chemistry and was recruited from industry. His reminiscences are quite revealing with regard to the challenges of his task, as well as the culture of the two universities and his *modus operandi.* He conceived his task as "try to pull the right people together, not only in terms of expertise and skills, but also personality: compatible and willing to work together."

> I actually found the Harvard Medical School professors easier to work with than the MIT professors. . . . I think the basis is, when you're a physician you've got to deal with an awful lot of realities every day. It's close up. Patients are sick; they would not be patients if they weren't sick. They are either slightly sick or very sick, and there are all kinds of judgments and human interactions that are part of the whole process of being a physician. Not so much in science, although as a professor, a teacher, you have requirements like that, the human interaction, they are never as demanding . . . Universities are very different than companies. Universities are probably one of the last bastions of the true free enterprise system, where you come down to individuals who are creating and performing on an individual basis. Companies and large organizations are teams . . . [in academia], you just can't get interesting, interested people involved—they have to be willing to submerge some of their expertise, some of the things they know so much about, to a common goal, and work along with people who are much more expert than they are in another field. So they're no longer literally one of the world's leading experts. They are now a little bit of a student, and a team player, you see, and that's a big personality demand on most peo-

ple . . . And one of the things I learned was that if I were going to make a success on this thing, and that really means making these programs come together and get funded, that I had to pitch in wherever the need was. I just couldn't run this by some handbook. What I mean by that is, if we found a great program director who was a wonderful writer and had the energy and time to do things, that's great. But if we found a great program director who either didn't have the time or wasn't interested in writing up a lot of the text, then I darn well better write up that text with all the input from him and other people. So my style, frankly, was to pitch in wherever it was needed and, frankly, different skills were needed for different programs.

Dr. Berstein saw his task to first identify special fields or areas, then identify people already interested, bring them together for a symposium, including lunch or dinner. This was an entrepreneurial effort. The goal was new initiatives, new creative projects which would be fundable (mainly by NIH). Exploration was broad and most endeavors were eminently successful. However, a number of efforts did not come to fruition, including left ventricular assist devices, linguistic disability, renal and pulmonary research areas.

Dr. Berstein remained in this position until 1980. Although he was succeeded by two short-term staff appointees, neither of them matched his success at putting together major projects. After 1988, no further efforts were made to continue this position. By then, the HST program had become quite well known in both universities, and the Joint Faculty had been expanded to over 150 members. Therefore, a number of collaborative projects were initiated by investigators themselves. At the same time, governmental support for large-scale projects was becoming more difficult to obtain. In retrospect, several long-term members of the HST faculty deplored the loss of the Director of Development, and some expressed the views that opportunities were missed, especially in material science, tissue engineering, neurosciences, molecular biology and genetics.

Members of the core faculty continued to consider research a major goal of the HST Division. To quote one commentator:

Collaborative research projects I considered to be one of the cornerstones of the HST Division. Having these collaborative kinds of interactions is a key element in staying at the cutting edge. We have to have faculty members from different disciplines working together in a productive manner. If we were able to bring together people who could get excited about working together on a research level, then there would be greater enthusiasm for bringing those same people together to develop new educational offerings, particularly at the interface of technology with engineering, medicine and biology.

A major if not key factor which launched the HST Program was the belief that progress in medical research and development was most likely at the interface of quantitative sciences and medicine and that optimal progress would require collaboration of scientists in different fields, as well as demand the education of a new class of physician/scientists conversant with both fields. While this perception was well conceived and borne out amply, one may well hold the opinion that progress has been considerably broader and more spectacular in other fields; namely, molecular biology and neuroscience. Indeed, the HST Program may be faulted in its limited and delayed emphasis upon these fields. Recognition, however, must be given to ongoing efforts from the earliest days to include molecular biology in the teaching program, facilitated by the personal interests and ongoing research of the founder and first director, Dr. Irving London. Thus a series of lectures in molecular biology and immunology were offered to first-year students, and later a fine, albeit brief, course in genetics was offered by Dr. Samuel Latt, which unfortunately was discontinued after his untimely death in 1988.

Why did it take until 1991 for a course in molecular biology and genetics to be reintroduced as a full semester course? Here we must consider the failure of HST to secure the collaboration of MIT's biology department, a leader in molecular biology and genetics. Although nominally a member of that department, Dr. London remained rather uninvolved, and the department in turn remained faithful to its disinterest in applied biology, human biology and medicine. Members of the biology department had the primary obligation to teach at MIT, and, unlike some other departments, this department did not release its members from that obligation if they wished to teach in HST. Fortunately, the department of genetics at HMS was more sympathetic and helpful.

The situation with regard to neuroscience was more complex. Although the initial full semester second year course in neuroanatomy did include some neuroscience, a subsequent pathophysiology offering in this field was not well attended, and it was not until 1991 that the Chairman of the Department of Neurosciences at HMS instituted a full neuroscience course taken by all HST students. This delay in offering first-class, essentially obligatory courses in these two areas may also have, at least in part, been responsible for a relatively lesser role of these fields in collaborative HST sponsored research. Notable, however, is the fact that the students recognized the importance of these fields, as seen in Figures 1 and 2 as well as in the list of topics of their research (See Appendix E).

Notes

1. The author of this chapter has been associated with the HST program from its inception, was course head of a major pathophysiology course (cardiovascular pathophysiology) and served on most committees, often as chair. Thus, he was in an advantageous position with regard to the selection of and access to interviewees. His familiarity and personal acquaintance with all interviewees was most valuable in guiding questions and eliciting views and critiques. Notwithstanding these advantages over a personally uninvolved outsider, the possible disadvantages of interviews by an "insider" must be considered. Bias cannot be completely ruled out.

2. Interviews were carried out with the following individuals:
   William S. Beck, M.D., Professor of Medicine, HMS
   George B. Benedek, Ph.D., Alfred H. Caspary Professor of Physics, MIT
   Irving A. Berstein, Ph.D., Assistant Director for Research Program Development, HST
   H. Frederick Bowman, Ph.D., Senior Academic Administrator, HST
   Deborah Burstein, Ph.D., Associate Professor of Radiology, HMS
   Martin C. Carey, M.D., D.Sc., Professor of Medicine, HMS, Lawrence Henderson Associate Professor of Health Sciences and Technology
   Cecil H. Coggins, M.D., Associate Professor of Medicine, HMS
   Herman N. Eisen, M.D., Professor of Biology, Emeritus, MIT
   Lee Gehrke, Ph.D., Associate Professor of Cell Biology in the MIT Division of HST
   Harvey Goldman, M.D., Professor of Pathology, HMS
   Robert A. Greenes, M.D., Ph.D., Associate Professor of Radiology, Associate Professor in the Department of Biostatistics, HSPH
   Farish A. Jenkins, Jr., Ph.D., Professor of Biology, Alexander Agassiz Professor of Zoology, HU
   Richard J. Kitz, M.D., Henry Isaiah Dorr Professor of Research and Teaching in Anesthetics and Anesthesia, HMS
   Walter L. Koltun, Ph.D., Assistant Director for Resources, HST
   Robert S. Lees, M.D., Professor of Health Sciences and Technology, HST
   Boris Magasanik, Ph.D., Professor of Biology, Emeritus, MIT
   Robert H. Mann, Ph.D., Whitaker Professor Emeritus of Biomedical Engieering, MIT
   Henry C. Meadow, Dean, HMS
   Alan Natapoff, Ph.D., Research Affiliate, Department of Aeronautics and Astronautics, MIT
   Walter A. Rosenblith, Ph.D., Provost and Institute Professor, Emeritus, MIT

Daniel C. Shannon, M.D., D.Sc., Professor of Pediatrics, HMS

Eleanor G. Shore, M.D., Dean for Faculty Affairs, HMS

Felix H.M. Villars, Ph.D., Professor of Physics, Emeritus, MIT

Richard J. Wurtman, M.D., Professor of Brain and Cognitive Sciences, Director Clinical Research Center, MIT

The original tapes, as well as the transcripts of twenty-four interviews conducted between April, 1993, and May, 1995, have been deposited in the Archives of the Harvard Medical School.

3. Examples of informal courses taught by students, usually as January courses:

(a) "Health Policy," Stan N. Finkelstein '75

(b) "Pharm for the Boards," Frank Rybicki '92

(c) "Survey of Medical Biochemistry," Mykol Larvie '91, Mark Mullins '91 and Whitney Edmister '93

Most of these students were M.D./Ph.D. candidates, and thus were able to offer these courses over several years. (a) and (c) eventually became formal curricular offerings.

4. R.A. Greenes, B.P. Bergeron, M.S. Dichter and J.T. and Fallon, "Clinical Problem as an Educational Paradigm in Teaching Preclinical Cardiac Pathophysiology, in F. Pinciroli and G. Meester eds. *Databases for Cardiology* (Dordrecht, The Netherlands: Kluwer Academic Publishers, 1991), pp. 113–140.

5. Abraham N. Morse, "Evaluating the Effectiveness of Nephromancer: A Renal Pathology Tutorial for the Macintosh Computer," Harvard-MIT Division of Health Sciences and Technology, 1993.

6. For further discussion of evaluation of the curriculum and courses, see Chapter 10.

7a. G.B. Benedek and F.M.H. Villars, *Physics with Illustrative Examples from Medicine and Biology,* Volume I, *Mechanics.* (Reading, Massachusetts: Addison-Wesley Publishing Co., 1973).

b. F.M.H. Villars and G.B. Benedek, *Physics with Illustrative Examples from Medicine and Biology,* Volume 2, *Statistical Physics.* (Reading, Massachusetts: Addison-Wesley Publishing Co., 1974).

c. G.B. Benedek and F.M.H. Villars, *Physics with Illustrative Examples from Medicine and Biology,* Volume 3, *Electricity and Magnetism.* (Reading, Massachusetts: Addison-Wesley Publishing Co., 1979).

8. Catalog 1979–1980, Harvard-MIT Division of Health Sciences and Technology (Cambridge, Massachusetts: MIT, 1979–1980, p. 14).

9. Some of these citations have been reported in L. Wilkerson and W.H. Abelmann, "Producing Physician-Scientists: A Survey of Graduates from the Harvard-MIT Program in Health Sciences and Technology," *Academic Medicine* 68 (1993): 214–218.

10. Harvard-MIT Program in Health Sciences and Technology, proposal dated February 26,1970.

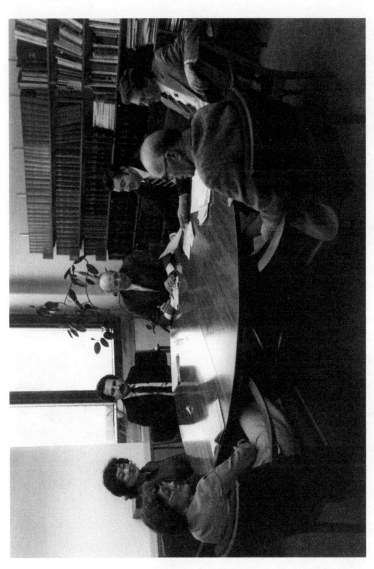

1. Meeting of the Administrative Council at MIT, ca. 1973. *Clockwise:* Eleanor G. Shore, M.D., M.P.H.; Keiko F. Oh, M.A.; Ernest G. Cravalho, Ph.D.; Irving A. Berstein, Ph.D.; Walter L. Koltun, Ph.D.; H. Frederick Bowman, Ph.D.; Irving M. London, M.D.

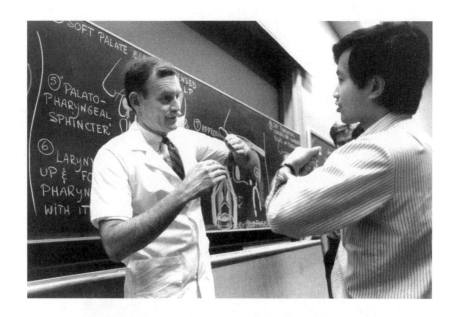

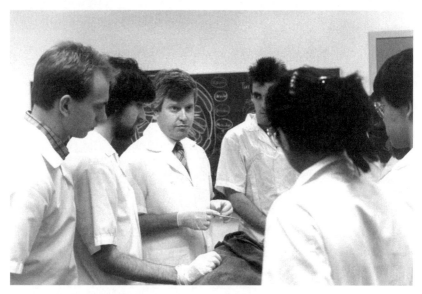

2. *Above,* Farish A. Jenkins, Jr., Ph.D., and Ming Xu Wang, M.D., 1991, in HST 010, Functional Anatomy, at HMS, 1988; *below,* Lee Gehrke, Ph.D., with Mark Albers, M.D., Ph.D., 1995, Seth J. Field, M.D., 1997 and Paul S. Cheney, M.S., 1988.

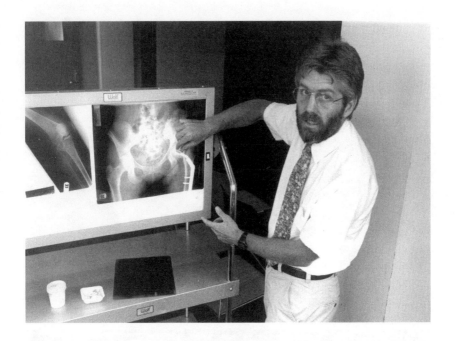

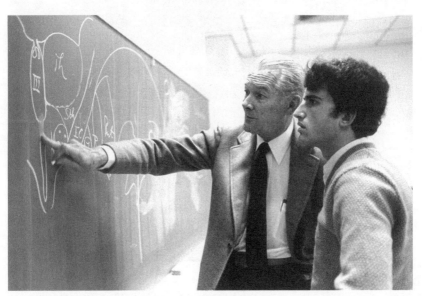

3. *Above,* Wilson C. (Toby) Hayes, Ph.D., HST 010, Functional Anatomy, ca. 1985; *below,* Walle J. H. Nauta, M.D., Ph.D., and Gilad S. Gordon, M.D., 1985, in HST 130, The Human Nervous System, ca. 1980.

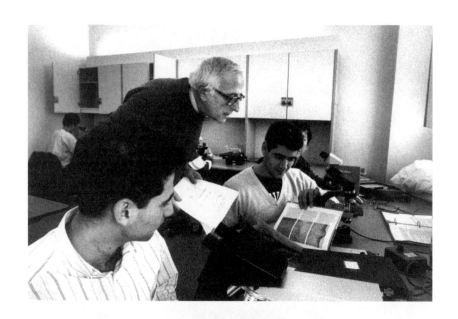

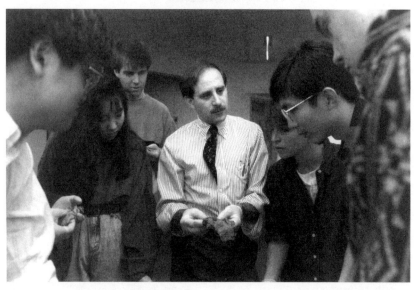

4. *Above,* Harvey Goldman, M.D., with Adel M. Malek, M.D., Ph.D., 1994, and Ralph de la Torre, M.D., 1992, in HST 030 Human Pathology, 1988; *below,* Frederick J. Schoen, M.D., Ph.D., with Volney L. Sheen, M.D., 1997, Charlene M. Chiang, M.D., 1996, Thomas J. Mullen, Ph.D., 1998, Nada Boustany, Ph.D., 1997, Robert Hurford, M.D., 1994, and Tai Sing Lee, Ph.D., 1993, in HST 030, Human Pathology, 1990.

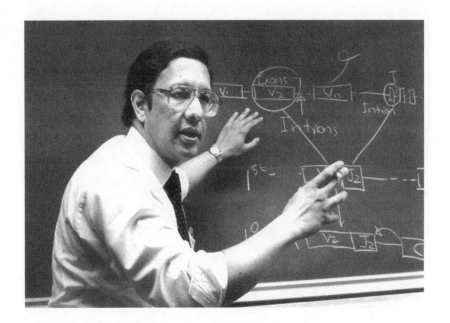

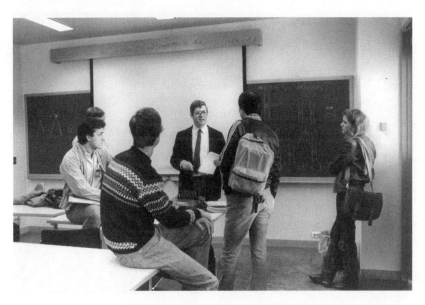

5. *Above*, Abul K. Abbas, M.D., in HST 175, Cellular and Molecular Immunology, ca. 1988; *below*, Samuel A. Latt, M.D., Ph.D., George Q. Daley, M.D., 1991, and other students in HMS 700, Genetics, 1987.

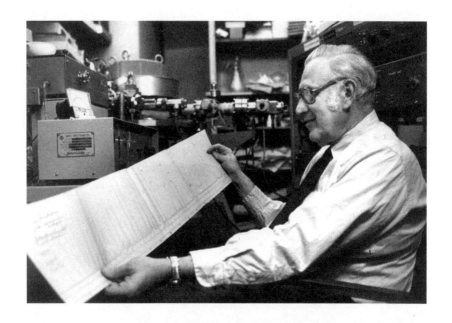

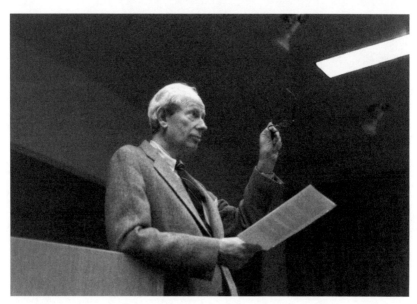

6. *Above,* Paul M. Gallop, Ph.D., HST 141, Molecular Basis of Some Clinical Disorders, in his laboratory at Children's Hospital, ca. 1988; *below,* Walter H. Abelmann, M.D., in HST 090 Cardio-vascular Pathophysiology, ca. 1988.

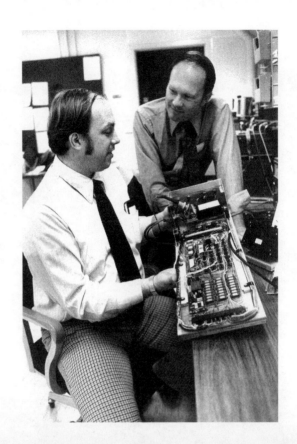

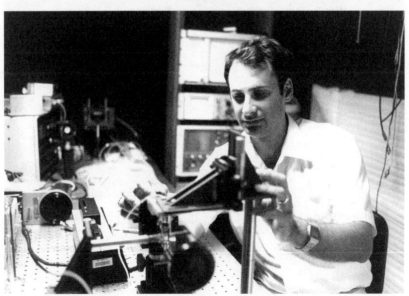

7. *Above,* Walter H. Olson, Ph.D., and Roger G. Mark, M.D., Ph.D., in the Biomedical Engineering Center, ca. 1979; *below,* Richard J. Cohen, M.D., Ph.D., 1976, in his laboratory, ca. 1985.

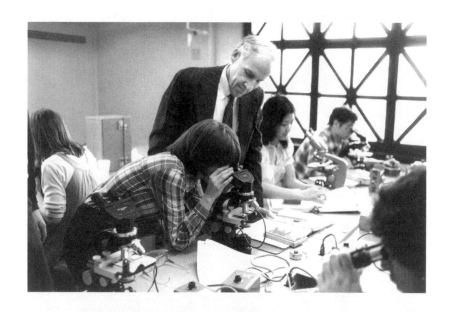

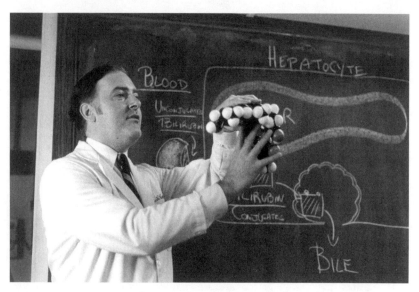

8. *Above,* William S. Beck, M.D., with students in HST 080, Hematology, ca. 1979; *below,* Martin C. Carey, M.D., D.Sc., in HST 120, Gastro-entrology, 1984.

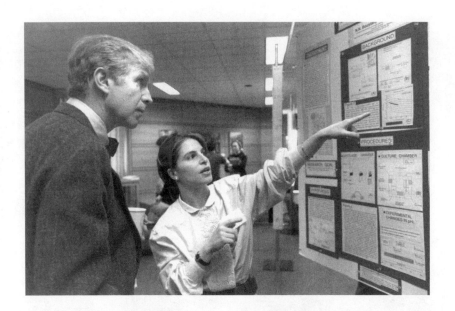

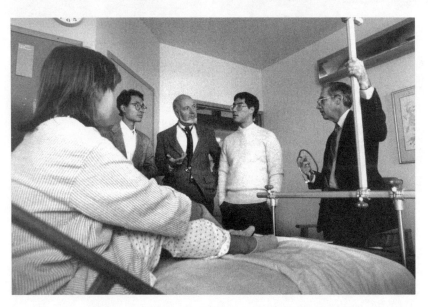

9. *Above,* Cecil H. (Pete) Coggins, M.D., with Nada Boustany, Ph.D., 1997, at the HST Forum of 1991; *below,* Arnold N. Weinberg, M.D., and John M. Moses, M.D., with Kenneth S. Hu, M.D., 1994, and Jack Tsao, M.D., Ph.D., 1997, in HST 220, Introduction to Patient Care and the Profession that Cares in 1990.

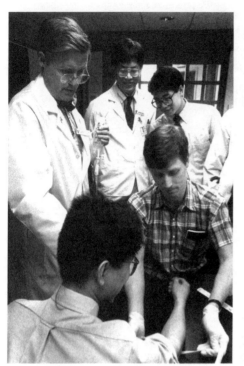
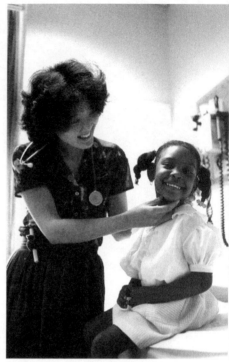

10. *Left,* W. Hallowell Churchill, Jr., M.D., with students in HST 200, Introduction to Clinical Medicine at Brigham and Women's Hospital, ca. 1990; *right,* Annabelle Okada, M.D., 1988, in HST 200, Introduction to Clinical Medicine, in 1986.

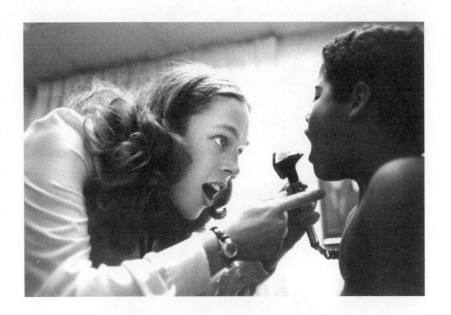

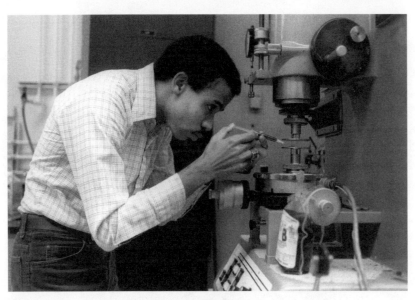

11. *Above,* Martha L. Gray, Ph.D., 1986, in HST 201, Introduction to Clinical Medicine and Medical Engineering, ca. 1982; *below,* James Oliver, M.D., Ph.D., 1994.

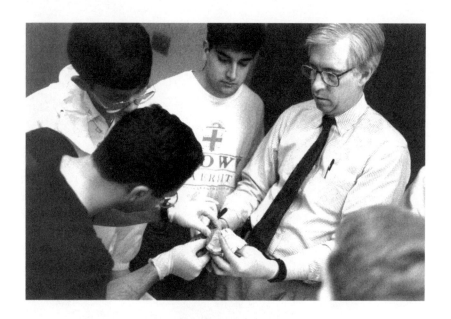

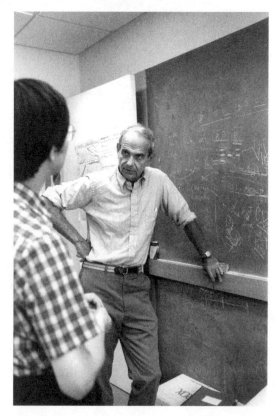

12. *Above,* John T. Fallon, M.D., Ph.D., HST 090, Cardiovascular Pathophysiology, 1980s; *below,* Herman N. Eisen, M.D., Immunology, 1970s.

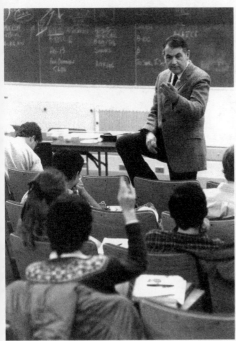

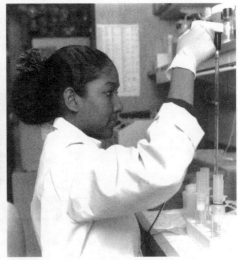

13. *Above,* Ronald A. Arky, M.D., HST 060, Endocrinology, 1980s; *below,* Cassandra Hall Walcott, M.D., 1992.

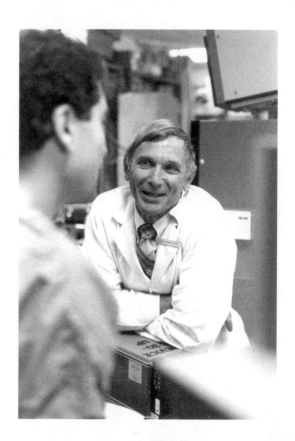

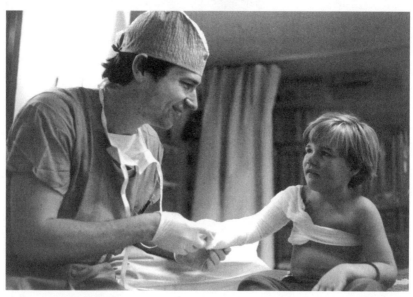

14. *Above,* Richard J. Kitz, M.D., late 1980s; *below,* Dennis Orgill, Ph.D., 1983, in HST 201, Introduction to Clinical Medicine and Medical Engineering, 1981.

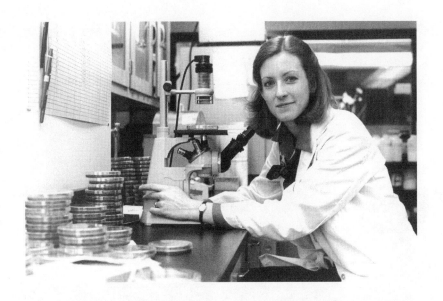

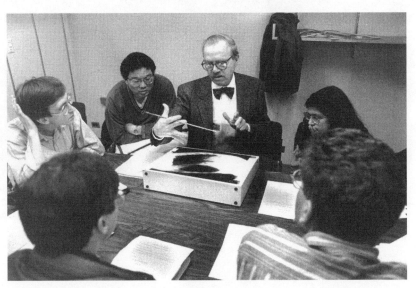

15. *Above,* Barbara L. Smith, M.D., Ph.D., 1983; *below,* Daniel C. Shannon, M.D., in HST Respiratory Pathophysiology, late 1980s.

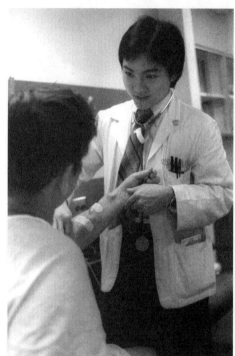
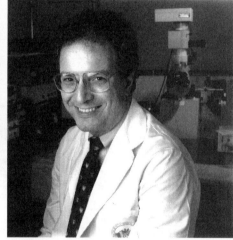

16. *Above,* Henry C. Chueh, M.D., Ph.D., 1989, in HST 200, Introduction to Clinical Medicine, 1986; *below,* Joseph V. Bonventre, M.D., Ph.D., 1976, early 1990s.

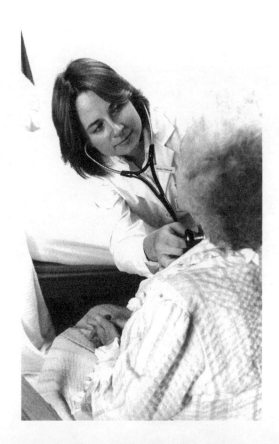

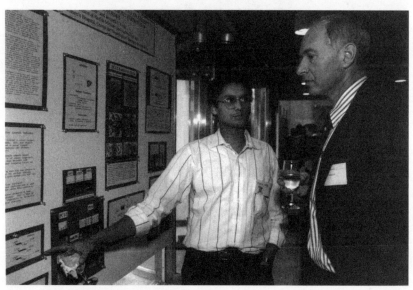

17. *Above,* Marilyn L. Yodlowski, M.D., Ph.D., 1984, in HST 200, Introduction to Clinical Medicine, 1982; *below,* Michael Rosenblatt, M.D., with Manish Shah, M.D. 1996, at the HST Forum 1994.

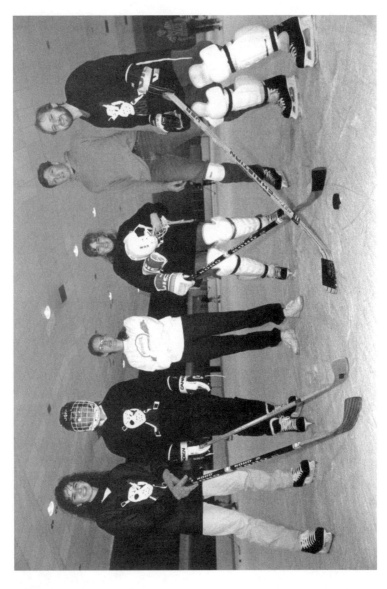

18. The 'Ice Jasons' HST Medical Engineering and Medical Physics Students' extramural ice hockey team in 1991.

Chapter 9

THE MEDICAL ENGINEERING/MEDICAL PHYSICS (MEMP) DOCTORAL PROGRAM 1978–1996

Roger G. Mark, M.D., Ph.D.

I. The Formative Years, 1970–1978

Program Design

The concept of a Ph.D. program at the interface of engineering and medicine was first espoused by President Jerome Wiesner during the very earliest days of the HST program in 1970. His rationale was that Harvard and MIT should collaborate not only to develop new strategies for the education of physicians, but also should work jointly to produce a new breed of physical scientists and engineers with in-depth training in the medical and clinical sciences so that they could function as independent investigators on important problems at the interface of technology and clinical medicine. Wiesner reasoned that the collaborating institutions would be particularly well positioned to provide selected graduate students with both a superb scientific and engineering education and a deep exposure to the unique medical and clinical courses designed for HST medical students. The concept of a doctoral program in Medical Engineering and Medical Physics was endorsed not only by President Wiesner and Provost Walter Rosenblith at MIT, but was also very high in priority for Henry Meadow who was Senior Associate Dean of the Harvard Medical School. The HST Administration was enthusiastic and began to organize planning efforts.

Despite the strong support for this educational goal from the top administrations of both universities, however, there was slow initial progress by the faculty toward designing such a program. Much of the creative energy of the biomedically-oriented engineering faculty at MIT was focused on the newly evolving HST/MD curriculum. Another factor, however, was the fact that some engineering faculty at MIT had definite reservations about the proposal. In fact, a few senior faculty were categorically opposed to the concept of an interdisciplinary biomedical engineering track, and they felt strongly that graduate engineering education at MIT should remain based solidly within traditional departments. Sentiments were expressed, such as:

> There is no such thing as a separate discipline of biomedical engineering . . . Biomedical engineering represents applications of traditional engineering disciplines to specific problems in medicine and biology, and thus biomedical engineering should remain within traditional departments . . . An interdisciplinary program such as MEMP couldn't possibly have rigorous quality control, and would by necessity be inferior to a departmental program.

A sequence of *ad hoc* faculty planning committees were appointed by the HST Administration to design a suitable educational program, but they repeatedly failed to reach consensus, and forward momentum never developed. The HST Administrative Committee[1] reviewed the planning process on a monthly basis and was generally disappointed that progress was not more rapid. After four or five rather fruitless years went by, Provost Rosenblith and President Wiesner pushed hard for a renewed high-priority faculty planning effort, and in 1975 a senior faculty Task Force on Medical Engineering was formed which was chaired by Professor Laurence Young of MIT's Department of Aeronautical and Astronautical Engineering.[2] The majority of its members were from Harvard Medical School, possibly reflecting the Administrative Committee's disappointment with the previous lack of productivity of senior MIT engineering faculty! The task force had a number of important issues to consider, including:

- How broad should the MEMP program be in terms of engineering disciplines? (President Wiesner favored wide breadth, to include engineering, chemistry, physics, mathematics, etc.)

- How should students be qualified?
- How could the new program design assure that department-based MIT faculty would accept MEMP students without considering them "second class"?
- How would the MEMP program be different from the existing interdepartmental BME (Biomedical Engineering) doctoral program at MIT?
- Should there be a core engineering curriculum? Would there be a common track for all or elective options?
- What options would there be for students desiring both a Ph.D. and an M.D. degree?
- What should be the appropriate requirements in the medical sciences?
- What kind of clinical experiences should be included in the curriculum?

The Medical Engineering Task Force appointed two major subcommittees: one for curriculum design and one to develop clinical clerkships. The **Curriculum Subcommittee** was comprised of MIT engineering and physics faculty members and was chaired by Professor Laurence Young.[3] It was charged with the responsibility of defining the formal course requirements and examination structure for the new doctoral program.

The **Subcommittee on Clerkships** was charged to define a series of clinical experiences for students in the new medical engineering/medical physics track. This committee was chaired by Dr. Richard Kitz (Anesthesiology, MGH).[4]

H. Frederick Bowman, Ph.D., the Administrative Officer of HST, functioned as executive secretary and was an active participant in the main task force and both of its subcommittees. In 1976 Professor Ernest Cravalho, then the Associate Dean of Engineering at MIT, made a major commitment to the HST Program and was appointed Associate Director of HST with responsibility for the MEMP program. He and Fred Bowman assumed major leadership in guiding the work of the committees in designing the program during 1975–76.

On November 23, 1976, the Medical Engineering Task Force issued a final report entitled "A Proposed Program in Medical Engineering and Medical Physics." It proposed the establishment of a doctoral program which would draw upon the resources of existing graduate departments at MIT and Harvard, the medical curriculum of the HST Program, and the clinical teaching resources of the Harvard-affiliated hospitals. The new degree program consisted of three major components:

1. A set of formal courses and examinations to guarantee that each student would achieve doctoral-level competence in his/her basic discipline of engineering or physical science, and a modest "core curriculum" of three biomedical engineering subjects required of all students;
2. A substantial set of preclinical medical courses and clinical experiences designed to provide students with a deep understanding of human pathophysiology and of clinical medicine; and
3. Thesis research, done at the university campuses or in the teaching hospitals under the direction of MIT or Harvard faculty on topics at the interface of technology and medicine.

The program design was based on the following principles:

1. In order to assure thorough grounding in a basic discipline, and in order to assure the support of collaborating MIT departments, MEMP students were to be required to meet the same quality standards as all other graduate students in the same discipline. The engineering/physical science credentialing was to be delegated primarily to collaborating departments at MIT or at Harvard. Quality control would begin at admission: MEMP students would have to be admitted by both a collaborating department and by HST. The engineering/physical science component of the MEMP curriculum was designed to follow closely the patterns established by collaborating departments. MEMP students would be required to fulfill the graduate course requirements and to pass the doctoral qualifying exams of their departments.[5] These procedures guaranteed that MEMP graduates would be fully competent in a defined discipline—sufficiently so that they could compete successfully for faculty appointments in such disciplines. The curriculum design also guaranteed that MEMP students would not be viewed as "second class" by discipline-oriented MIT faculty members, who generally were skeptical about the rigor of biomedical engineering degree programs. The Curriculum Committee also felt that all graduates, independent of their basic discipline, should receive instruction in several "core" biomedical engineering subjects, including instrumentation, electronics, and medical engineering measurements.

2. MEMP students were to be deeply immersed in the medical sciences, both in the classroom and in clinical environments. MEMP students were to join HST/MD students to participate in a significant portion of the pre-clinical curriculum in medical sciences. During this class-work, the MEMP students would acquire specific knowledge and also would develop friendships and shared experiences with medical colleagues which would facilitate later interdisciplinary research. Later in the program, MEMP students were to receive almost a full year of clinical training in the teaching hospitals. The teaching was to be done by collaborating HMS physicians and hospital-based biomedical engineering faculty, with the objective of teaching the students the basic skills of physical diagnosis, the principles of clinical care of patients and medical decision-making, and also a number of significant clinical applications of technology.

3. Thesis research opportunities were not restricted to the university campuses but also included projects at the teaching hospitals. Although no limitations were ever placed on the choice of thesis topics, it was hoped that students would choose projects with potential clinical relevance. Supervision was to be by a Harvard or MIT faculty member associated with the HST Program, and by a committe of faculty, at least one of whom was to be from the student's basic discipline.

Formal Approval Process at MIT

In order for the proposed new program to be implemented, it had to be formally reviewed and approved by the MIT faculty. The initial scrutiny was conducted by the Committee on Graduate School Policy (CGSP), which included representatives from each department. It was obviously important that HST secure the support of interested departments before the CSGP met, and therefore an extensive "selling" effort was instituted. Dr. Bowman and Prof. Cravalho were dispatched to visit all department heads in the School of Engineering and the Department of Physics to explain the program and to solicit each department's support for the new initiative. Because of the careful design of the curriculum, and the high standards expected of the students, there were no departmental objections. The CGSP approved the concept, and it was scheduled to be considered by the entire MIT faculty at its regularly scheduled meeting on February 16,

1977. That faculty meeting was rather poorly attended (about forty members at the start of the meeting and about fifty-five at the end), which was not unusual for non-controversial meetings. The faculty first voted on graduate and undergraduate degrees and an addition to the General Institute Requirements. They next discussed expanding the duties of the Committee on Industrial Liaison and considered issues relating to use of human subjects in social science research. Finally, the MEMP Program discussion was launched by Dean Jean Richard who moved, on behalf of the CSGP, that:

> The Faculty recommend to the Corporation the establishment of the following degrees:
>   Sc.D. in Medical Engineering, Ph.D. in Medical Engineering, Sc.D in Medical Physics, Ph.D. in Medical Physics, under the Joint Harvard-MIT Program in Health Sciences and Technology.[6]

Provost Walter Rosenblith spoke strongly in favor of the motion, and provided the faculty with a detailed review of the formation and mission of HST. He emphasized the importance of the newly proposed degree program in preparing engineers and physicists to effectively apply technology to the understanding, prevention, and control of human disease and disability. Professors London and Cravalho discussed the proposed curriculum; the former in a general way, the latter in detail. They explained that the program proposed to admit approximately ten students per year, which predicted a steady-state number of approximately fifty students. A number of questions were raised by the faculty which explored the possibility of Ph.D.-M.D. options, the details of doctoral qualifying exams, the breadth of the program with respect to collaborating departments and the responsibility of collaborating departments. Additional questions were raised about the administration and faculty of the HST Program, which were answered by Professors London, Cravalho, and Rosenblith. President Wiesner reviewed the growth of HST, emphasized its importance to MIT, and strongly endorsed the MEMP proposal. After some further brief discussion, President Wiesner called for a vote on Dean Richard's motion, which had been seconded. There were thirty-one votes in favor, and none opposed. The motion involved a change in the Regulations of the Faculty, and the vote was sufficient to effect the change.

That faculty vote, and its subsequent endorsement by the MIT Corporation, constituted a major forward step in the development of HST. For the first time, the Program was authorized to admit its own graduate students and to recommend its own doctoral degrees to be awarded by MIT!

The Program at Harvard

It was always recognized and agreed among the planning faculty and the inter-institutional administrators that Harvard's Graduate School of Arts and Sciences (GSAS) would participate in the MEMP program. However, the number of students enrolling via Harvard was expected to be low—perhaps one or two each year. Thus, it was decided not to define a new degree track through Harvard. Rather, students would apply to GSAS and to HST and indicate their interest in the MEMP program. If accepted by both, the students would be admitted, would be obligated to fulfill the MEMP requirements, would receive MEMP financial support, would pay all tuition to MIT, and would ultimately receive a doctoral degree from Harvard.[7]

Financing the Program

The HST administration, and also the MIT Provost, Walter Rosenblith, recognized that the new doctoral program would be unusually demanding on student time. In order to permit students to complete the program requirements in a reasonable time period they would need to spend essentially full time in course work for the initial three to three-and-a-half years. Thus no time could reasonably be allocated to a part-time work position such as teaching or research assistant—the traditional means of providing financial support to graduate students. Rosenblith felt that the MEMP program was a bold and important experiment and that student funding was an essential part of the commitment of the Institute. The availability of student support was felt to be essential to attract first-rate graduate students and to allow them to concentrate fully on their academic work. Therefore, he authorized seven semesters of fellowship support for each student admitted. This support would normally be adequate to bring students through the initial course-intensive part of the program. The research years were to be supported via research assistantships provided by the faculty. The institutional funding provided by the MIT administration represented a major commitment to the new program. At the time, tuition costs were $4,000 per year, so the total first year cost for ten students would be $40,000. In steady state, however, the annual budget for student support would grow to more than $140,000!

II. Launching MEMP and the Early Years,

1978–1985 Launching the Program—1978

Professor Ernest Cravalho assumed leadership of the new program and guided the efforts of collaborating faculty members. An admissions committee was formed, and plans for recruiting the first class began. The objective was to move quickly and try to admit the first class by September of 1978. Faculty members were encouraged to visit other universities and to present the new program to students interested in biomedical engineering. The admissions committee also sought the assistance of collaborating MIT and Harvard departments to identify individuals whose application essays suggested a possible interest in the new curriculum. MEMP was unique among biomedical engineering graduate programs because of its heavy medical sciences component. It was the only engineering program in the country which included clinical training. Thus, it was particularly attractive to students with a strong commitment to research careers at the interface of physical science with clinical medicine, but who did not wish to become physicians. Fortunately, by early spring an excellent group of applicants had been identified, interviewed, and invited into the new program. A class of thirteen individuals finally was admitted. The initial class included four women and nine men, and the departmental affiliations (all at MIT) were as follows: two in chemical engineering; four in electrical engineering, five in mechanical engineering, and two in physics.

Before the new class arrived, the faculty made some minor modifications to the proposed MEMP curriculum. In particular, it was decided that the core biomedical engineering courses should include biomedical signal processing. To free up the necessary space in the schedule, the requirement for one of the medical science courses (endocrinology) was dropped. Intensive planning began for the new biomedical signal processing course, and the faculty benefitted by the contributions of Dr. Dan Adam, a visiting assistant professor from Israel, who took primary responsibility for it. Planning for the clinical portion of the curriculum intensified. The description of the MEMP curriculum as it appeared in the 1979–80 catalog is reproduced in note 8.[8]

The new class arrived in September and moved into a newly outfitted student cluster in Building 20 on the MIT campus. That building was the old home of the WWII Radiation Laboratory; it had been constructed at that time as a "temporary" wooden structure. It was "full of character" and easy to modify as well! Desks, refrigerator, sink, etc., were provided for the students in an area near the HST Biomedical Engineering Center, and they quickly bonded as an excited and highly motivated group.

The Curriculum in the Early Years

The students were advised to begin their graduate work with medical courses taught at the Harvard Medical School. All students accepted that advice, and they quickly became immersed in Human Anatomy and Pathology, studying together with their HST/MD student colleagues. Taking medical courses at the outset of the program was highly effective as a "bonding" experience for the students, and it helped them to solidify their medical engineering/medical physics identity and commitment. A weekly MEMP seminar provided additional opportunities to meet faculty and begin to learn about biomedical engineering research opportunities in the Harvard-MIT community. In addition, the students received enormous personal support and counseling by the faculty, particularly from Prof. Cravalho. All found master's thesis projects, and they were able to complete them within two to three years in addition to the required course work. It was not easy for some of the students to re-enter the engineering mode and prepare for qualifying examinations, but eventually all of the inaugural class passed.

In 1981, the first MEMP students began their introduction to the world of clinical medicine. The new course, "Introduction to Medicine and Medical Engineering" (ICM) was offered for the first time in 1981 and was open to MEMP students from the first several classes who had completed the required medical science courses and had passed doctoral qualifying examinations. The new semester-long course was designed and organized at the Beth Israel Hospital under the direction of Drs. Walter Abelmann and Roger Mark. It was designed to teach MEMP students the skills of history-taking and physical examination; to introduce them to the role of the physician and the medical decision-making process; to train them to organize and communicate clinical information in written and oral form; and to integrate history, physical exam and laboratory data to form pathophysiological hypotheses. In addition, the course investigated a variety of important diagnostic and therapeutic technologies from both the engineering and clinical perspectives. The initial version of the course was quite successful. In particular, the instructors noted that the rate and quality of clinical skill development in MEMP students was indistinguishable from that of HST medical students.

After ICM was completed, the students began a series of three clinical clerkships. The first was a six-week rotation in medicine, held at the Mt. Auburn Hospital in Cambridge. The students joined regular ward teams and assumed the role of third-year medical students. They admitted patients, followed them daily, wrote orders under supervision, and took on-call with the supervising house officer. After completion of the medicine clerkship, the MEMP students had acquired substantial clinical experience and were ready for the more individualized elective clerkships.

Six-week clinical electives had been designed in surgery (BWH), cardiology (BWH), and anesthesia (MGH), each of which focused on both clinical patient care and relevant technical and engineering clinical interfaces. Students were free to choose any two existing electives or to propose and design their own in conjunction with clinical faculty members. In general, students were to spend about half of their time participating in the clinical care of patients and half of their time preparing a "term paper" on an area of active research and development in a biomedical technology related to the clinical specialty.

The clinical experiences were highly successful and were generally very popular with the students. The students experienced a dramatic enhancement in their level of understanding of the processes, institutions, and professionals associated with medical care. They became comfortable and confident in working in the clinical setting, and in interacting with physicians as colleagues. Following the year of clinical rotations, students spent essentially full time on doctoral research.

Highlights of the Early Years, 1978–1985

The first seven years of the MEMP program were largely successful, and the program benefitted from the active participation of both faculty and students in a continuous process of evolution and "tuning" of the curriculum and policies. The strong clinical focus of the program was maintained, and indeed was felt by faculty and students alike to be a critical defining characteristic of MEMP. A number of issues arose during the first seven years which deserve mentioning.

1. Admissions

Because of the demanding nature of the MEMP program, and its heavy medical component, it became clear that the admissions process was of critical importance in identifying students who had both the academic excellence and the clear-cut career commitment needed for success. MEMP students would quickly discover that there were more direct (and probably easier) pathways to a Ph.D. degree in standard (well-defined) departmental programs. In addition, the M.D. route might also be a strong temptation to some MEMP students because of its clear academic path with less demand on original research creativity and a highly rewarding and secure career path at the end. The Admissions Committee was responsible for screening, interviewing, and selecting individuals who would have a maximum probability of completing the program without dropping out to an alternative route! The task of the Admissions Committee was complex:

- Find students with outstanding academic credentials and a strong research interest/aptitude.
- Find students who have solid engineering credentials, who will do well in their departmental graduate course work and qualifying exams.
- Find students who are strongly committed to the clinical emphasis of the program, but who want a Ph.D., not an M.D., as the primary goal.
- Avoid students who are looking for a partly funded "back door" to medical school!
- Find students whose personality is compatible with the clinical environment.
- Expedite the admissions process if possible in order to be able to have success in recruiting the best students.

In the early years, many applications were specifically solicited from collaborating departments. As time went on, however, the MEMP program became more widely known to students at MIT/Harvard and elsewhere, and more students applied directly to HST. The percentage of applications solicited from collaborating departments decreased. The Admissions Committee found that the probability of a student's successfully completing the MEMP program was much higher among those who had applied directly to HST, probably reflecting those candidates' stronger degree of commitment to a career at the interface of engineering and medicine. The annual rate of matriculation of new students has been ten to twelve throughout the program's history (Figure 1).

2. Evolution of the Curriculum

One of the earliest debates concerning the organization of the curriculum was the specific ordering of the course work. The initial strategy

MEMP ADMISSIONS

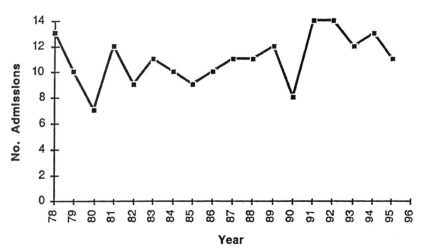

Figure 1.   Number of students admitted to the MEMP program each year.

of encouraging students to begin taking medical courses immediately had the great advantage of providing a strong bonding experience for the students, and strengthening their identity as MEMP students. Building enthusiasm for their chosen career direction was important. However, while taking a heavy course load of medical subjects, students had little opportunity to develop academic links with their engineering/physics departments. Preparation for doctoral qualifying exams was slow. Some MEMP students experienced difficulty with MIT departmental qualifying exams, although others did very well. After a few years the faculty began to advise students to focus first on their engineering/physics commitment, identify a master's thesis, begin to prepare for departmental qualifying exams and postpone life sciences until the second year. The change in the published curriculum occurred by 1980. The change probably did improve the performance of MEMP students on departmental qualifying exams. But the change also meant losing the unifying effects of a set of common courses for all incoming students, and the motivating early glimpse of the world of medicine. The loss of student body cohesion was significant since their only common experience was the graduate seminar required of all students.

Early in the history of the program there was considerable student disagreement with the strict requirement for the core set of three specific biomedical engineering subjects: Biomedical Signal Processing, Medical Engineering Measurements, and Medical Engineering Measurements Laboratory. Some students felt that the courses were too restrictive, or irrelevant to their own career interests, and students with little EE background found the courses particularly intimidating. Students argued for more flexibility in meeting the Biomedical Engineering requirement by choosing three subjects more related to their research interests. By 1985 the faculty had agreed with this request, and students were allowed to select their own subjects with the approval of faculty counselors.

3. M.D. Options for MEMP Students

Not surprisingly, a number of MEMP students entered the program with an interest in a combined Ph.D.-M.D. program, and others developed such an interest after studying medical and clinical subjects. It was necessary to develop a clear policy and procedure regarding medical school options for MEMP students. On the one hand the faculty and administration recognized the desirability of an M.D. degree for individuals who wished to engage in clinical investigation. On the other hand, they were concerned that the availability of an M.D. degree might sidetrack students from medical engineering/medical physics fields into a more traditional practice of medicine. They felt it was important to guard against MEMP being perceived as an alternative route into medical school for engineers. The faculty concluded that the choice of an M.D. option should be an individual one, and the following policies were adopted:

- Students desiring an M.D./Ph.D. at the time of application to graduate school were encouraged to apply simultaneously for admission to the HST/MD and MEMP programs. If admitted to both tracks, the two programs could be optimized for efficiency.
- MEMP students deciding later to seek a medical degree were specifically barred from applying to Harvard Medical School until the final year of doctoral research. An agreement was reached between the HMS and HST administrations that up to three transfer positions would be made available in the third-year M.D. class for MEMP graduates. A formal admission process was required (without MCATs), with admission decisions made by a small subcommittee including the director(s) of HST, the Dean of Academic Programs at HMS, and the Director of Admissions at HMS. MEMP students accepted into HMS were

not permitted to matriculate for the M.D. until the Ph.D. thesis was completed and accepted. All medical course work completed satisfactorily as part of the MEMP curriculum was accepted for credit toward the M.D. degree. Generally an additional two years were required to complete the M.D. requirements. National Board exams Part I were taken before starting clinical rotations. Similar arrangements were negotiated with Tufts University School of Medicine.

MEMP students who dropped out of the MEMP Ph.D. program to seek an M.D. degree were not permitted to enroll at HMS but were encouraged to apply to other medical schools, some of which granted advanced standing on the basis of medical courses taken at HST.

Over the first ten years of the MEMP program, four students left HST to pursue medical studies elsewhere. Of the twenty-four MEMP graduates during that decade, ten (42%) earned an M.D. as well (three entered MEMP with a previous M.D., three were enrolled simultaneously for both degrees, and four earned an M.D. at HMS after earning the MEMP Ph.D).

III. Changes and Evolution

The Stress of Administrative Changes at MIT and in HST

In 1980, ten years after the founding of HST with the enthusiastic support of President Wiesner and Provost Rosenblith at MIT, these leaders retired from their positions. A new President, Paul E. Gray, and a new Provost, Francis Low, took office, and among other things they began to assess existing MIT programs, including HST. The special relationship between HST and the top MIT administration was no longer as intimate and supportive as it had been. The Provost no longer attended weekly planning meetings with the HST Administrative Committee and delegated management of HST to Professor Kenneth Smith, the Associate Provost. Communication between the HST administration and the MIT administration faltered, and the Provost began to struggle to define a new organizational structure for the Division. Over the next few years, relationships between HST and the MIT administration did not improve and, in fact, became more difficult. Furthermore, the time was drawing close for Dr. Irving London's mandatory retirement as the Director of the HST Division, and at that time a new organizational structure and new leadership would be required. The period 1980–84 was one of increasing uncertainty and anxiety about the future of HST in general. Morale decreased, and there was a measurable negative impact on student behavior as well. In the MEMP program, there was an increase in the number of students leaving the program to pursue other options (Figure 2).

The Johnson Committee Review of HST

In June 1984 an *ad hoc* committee was appointed by Presidents Derek C. Bok and Paul E. Gray to review the HST Division. This high level committee was chaired by Howard W. Johnson, Honorary Chairman of the MIT Corporation and past president of MIT. The other eight committee members were senior faculty members of Harvard Medical School and MIT.[9] The committee was charged to make a full review of the academic and research programs of the Division, to document its strengths and weaknesses, its accomplishments, and its costs in terms of money, space and other resources. The committee was asked to assess the value of the Joint Division to each of the two universities and to advise the presidents on the future of the Division—specifically about the possibilities for selective expansion, contraction, or termination of its various programs. The committee met for two- and-one-half days in July of 1984, reviewed written documentation and letters which had been solicited from faculty and others, interviewed a number of witnesses, and prepared their report. The final written report was submitted on September 10, 1984, and its detailed findings are discussed elsewhere (Chapters 10 and 11). For HST, one of the most distressing recommendations of the Johnson Committee was that "the MEMP program as it stands be terminated, and that its purposes and goals be pursued in a different manner." The Committee suggested that "at least three and possibly five additional students be accepted into the Biomedical Sciences educational program. These students should be committed to a Ph.D. in engineering or physics, as well as to the M.D. degree." The committee was careful to insist that "the students enrolled in the current MEMP program be allowed to complete this program."

The Johnson Committee felt that the medical and clinical content of the MEMP program was so extensive that with relatively little additional effort students could earn both the Ph.D. and the M.D. degree. They felt that students entering MEMP were already ambiguous about the issue of an M.D. and that it would be wise (and more cost-effective) to develop two separate graduate programs for biomedical engineers: one a formal Ph.D./M.D. track with a total of six to eight

DROP-OUTS

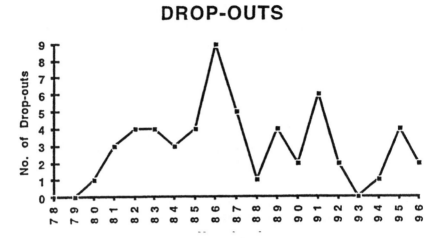

Figure 2. Number of students leaving the MEMP program without the doctoral degree, plotted by year in which they left.

specific positions reserved in the M.D. program for such individuals, and the other an interdepartmental graduate program supplemented by some hospital-based experiences organized through HST. The report continued: "The committee believes that the training of engineers and physicists to work at the interface of these disciplines with medicine is important, but believes that a refocused effort as described above would be more cost efficient and more productive of graduates with the necessary training."

Shortly after the Johnson Committee report was submitted, Provost Low resigned, and Professor John Deutch was identified as the new MIT Provost, effective July, 1985. Associate Provost Kenneth Smith remained in his post with continued responsibility for HST. Needless to say, a period of intense political activity began, together with much anxiety. What would happen to the HST Division in terms of its organizational structure and leadership? What would be the future of the MEMP program given the Johnson Committee report? MEMP students were particularly active in vociferously defending the value and uniqueness of the MEMP doctoral program. Deborah Burstein '86 and Martha Gray '86 were particularly effective in rallying support for MEMP and were definitely heard by the MIT administration. Many members of the faculty as well were distressed at the proposal to terminate the MEMP program and rose to its defense.

By late spring 1985, the administrations of MIT and Harvard Medical School had selected Drs. Richard J. Kitz (HMS) and Roger

G. Mark (MIT) to lead HST as co-directors beginning in July, 1985. Both individuals were strongly supportive of the MEMP program, and they won the agreement of the MIT provost that MEMP would be continued, but with the stipulation that a careful analysis of the program be conducted, with a view toward streamlining it. In addition, MIT institutional support for student fellowships would be cut from three-and-one-half years to three semesters.

Redesign of the MEMP Program, 1985

The new administration of HST placed high priority on addressing the issue of redesigning and stabilizing the MEMP program. A first step was to recruit a committee of faculty members and student representatives to take responsibility for the graduate programs in HST, particularly MEMP. This graduate committee was known as the Biomedical Engineering/Physical Science (BEPS) Committee. It was representative of the collaborating engineering and physics departments at MIT and Harvard.[10] It had overall responsibility for policies and procedures affecting the MEMP program including curricular changes, review of new course proposals, tracking and advising of students, approving thesis proposals and thesis committees, acting on student petitions, etc. It was chaired by the MIT Co-director of HST, Professor Mark, and reported to the HST Joint Faculty Committee.

The BEPS Committee and the HST administration wished to maintain the MEMP program's educational objectives and its priorities of solid discipline-oriented graduate education, strong medical and clinical training and research experiences at the interface of technology and medicine. However, the boundary conditions imposed by the MIT provost meant that a careful redesign of the MEMP curriculum was critical. After considerable deliberation, the BEPS Committee approved the following specific changes in the program:

1. The number of MEMP admissions per year would be limited to ten for budgetary reasons.
2. Students admitted to the program, beginning in 1986, would be guaranteed three semesters of departmental support. To optimize the judicious use of these moneys, students were permitted to consider their fellowship as "money in the bank," which could be drawn upon as needed at whatever rate was needed. Students were encouraged to find outside fellowship support and/or teaching

and/or research assistantships to supplement their HST fellowships.

3. The curriculum was modified in several important ways which were designed to decrease the length of the program while retaining its major components:

- The master's degree requirement was made optional for students in departments which did not normally require a master's degree as a prerequisite for the Ph.D. (Chemical Engineering, Nuclear Engineering, Physics, Harvard's Division of Engineering and Applied Sciences). The master's requirement was maintained for MEMP students in departments normally requiring the masters degree (Electrical Engineering and Computer Science, Mechanical Engineering).

- A change was made in the three-subject biomedical engineering core requirement to add flexibility and increase efficiency. Students, with the approval of their faculty advisor, could now select their own three subjects. These courses could also be credited toward the departmental graduate program if appropriate. The subjects did not have to be strictly "biomedical," but did have to have relevance to the student's research work. For example, if a student were working on research in biomedical applications of laser spectroscopy, subjects in optics, laser physics, or spectroscopy could be justified as fulfilling the requirement.

- A major change was made in the duration of the clinical content of the program. All students were required to take "Introduction to Clinical Medicine and Medical Engineering," which was now taught at the Mount Auburn Hospital with the additional guidance of Dr. Charles J. Hatem. That course was redesigned to be taught in a very intensive manner in a six-week period starting in January, the "Independent Activities Period" at MIT between fall and spring terms. Thus, this course would not interfere significantly with regularly scheduled subjects or with research progress. The six-week clerkship in medicine was scheduled during the summer—again to avoid significant conflict with other courses. The additional clinical experience was reduced from a full semester to a one-month, individually designed student/faculty preceptorship, combining experience in patient care and clinical research.

- In an effort to provide early exposure of all MEMP students to issues and research opportunities in medical engineering/medical physics, and to provide a common "bonding" experience for them while they were focusing most of their efforts on departmental course-work, two hospital-based tutorials were designed and led by Professor Ernest Cravalho. Students were required to complete both of these tutorials by the end of the fourth term. Tutorials met for one to two evening hours every one to two weeks for two terms total. The first tutorial presented an introduction to the scope of medical engineering/medical physics, examples of important research activites in the hospital settings, discussions of career options, biomedical ethics, etc. The second tutorial experience exposed the students to a number of real-life applications of technology in clinical settings. Students visited hospital clinical laboratories, imaging facilities, high-tech surgical procedures, intensive care areas, etc., and had opportunity to consider the impact and cost-effectiveness of the clinical technology.

- Only minor changes were made in the doctoral examination structure. All students were required to pass the doctoral qualifying examinations given by their departments as the first component of the general exam. The second component was a thesis proposal examination described below.

- The BEPS Committee tightened the procedures relating to doctoral thesis supervision. This was felt to be particularly important given the wide range of faculty supervisors and laboratories available to the students. In addition to the thesis supervisor (who could be a faculty member at either Harvard or MIT), a thesis committee of at least three faculty members was required. The chairperson of the thesis committee was to be a faculty member of the institution granting the degree. At least two committee members were to be from the student's basic engineering or physical science discipline. Representation from the medical or biological sciences was expected as well. Students were required to meet with their committees at least once per semester. A formal thesis proposal examination was established. After submitting a written thesis proposal to the committee for review, the student was required to defend it orally. The thesis committee was responsible for assuring the adequacy of the proposal and the preparation of the student. The BEPS Committee reviewed the results of thesis proposal defenses and approved the make-up of the thesis committees.

The new revision of the MEMP program was described in the HST catalog of 1985–86.[11] The new procedures and policies did shorten the length of the MEMP program by about a year, and experience showed that it was possible for the students to find adequate support, although with some increase in fiscal anxiety. The rate of application to the MEMP program steadily increased, and the Admissions Committee found that the percent of students admitted upon referral from other departments decreased. The esprit and morale of the student body improved after the HST administrative uncertainty was resolved, and the number of drop-outs decreased. The curricular changes seemed successful and remained in effect from 1985–1994.

MEMP Curriculum Review and Revision, 1994

In keeping with the HST tradition of periodically reviewing courses and programs, a comprehensive internal evaluation of the MEMP curriculum was undertaken in early 1994 by a BEPS subcommittee headed by Professor Martha Gray.[12] The charge to the committee was to review the entire curriculum and make appropriate recommendations for modifications, with particular attention to the following issues:

- Evaluate the departmental requirements and qualifying exam procedures. Should HST administer its own qualifying exam?
- What should be the correct amount of molecular biology and biochemistry in the curriculum?
- What policy should govern the specific preclinical courses required? How much flexibility should there be in the choice of these subjects?
- How effective are the clinical courses? Should there be modifications?
- Carefully assess the clinical preceptorship—is it meeting an important need? Should it be eliminated?

The committee presented its report in spring 1994 and made the following important points and recommendations:

1. Given the increasing importance of molecular biology to biomedical engineers, the Gray committee felt that all MEMP students should be required to take HST-160 "Molecular Biology and Genetics in Modern Medicine" or an equivalent. The requirements for Human Functional Anatomy and Human Pathology were retained. Three additional pathophysiology courses were required, chosen from a list of four, but with added flexibility if approved by the faculty advisor.

2. The clinical program was not changed. The one-month preceptor-ship was examined in detail, including considerable feedback from students who had taken the course in the past. The committee decided to retain that requirement, but to urge that it be met within a year of the other clinical subjects to take advantage of the students' clinical skills and to assure that its impact would be related to thesis research.

3. The requirement for a core set of three biomedical engineering subjects was dropped in recognition of the fact that the flexible interpretation of the requirement had essentially eliminated it as a separate requirement already.

4. The subcommittee recommended that department-based qualifying examinations be continued in order to guarantee thorough, discipline-based preparation of MEMP students.

The recommendations of the Gray Committee were discussed by the BEPS Committee and were accepted unanimously and with appreciation. They were implemented as of July 1, 1995. The revised MEMP program curriculum was published in the HST 1994–95 catalog.[13]

IV. Quantitative Review and Summary Statistics, 1978–199

Admissions

Over the seventeen-year period 1978 through 1995, a total of 198 students, 140 (71%) men and fifty-eight (29%) women, were admitted to the MEMP program. Admissions averaged about eleven per year (Figure 1). The number of applications per year typically was at least an order of magnitude higher than the number of students finally admitted. As might be expected, the application rate rose steadily as the program became better known throughout the country. The number of applications screened by the Admissions Committee was 166 and 146 in 1994 and 1995, respectively.

Departmental Affiliations

The MEMP students were admitted jointly by a wide variety of departments, primarily in the School of Engineering at MIT, but with significant representation of the MIT Department of Physics and the Harvard Graduate School of Arts and Sciences (HGSAS), primarily the Division of Engineering and Applied Sciences. Table 1 shows the statistics over the entire seventeen-year history of the program. The largest engineering departments at MIT, EECS and Mechanical Engineering attracted the majority of MEMP students, accounting for more than half of all MEMP students. Table 2 compares the departmental distribution of students during the initial seven years (1978–1985) to that during the last ten years (1986–1995). There was little change in the major roles of Mechanical and Electrical Engineering, but surprisingly there was a significant decrease in the percentage of MEMP students in chemical engineering. There was also a noticeable increase in the number of students in the HGSAS.

Drop-outs

The MEMP program was a demanding and highly focused one, and it is not surprising that a significant number of students dropped out before completing the doctoral degree requirements. Over the seventeen-year period (1978–1995), a total of fifty-five students dropped out—28% of all those admitted. Thirty-five were men and twenty were women. Thus, approximately 26% of the male students left without completing the degree, and 35% of the female students dropped out.

Figure 2 plots the number of students leaving the program without a doctoral degree as a function of the year in which they left. Notice the increase in drop-outs in the period of 1985–1987. This was the time of greatest administrative stress and uncertainty in the program, corresponding to the change in administrations of both MIT and HST.

Reasons for drop-out were classified as follows:

1. *Unknown*—insufficient information available to make determination.
2. *Personal Reasons*—Change in career direction, family problems, psychological problems, etc.
3. *Academic Difficulty*—Poor grades, failing qualifying exams, poor research aptitude, etc.
4. *Another Ph.D. Program*—student changed registration to another doctoral program at MIT or Harvard.
5. *Medical School*—student dropped out to enter a full-time M.D. program.

Table 3 shows the breakdown of reasons for drop-outs in the entire group of fifty-five individuals who left the program over the seven-

Table 1.   Distribution of MEMP student departmental affiliations during the period 1978–1995. The total number of students was 197.

Department	Number of Students	Percent of Total
Electrical Engineering and Computer Science	67	34.01
Mechanical Engineering	56	28.43
Chemical Engineering	23	11.68
Physics	22	11.17
Harvard Graduate School of Arts and Sciences	13	6.60
Nuclear Engineering	6	3.05
Aeronautics and Astronautics	3	1.52
Materials Science and Engineering	2	1.02
Chemistry	2	1.02
Applied Biology	1	0.51
HST	2	1.02
Total	197	100.00

Table 2.   Percent Distribution of MEMP students in the major affiliation departments during the early years (1978–1985) and the more recent period (1986–1995). N=81 students in the early period, and N=116 in the later period.

Department	Early Period%	Late Period%	Percent Change
Electrical Engineering and Computer Science	33.3	34.5	+/−
Mechanical Engineering	24.7	31	+
Chemical Engineering	19.8	6.0	− −
Physics	11.1	11.2	+/−
Harvard Graduate School of Arts and Sciences	2.5	9.5	+++
Nuclear Engineering	2.5	3.5	+

teen years reviewed. In contrast with doctoral programs in science, engineering students (including MEMPs) have a number of viable options after they earn the master's degree. Changes in career direction are not uncommon at this point. The majority of dropouts were for academic or personal reasons, and these causes are often linked. The percent of dropouts who left to go to medical school was substantial (particularly among the women) but is not surprising given the strong interest in medicine of the students attracted to the MEMP program.

Table 3.   Reasons for Student Drop Out over the Period 1978–1995

Reason	ALL (N=55)	Percent	Men (N=35)	Percent	Women (N=20)	Percent
Personal Reasons	15	27	10	29	5	25
Academic Difficulty	13	24	10	29	3	15
Went to MD Program	13	24	5	14	8	40
Different PhD Program	7	13	5	14	2	10
Unknown	7	13	5	14	2	10

The overall drop-out rate of almost 30% is quite high compared to departments in the MIT School of Science but is more comparable to the experience in the School of Engineering. It is also clear that the drop-out rate has decreased somewhat in more recent years, perhaps reflecting more careful sifting of applicants by the Admissions Committee. The decrease in attrition rate may also reflect the streamlining of the curriculum, better faculty support of the students and the recognized commitment of both MIT and Harvard to the program.

Graduates

The first MEMP doctoral degree was awarded in June 1981 to an individual after only three years in the program. However, he had entered with advanced standing, having already completed the S.M. degree in electrical engineering. The first of his classmates and others began to finish two years later in 1983. The number of MEMP graduates per year is shown graphically in Figure 3. Of interest is that the number of graduating students averaged four to five per year until 1991, after which the numbers began to rise significantly. In 1996 there was an all-time high of fourteen students who completed the program.

Duration of the Program in Years

The MEMP program was designed to require five to six years of graduate work. The time actually taken by the eighty-three graduates ranged from one to eleven-and-a-third years! The distribution of program durations is shown in Figure 4. The mean duration was 5.95 ± 1.8 years. Those students whose formal registration lasted only one

MEMP Graduates

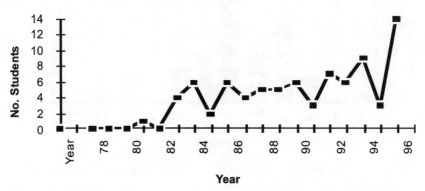

Figure 3.   MEMP graduates per year as a function of the year graduating. (N=83)

DURATION OF DOCTORAL PROGRAMS 1978-1995
(N=83)

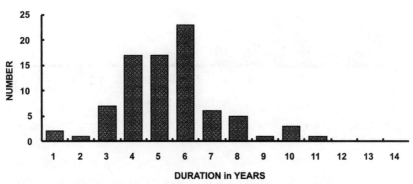

Figure 4.   The distribution of durations of MEMP doctoral programs over the period 1978–1995. Mean = 5.95 years, with standard deviation of 1.8 years. (N=83)

to three years came into the program with considerable advanced standing. At the other extreme, of the seven students whose programs lasted more than eight-and-a-half years, five (71%) were enrolled for both the Ph.D. and M.D. degrees.

There was a discernable shortening of the MEMP programs after the streamlining of the curriculum introduced for the class entering 1986. Figure 5a shows the distribution of program durations for the forty-eight students in the earlier classes (1978–1985). The mean duration was 6.3±1.95. Figure 5b shows the distribution of program

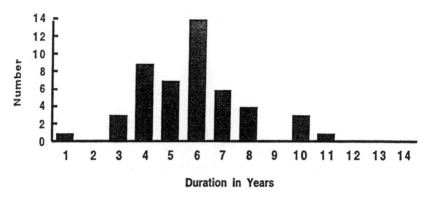

Figure 5a. Doctoral Program durations for MEMP graduates who entered the program between 1978–1985 (N=48)

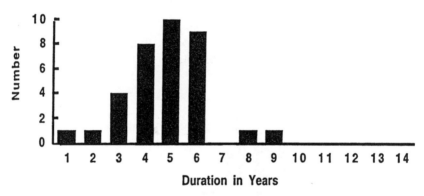

Figure 5b. Program durations for MEMP graduates who entered the program between 1986 and 1995. (N=35)

durations for the thirty-five students entering later (1986–1995). The mean duration for this period was 5.47±1.54 years.

Doctoral Research

MEMP students pursued graduate research in laboratories at MIT, Harvard, and the teaching hospitals. Their work ranged from basic to applied projects, and the subject matter ranged from highly biological to physical science and technology. A list of thesis topics and faculty supervisors of all eighty-three graduates is contained in Appendix E2.

Table 4 documents the primary sites of the doctoral research and demonstrates that, while more than half of the projects were sited in MIT laboratories, under the direction of MIT biomedical engineering

Table 4.   Primary Sites of the Thesis Research of MEMP Graduates (1978–1995)

Site	No. Student Theses
MIT	44 (53%)
Harvard College	2 (2%)
Massachusetts General Hospital	11 (13%)
Beth Israel Hospital	8 (10%)
Brigham and Women's Hospital	4 (5%)
Massachusetts Eye and Ear Infirmary	1 (1%)
Harvard Medical School	2 (2%)
Collaborative Projects with Two Sites	
MIT/Massachusetts General Hospital	2 (2%)
MIT/Brigham and Women's Hospital	3 (4%)
MIT/Beth Israel Hospital	2 (2%)
MIT/Other	1 (1%)
MIT/Harvard Medical School	1 (1%)
Harvard Graduate School of Applied Sciences/Beth Israel Hospital	2 (2%)
Total	83

Table 5.   Categories of Doctoral Research of MEMP Students

Category of Project	Number
Biomedical Imaging and NMR Spectroscopy	13
Orthopedic Biomechanics	12
Diagnostic Techniques/Instrumentation	10
Quantitative Cellular/Tissue Physiology	9
Quantitative Systems/Organ-Level Physiology	9
Therapeutic Systems, Methods, Instrumentation	9
Cellular and Molecular Biophysics	6
Quantitative Neurobiology	6
Biomedical Fluid Mechanics	5
Artificial Cell-Based Tissue/Organs	3
Total	82

and physics faculty, the remaining 47% were sited primarily in hospital-based laboratories.

The projects have been enormously varied, and are difficult to characterize. However, a crude summary of broad categories of work is shown in Table 5.

V. Summary

The MEMP doctoral program was designed to produce well-trained physical scientists and engineers with in-depth knowledge of the medical sciences and first-hand experience of the world of clinical medicine. This unique opportunity has been made possible by combining the teaching, research, and administrative resources of both MIT and Harvard under the auspices of the Harvard-MIT Division of Health Sciences and Technology. The initial design and organization of the program was complex and difficult, primarily in obtaining the necessary faculty agreement and support. The gestation period was eight years long and the "birth" might never have materialized without the vigorous advocacy and support of the top administrations of both MIT and Harvard Medical School. The program was launched in 1978, and it was particularly rigorous and demanding in both physical science/engineering and in medicine. The academic requirements were streamlined somewhat in 1985, but there was no compromise in the high academic expectations. The program has continued to be modified by the faculty in response to changing research needs and opportunities. Its emphasis on basic biology has grown in recent years, and some course requirements have been liberalized to allow students more flexibility. However, its major focus on preparing students to address research problems relating to clinical medicine has not changed. Faculty are currently considering new educational tracks at the interface of engineering and the biological sciences; these would be in addition to, not a replacement of, the MEMP program.

MEMP involves engineering and medical faculty of the Harvard Medical School in addition to faculty from virtually all of MIT's engineering departments and the Harvard Division of Engineering and Applied Sciences. MEMP student thesis research, done on the university campuses or in the teaching hospitals, has ranged from fundamental science to applied engineering and has covered subjects from biology to clinical medicine.

Over the seventeen-year history of the program reviewed here, a total of 197 students have been admitted. Eighty-three (41%) of these have received the doctoral degree; fifty-five (28%) left the program for a variety of reasons without completing it; and the remaining fifty-nine (30%) students are still enrolled. The average length of the doctoral program has been approximately six years, which compares favorably with other engineering doctoral programs.

Evaluation of the MEMP program has been done in a series of external reviews by HST's Visiting Committee (the HST Advisory Committee), and by analysis of the careers of MEMP graduates. This subject is covered in Chapter 11.

Notes

1. The HST Administrative Committee included: Provost Walter Rosenblith (MIT), Dr. Eleanor Shore (representing President Bok of Harvard), Mr. Henry Meadow (Dean's office, HMS), Dr. Robert Blacklow (HMS), Dr. Irving London (HST), Prof. Ernest Cravalho (HST), Dr. H. Frederick Bowman (HST), and Dr. Irving Berstein (HST).
2. Members of the Task Force for Medical Engineering: Laurence Young, Sc.D. (MIT: Aeronautics and Astronautics); S. James Adelstein, M.D. (HMS: Radiology); William Berenberg, M.D. (HMS: Pediatrics); John F. Burke, M.D. (HMS: Surgery); Franklin H. Epstein, M.D. (HMS: Medicine); Samuel Helman, M.D. (HMS: Medicine); Alain Rossier, M.D., Ph.D. (HMS: Medicine); Clement Sledge, M.D. (HMS: Orthopedics); and Wilbur B. Davenport, Sc.D. (MIT: Electrical Eng.).
3. Members of the Curriculum Subcommittee: Laurence Young, Sc.D. (MIT: Aeronautics and Astronautics); Gordon Brownell, Ph.D. (MIT: Nuclear Engineering); Clark Colton, Ph.D. (MIT: Chemical Engineering); Ernest Cravalho, Ph.D. (MIT: Mechanical Engineering); J. David Litster, Ph.D. (MIT: Physics); Irving London, M.D. (MIT/HMS: HST); Roger Mark, M.D., Ph.D. (MIT: Electrical Engineering); Charles Oman, Ph.D. (MIT: Aeronautics and Astronautics); Robert Rose, Ph.D. (MIT: Materials Science and Engineering).
4. Members of the Subcommittee on Clerkships: Dr. Richard Kitz (MGH: Anesthesiology), Professor Gordon Brownell (MIT: Nuclear Engineering), Dr. John Burke (MGH: Surgery), Professor Ernest Cravalho (MIT: Mechanical Engineering), Dr. Robert Leffert (MGH: Orthopedics), Professor Irving London (MIT/HMS: HST), Dr. Dwight Robinson (MGH: Medicine), and Professor Laurence Young (MIT: Aeronautics and Astronautics).
5. The original curriculum design called for all MEMP students to qualify for a master's degree in their departments (with thesis if required).
6. MIT doctoral candidates in engineering normally may choose either the "Doctor of Science" (Sc.D.) or the "Doctor of Philosophy" (Ph.D.) degree. There is no difference in requirements for the two degrees.
7. This policy was designed to provide approximate equity in the flow of funds between the two universities. All tuition income would accrue to MIT, but MIT would be responsible for student financial support and program administration. In addition, HST made a long-term financial commitment to the

support of some faculty effort at Harvard for developing biomedical engineering subjects.

8. Description of the Medical Engineering and Medical Physics curriculum, as it appeared in the 1979–80 catalog of the Harvard-MIT Division of Health Sciences and Technology (page 8):

This curriculum is a five-year program leading to the Ph.D. or Sc.D. Degree awarded by Harvard University or MIT. The objective of this program is the education of individuals who will be well qualified as engineers and/or physicists and will have an extensive knowledge in the medical sciences so that they may engage in investigation of important problems in human biology and clinical medicine.

During the first two years of the program, students are registered in both an engineering or physics department and the Division of Health Sciences and Technology. By the end of the second year, students should have completed both the departmental requirements for the S.M. degree, including a thesis, and the medical science and medical engineering subject requirements of the doctoral program. In order to continue in this program beyond the second year, students must pass a qualifying examination comprised of three parts: one part set by the department awarding the S.M. degree to test competency in engineering or physics; one part set by the Harvard-MIT Division to test competency in the medical science and medical engineering requirements; and one part designed to evaluate research ability through presentation and defense of the S.M. thesis.

Students judged qualified will enter the third year, the clinical year, and be registered only in the Harvard-MIT Division. In this clinical year students will be involved in four clinical experiences, one in medicine required for all students, the other three to be selected by the student. The purpose of the clinical work is to develop an understanding of the practical constraints as well as the opportunities for applying science and technology to health needs. Students will participate in both patient care activities and clinical research activities under the supervision of engineer/physicist-physician teams. At the end of the third year, students will begin doctoral research under the supervision of faculty from HST and the appropriate engineering or physics department. This research, usually identified during one of the clinical experiences, would normally be completed and defended before the Harvard-MIT Division and department faculty by the end of the fifth year.

Students in this program can earn the degree through either MIT or Harvard. To be considered for admission, students must have completed a baccalaureate degree in engineering or physical science. Recommended preparation includes at least one undergraduate subject in each of the following areas: biology, organic chemistry, physical chemistry, and advanced calculus. Also required are the GRE Aptitude test and one Advanced test.

Students who apply to the Program through MIT must also apply as regular graduate students in an S.M. degree program in one of the engineering departments or in physics (normally the department most closely related to the field of the undergraduate major).

9. Members of the Johnson Committee included: Howard W. Johnson, Honorary Chairman of the MIT Corporation (Chairman); Dr. S. James Adelstein,

Dean for Academic Programs HMS (ex officio); Dr. Harold Amos, Prof. Microbiology & Molecular Genetics, Chairman of the Division of Medical Sciences, HMS; Dr. W. Gerald Austen; Dr. H. Franklin Bunn; Dr. Herman Eisen; Prof. Morton Fleming; Prof. Jerome Friedman; Prof. Kenneth Smith (ex officio).

10. Departments represented on the BEPS Committee, 1985: Applied Biological Sciences (MIT); Aeronautical/Astronautical Engineering (MIT); Chemical Engineering (MIT); Electrical Engineering/Computer Science (MIT); HST; Mechanical Engineering (MIT); Nuclear Engineering (MIT); Physics (MIT); and Division of Engineering and Applied Sciences (Harvard).

11. The revised MEMP Program as described in the HST catalog 1985–86 (page 21): This curriculum is a nominal five-and-a-half year program leading to the Ph.D. or Sc.D. degree in Medical Engineering or in Medical Physics awarded by MIT or the Ph.D. degree awarded by the Harvard Faculty of Arts and Sciences. The objective of this program is the education of individuals who will be well qualified as engineers or physicists with extensive knowledge in the medical sciences so that they may engage in investigation of important problems in human biology and clinical medicine.

To be considered for admission, students must have completed at least a baccalaureate degree in engineering or physical science. Recommended preparation includes at least one undergraduate subject in each of the following areas: biology, organic chemistry, physical chemistry, biochemisty, and advanced calculus. The GRE Aptitude Test and one Advanced Test are also required. Admission to the Program is highly competitive. A maximum of ten students is admitted each year. Students can be admitted only for the fall semester; there are no admissions in midyear.

Throughout the program the students are registered either at MIT or in the Harvard Graduate School of Arts and Sciences. Students registered at MIT who enter the program with the bachelor's degree spend the first five semesters completing the departmental requirements for the S.M. degree, including a thesis, and the medical science and medical engineering subject requirements of the doctoral program. During this time, these students are registered in both an engineering or physics department and the Division of Health Sciences and Technology. Students who enter the Program with the master's degree must, as a minimum, complete the medical science and medical engineering subject requirements during the initial phase of the program. During this time, these students are registered only in the Division of Health Sciences and Technology.

The students registered in the Harvard Graduate School of Arts and Sciences should satisfy the medical science and medical engineering subject requirements and the departmental requirements for the Ph.D. except for those relating directly to the Ph.D. dissertation itself.In order to continue in this program beyond the initial phase, all students must pass qualifying examinations set by the academic department and the Harvard-MIT Division to test competency in engineering or physics, the medical sciences, medical engineering, and research.

Students who qualify are then engaged in three clinical experiences: two required of all students (introduction to clinical medicine and internal medicine), and one individually arranged by the students in consultation with faculty advisors. The purpose of the clinical work is to develop an understanding of the practical constraints of clinical investigation and to provide opportunities for applying science and technology to health needs. During these experiences, students participate in both patient care activities and clinical research activities under the supervision of engineer/physicist-physician teams.

After the clinical experiences, students begin doctoral research under the supervision of faculty from the Harvard-MIT Division and the academic department. This research should focus on a fundamental problem of clinical relevance and should normally be completed and defended before the faculty by the end of the eleventh semester.

12. The MEMP Curriculum Review Committee included the following members:

Dr. Joseph Bonventre, HMS
Dr. H. Frederic Bowman (Recorder)
Professor Ernest Cravalho, ME/HST
Profeessor Martha Gray (Chair) EECS/HST
Professor Wilson Hayes, HMS
Professor Roger Kamm, ME
Professor Robert Langer, ChE
Professor Roger Mark, EECS/HST (Ex-officio)
Professor Thomas McMahon, HFAS
Ms. Tobi Nagel, MEMP Student
Dr. Bruce Rosen, HMS
Professor Michael Rosenblatt, HMS/HST
Dr. Frederick Schoen, HMS
Dr. Mary Rose Sullivan, WRVAH

13. The revised MEMP curriculum as described in the HST 1994–95 catalog (page 19): The "MEMP" curriculum is a five to six year program leading to the Ph.D. or Sc.D. in Medical Engineering or Medical Physics awarded by MIT, or the Ph.D. degree awarded by the Harvard Faculty of Arts and Sciences. The objective of this program is to educate individuals who will be well-qualified as engineers or physicists, and who will have extensive knowledge of the medical sciences such that they may engage in productive, independent investigation of important problems at the interface of technology and clinical medicine. The program provides a thorough graduate experience in a classical discipline of engineering or physics, and also requires considerable study in the basic medical sciences. In addition, students are afforded a unique opportunity to learn important clinical skills and to acquire an in-depth understanding of the process of clinical care and medical decision-making and of the role of technology in patient care.

Throughout the program students are registered either at MIT or in the Harvard Graduates School of Arts and Sciences. During the initial phase of the program, students are registered in both a graduate department and in HST and concentrate on developing strength in their basic engineering or physical science disciplines. Students also take subjects in human anatomy, pathology, and pathophysiology together with the medical students. In order to continue to the second phase of the program, MEMP students must satisfactorily pass the doctoral qualifying examination administered by their graduate department. This examination tests competency in engineering or physics and also reviews the student's progress in independent research.

After passing the qualifying examination, students are eligible to participate in the clinical courses. These include HST 201, a six-week, full-time course in Introduction to Clinical Medicine (history-taking and physical examinations); and HST 202, a six-week rotation in medicine at Mt. Auburn Hospital where students participate in longitudinal patient care.

Later, usually in association with doctoral research, students engage in an individually arranged, interdisciplinary preceptorship during which time they study, in depth, a particular biomedical technology and its application to patient care or clinical research. The preceptorship is generally based in a teaching hospital and is supervised by both a clinical and a technical preceptor. The clinical experiences provide the student with an intimate understanding of the world of medicine and of the practical constraints and the opportunities for applying science and technology to health needs.

Doctoral thesis research is conducted under the direction of faculty members from MIT or Harvard and should focus on a fundamental problem of medical relevance. The thesis, when completed, is publicly defended before HST and departmental faculty.

Degree Requirements

The MEMP program requires the successful completion of the following general requirements:

A. An approved graduate program in the student's basic engineering/physics discipline. This consists of at least 42 units of graduate "H" courses approved by the departmental faculty counselor. This requirement may be waived at the discretion of the departmental faculty counselor for students entering with a master's degree in the departmental discipline.

B. Regular participation in the Biomedical Engineering Seminar (HST 590) and completion of the hospital based Tutorials in Medical Engineering and Medical Physics (HST 595, 596) are required during the first two years of registration.

C. Successful completion of the doctoral qualifying examination administered by the student's disciplinary department.

D. Completion of a master's thesis for students in departments which normally require a master's degree as a prerequisite for doctoral study.

E. Completion of a two-part preclinical requirement. Part one, a basic requirement, includes:

Anatomy (HST 010 or HST 510)
Pathology (HST 030)
Molecular Biology (HST 160 or other)

Part two, a pathophysiology requirement, includes three courses from the following list:

    Cardiovascular Pathophysiology (HST 090)
    Respiratory Pathophysiology (HST 100)
    Renal Pathophysiology (HST 110)
    Introduction to Neuroscience (HST 130)
    (Substitutions may be permitted with the approval of the MEMP faculty advisor.)

F. Completion of a structured clinical training program in the teaching hospitals, which provides students with a unique opportunity to participate in patient care and to understand, firsthand, the issues involved in medical decision-making and the potential and limitations of technology. Required courses include HST 201, 202 and 203. HST 203 should be completed within one year following HST 202.

G. Independent doctoral thesis research guided by the following policies:

    1. The research supervisor must be a faculty member at MIT or Harvard. (In exceptional cases the Biomedical Engineering/Physical Science (BEPS) committee may approve a senior research staff member as a thesis supervisor.

    2. A thesis committee, approved by the BEPS Committee, must be identified to oversee and evaluate the research. The thesis committee must consist of three or more MIT or Harvard faculty members, at least two of whom must represent the student's basic engineering or physics discipline. It is strongly recommended that the committee also include representation from the relevant biological or clinical sciences. The chair of the thesis committee must be a faculty member of the institution granting the student's degree: either MIT or Harvard Faculty of Arts and Sciences. The committee chairperson is responsible for conducting the thesis proposal defense and for convening committee meetings to periodically review research progress.

    3. A formal thesis proposal must be presented and defended by the student to the thesis committee. After approval by the thesis committee, the proposal is forwarded, together with signed thesis supervision and reader agreements, to the BEPS Committee for final approval.

    4. It is expected that the student will meet periodically (at least once each semester) with the thesis committee to review and discuss research progress.

    5. The thesis must be successfully defended in public before the thesis committee. The written document must be approved by the thesis committee, signed by the research supervisor, and accepted by the Division.

Ph.D.-M.D. Options

Students who desire to pursue studies in the medical sciences leading to the M.D. degree together with studies in medical engineering or medical physics should apply to the two programs simultaneously. Note that the deadline for application to the medical sciences program precedes the deadline for application to the MEMP program by a substantial time period.

During the course of their studies in medical engineering or medical physics, some students develop an interest in pursuing the M.D. degree. Students in the first year MEMP class may apply for admission to Harvard Medical School in competition with other incoming students (application deadline is October 15). A second option is available to MEMP students who decide on Ph.D.-M.D. studies. When their doctoral program is nearing completion, these students may apply for a limited number of transfer positions at Harvard Medical School. (Some other medical schools have also indicated an interest in HST/MEMP transfer students. Completing the M.D. degree normally requires two years of additional study after completion of the doctoral degree in MEMP.

Chapter 10

EVALUATION OF THE M.D. PROGRAM

Walter H. Abelmann, M.D.

There are two general categories of evaluation: process evaluation and outcome evaluation. At the inception of the HST Program, it was considered important to build ongoing evaluation into the program. This chapter will summarize these efforts and their results.

PROCESS REVIEWS
Students' Evaluation of Individual Courses

In the preclinical M.D. curriculum, which also forms part of the MEMP curriculum, a course evaluation form is distributed to students at the end of each course. The returns are processed by a student committee at HMS, and the tabulated results are made available to the course faculties; summaries are also made available to students for future guidance.

Faculty Evaluation of Individual Courses and of The Curriculum

As described in Chapter 8, the curriculum committee appoints subcommittees to evaluate individual courses at regular intervals. Student evaluations (see above) are made available to these committees. The subcommittees report to the main curriculum committee which makes copies of these reports as well as their recommendations; these are made available to the respective course heads. The curriculum committee itself reviews overall aspects of the curriculum in an ongoing manner, at its meetings as well as at annual retreats, in which other members of the faculty participate. Students participate at all levels of these reviews.

The Johnson Committee

In June 1984, an *ad hoc* committee was appointed by Presidents Derek C. Bok and Paul E. Gray to review the Harvard- MIT Division of Health Sciences and Technology. This committee was chaired by Howard W. Johnson, honorary chairman of the MIT Corporation. The Presidents of the two universities charged the committee with making a full review of the three principal components of the Division: the Biomedical Sciences Educational Program; the Medical Engineering and Medical Physics Educational Program; and the Research Program. This review involved faculty from both institutions and engaged the two universities and the Harvard teaching hospitals. The committee was asked for advice on the future of the Division, specifically about possibilities for selective expansion, contraction or termination of each of the three programs.

The committee met at Endicott House for two-and-one-half days, from July 17–19, 1984. It reviewed a two-volume report of the HST Division prepared by the Director of the Division and his associates.[1] The committee also heard the testimony of several individuals who had been closely associated with the program as it developed. Dr. Howard Johnson also had written letters to many individuals who had an association with the program, requesting their opinions; their responses were made available to the committee during the meeting.

The review committee agreed unanimously that the record for the Biomedical Sciences Education Program (BSEP) is uniquely first rate, that it has proven itself, and that it should be continued.[2] They also agreed unanimously that one of the Division's greatest strengths and values lies in the quality of the students it attracts. The review committee endorsed the concept of the Harvard-MIT collaboration in the education of physicians with strong backgrounds in the quantitative and life sciences and found it fundamentally sound and even more important than ever because of the need for more physician-scientists. It was recognized that the integration of the physical and engineering sciences and the biological sciences into a single curriculum is difficult and generates tension, especially for extremely bright and demanding students. To realize the full potential of this program, the committee recommended that primary appointments in the HST Division be made of faculty members whose principal commitment is to the educational and research activities of the HST Division. Such appointments would require additional endowment. The committee also proposed more uniform requirements for a higher level of skill in the physical sciences, mathematics and engineering by students matriculating in the program. The further suggestion was made that the size of the student body be expanded by three to five students per year; i.e., to twenty-eight or thirty.

With regard to the Medical Engineering and Medical Physics (MEMP) Program, the review committee proposed that this program be terminated and that its goals and purposes be pursued in a different manner. They suggested that three to five additional students be accepted into the Biomedical Sciences Educational Program and that these students should be committed to a Ph.D. degree in Engineering or Physics as well as to the M.D. degree (see Chapter 11).

The review committee found that the HST Research Program plays a fundamental role in fostering collaboration between faculty members in the two universities and that this collaboration in research leads to greater interest in the educational program of the HST Division. The committee recommended that the research program be enhanced by the appointment of a research advisory council with membership selected broadly from the faculties of the two universities, that there should be special emphasis on fostering greater collaboration between the engineering faculty at MIT and the clinical faculty at Harvard, that a regular series of Harvard and MIT research seminars be held to provide further interaction for scientists in the two institutions, and that additional funding should be provided to underwrite new ventures and support new efforts.

Finally, the review committee noted that there is a special character about the HST Program that especially commends it to the two universities. "It remains the principal formal collaboration between Harvard and MIT and it represents a model for inter-university collaboration." The recommendations of the Johnson Committee, in general, were accepted by the Division. There was, however, serious objection on the part of the faculty and especially on the part of the students to the recommendation that the MEMP Program be terminated and melded with the M.D. program. Thus, this recommendation was not accepted (see also Chapter 11).

The Advisory Committee

In 1987, an Advisory Committee was established by the two universities. This Committee comprises twelve to sixteen members, drawn from faculties throughout the United States, and includes at least one alumnus. At intervals of two years, this Committee has met and visited the program, usually for two days. It acts as a visiting committee and reports to the director(s) of the program as well as to the Provost of MIT and the Dean of the Harvard Medical School. Special consideration, in turn, has been given to the admissions process, the M.D. and Ph.D. curricula, the research pursued by students, faculty appointments, and the structure and administration of the program. The Advisory Committee also reviewed the results of the 1990 follow-up study (see below). This Committee, then, may be considered as having used both process and outcome evaluation.

As is customary with regard to Visiting Committees, the preparations for the visit, comprising the progress report to the Committee, the agenda for the meeting, and the decision as to which aspects of the program are to be focused upon, constitute important exercises for the leadership to define and assess broad as well as specific aspects of the program, and to define present and future goals. Site visits have included presentations by HST faculty and administration, meetings in small groups with faculty and students, and executive sessions and feedback to the administration. The general format was proposed by the HST directors around specific questions posed and finalized by the chairperson of the visiting committee, after consultation with the members of the committee.

After its first visit in 1988, the Advisory Committee described the program as strong, successful and well-managed.[3] It recommended greater representation of molecular biology in the curriculum. It opined that opportunities in biomedical imaging, speech and hearing science, as well as clinical neurosciences, had not been fully exploited. The committee recommended evaluation of graduates of the program. It also urged that the balance of resources between the small primary and the large part-time faculty be reconsidered.

In 1990, the Advisory Committee judged student research to be of excellent quality. With regard to admissions to the program, the committee recommended broader institutional representation.[4] It also recommended that students be informed early of curricular as well as research options. Another recommendation addressed the need to re-inforce the physician-scientist concept as an objective of the program. This recommendation arose out of several M.D./Ph.D. candidates' decisions not to complete the M.D. portion of the curriculum after a successful research experience. Also, more students should be encour-aged to follow the five-year option or the M.S./M.D. option. The committee also recommended the solicitation of additional endow-ment to secure the stability of the program. An increase in the pri-mary faculty was recommended to contribute to the oversight and management of the program and to serve as role models for interdis-ciplinary research. The committee again suggested greater participa-tion of molecular biologists in the program, as well as more rapid expansion of the imaging program. With regard to the ongoing follow-up survey of HST graduates, it was recommended that the survey be repeated every five to ten years.

After its 1992 visit, the committee again reported that "the HST programs are strong, of high quality, and continue to attract excep-tionally well-qualified students." The committee approved, in gen-eral, the structure, function and governance of the Division, but ex-pressed several major concerns:

> Programs are implemented through a series of faculty committees. The Programs are implemented by a large cadre of HMS and MIT fac-ulty drawn from various departments. The faculty are motivated by a dedication to the HST mission and by the excellence of the students. These faculty contribute generously to the program despite a personal cost in time and effort and some risk to career advancement, since at that time all faculty had primary academic responsibilities to their par-ent departments at HMS or MIT. Our initial surprise was that a pro-gram as complex as this could be implemented primarily through beneficence.[5]

The committee was concerned that "the organizational arrange-ments, metastable at best, are now becoming unstable." This view was based, in part, upon concerns for the core faculty, who, although "all continue to have a deep commitment to the program," felt that they had no role in program planning and policy decision making, or in recruitment of new core faculty. There was also concern about lack of career guidance and mentoring through the Division. Core faculty also lacked contiguity of research space.

The committee looked with favor upon new educational programs in biological engineering/biological physics, in radiological sciences, and in speech and hearing sciences, as well as the proposed M.D./ M.S. program. They pointed out, however, that "these ventures will truly require the development of new physical resources and additional human resources," lest the current system of organization and governance be destabilized further. The committee recommended "a fresh, forward-looking vision of future HST activities and a careful reassessment of the administrative process that will enable HST to achieve its objectives." To this end, the committee's recommendations included updating the mission statement of the Division, empowerment of the core faculty to achieve an effective balance with the affiliated faculty, more attention to issues of contiguous research space and provision of "a valid academic career path for core faculty."

After its 1994 visit, the Advisory Committee stated that "the educational component of the program [is] outstanding . . . should be encouraged to continue the innovative spirit that led to the formation and evolution of the program."[6] The committee, however, expressed concern regarding the divisional status of HST and its dual relation with Harvard and MIT. It strongly favored that the focus of the HST program should be the combination of "a premier educational program and an outstanding interdisciplinary research program." It recommended that the core faculty be expanded and that its functional status be clearly defined. It suggested that the core faculty be built around well-defined research themes, such as modern imaging, and that contiguous space be provided for the core faculty.

The committee also considered it important to develop courses "that reflect ongoing changes in biomedicine (e.g., courses in outcome research and neurobehavioral sciences), as well as to apply innovative technological approaches to the HST teaching process." Greater participation of the MIT faculty in the HST teaching program was also suggested. With regard to the MEMP program, it was recommended that it consider expansion to more than twelve to fourteen new students per year. As to M.D. students, the committee took note of students' feelings that they were not integrated well enough in the Harvard Medical School. The committee also recommended that in the curriculum more emphasis be placed upon methods of outcome research; epidemiology and biostatistics; medico-legal, and ethical studies; and modern management philosophies.

OUTCOME EVALUATION

Students' Accomplishments

Most preclinical courses base evaluation of students upon written examinations, problem sets, and performance in sections and/or tutorial sessions. Although all preclinical courses are officially Pass/Fail, confidential records of students' performance are kept by individual course heads and the curriculum office. Narrative evaluations are available to individual students. These may include classification into excellent, satisfactory, marginal and unsatisfactory. The last two categories are rarely used. With the exception of Pass/Fail, these data are not available to the registrars and are mainly used as feedback to students, but become most valuable sources for descriptive aspects of the Dean's letter, which is prepared in the students' last year to support applications for residency training.

Students' research accomplishments are reflected in the annual Forum, at which students report on their research, either by presentation or in poster sessions. Similarly, HST students participate in the annual Soma Weiss Student Research Assembly at the Harvard Medical School. Most students author or co-author several publications based upon their research. HST M.D. students have consistently earned a larger number of M.D. degrees with honors, as well as prizes, than would be predicted on the basis of their proportion of the entire HMS class.

The houseofficerships secured by graduating students may also be considered a form of outcome evaluation. Consistently, the great majority of graduating students have been accepted by their first or second choice of hospitals, almost always leading teaching hospitals in the United States. A perusal of the membership directory of the American Society for Clinical Investigation, a most prestigious society of physician- scientists, reveals that, notwithstanding the relative youth of HST, nineteen alumni/ae have been elected to membership so far.

Failure to Complete M.D. Program

Another dimension of evaluation is the number of students who failed to complete the course of study and thus did not receive the M.D. degree. Of the 561 students admitted to the M.D. program in the years 1971 through 1991, only fifteen, or 2.7%, did not complete the program. They comprised three students who died, six students who completed the Ph.D. degree here and took up careers in basic sciences, one student who held a Ph.D. on entry, three students who did not complete their studies for medical or personal reasons, and two students who were asked to leave.

Follow-up Studies

Follow-up surveys of graduates from the Harvard-MIT Program in Health Sciences and Technology were initiated in 1990, when, after field testing, a questionnaire was sent out to the 234 graduates of the Classes of 1975 to 1985, with a 90% return. The four-page questionnaire comprised demographic information, academic appointments and responsibilities, involvement in research and teaching, and evaluative comments on the HST experience. The results of this first survey have been published.[7]

In 1995, a second follow-up study was completed.[8] A slightly revised form of the original questionnaire was sent to the fifty-nine graduates of the classes 1986 through 1988, and a one-page supplemental form went out to the graduates who had received the earlier full questionnaire. This section will review the results of the combined, updated follow-up of 293 living graduates of the classes 1975 through 1988. (Three alumni had died.)

The overall return of questionnaires was 92%. There were twenty-three non-responders. Some demographic information was available on twelve additional graduates of these classes, whereas eleven individuals were lost to follow-up.

Of all respondents, 230 (82%) were men. One hundred ninety-eight (70.2%) graduated with only the M.D. degree. Eighty-four (29.8%) graduated with M.D. and Ph.D. degrees; however, fifteen of these had obtained their Ph.D. prior to entering Medical School.

The sixty-nine alumni/ae who completed their M.D./Ph.D.s in the HST program took an average of 6.9 years to do so. The 199 M.D. graduates spent an average of 4.3 years in residence. Thirty (15.1%) took more than four years.

Table 1 presents the reported careers. More than a third of these (40%) were in internal medicine or one of its subspecialties; 13% selected surgery or one of its subspecialties. The remaining career choices comprised a wide spectrum of clinical and basic science disciplines. As indicated in the table, a number of students had entered careers outside, but usually related to, medicine. At the time of the survey, six graduates were still serving a residency and seventeen were in

Table 1. Career Choices*

No.	%	Field
59	21.9	Internal medicine subspeciality
48	18.4	Internal medicine
22	8.2	Surgery subspeciality
14	5.2	Surgery
13	4.8	Anesthesiology
12	4.5	Neurology
12	4.5	Radiology
12	4.5	Ophthalmology
8	3.0	Pediatrics
8	3.0	Pediatric subspecialty
6	2.2	Psychiatry
6	2.2	Pathology
6	2.2	Genetics/molecular biology
5	1.9	Emergency medicine
5	1.9	Family medicine
4	1.5	OB/GYN
4	1.5	Pharmacology
4	1.5	Cellular biology
4	1.5	Corporate executive
2	0.7	EENT
2	0.7	Dermatology
2	0.7	Biochemistry
2	0.7	Bioengineering
1	0.4	Immunology
1	0.4	Biology
1	0.4	Microbiology
1	0.4	Chemical and nuclear engineering
1	0.4	Molecular biophysics
1	0.4	Anthropology
1	0.4	Public policy analyst
1	0.4	Lawyer
1	0.4	Pastor

*A significant number of respondents whose primary career lies in basic science also have part-time clinical appointments.

fellowships. One hundred seventy-nine (66%) of the respondents described their primary preferred role as academic medicine; i.e., members of a medical school faculty with responsibilities for teaching and research, at times in combination with administration.

Table 2 presents the faculty ranks. Two hundred and ten (71.4%) held faculty positions, eighty at the level of professor or associate professor. They held appointments at sixty-four different medical

Table 2.   212 (75%) of Respondents (N=282) Reported Faculty
Positions in 64 Medical Schools (includes NIH)

Position	MD	(N=141)	MD/PhD	(N=71)	Total	(N=212)
	N	(%)	N	(%)	N	(%)
Professor	10	(7.1)	13	(18.3)	23	(10.8)
Associate Professor	30	(21.3)	14	(19.7)	44	(20.8)
Assistant Professor	44	(31.2)	29	(40.8)	73	(34.4)
Instructor	24	(17.0)	9	(12.7)	33	(15.6)
Clinical Professor	0	(0)	2	(2.9)	2	(0.9)
Clinical Associate Professor	9	(6.4)	2	(2.9)	11	(5.2)
Clinical Assistant Professor	14	(9.9)	1	(1.4)	15	(7.1)
Clinical Instructor	10	(7.1)	1	(1.4)	11	(5.2)
Totals	141	(100)	71	(100.1)	212	(100)

schools. Fifty-eight were on the faculty at either Harvard or MIT. Fifty (19%) reported being primarily in medical practice, with twenty-eight in private practice settings. Seven graduates described careers outside medicine or medical sciences, as listed in Table 1.

Two hundred or (73.5%) of the respondents reported being active in research (N = 272); they spent an average of 47% of their time on this activity; 104, or 38%, spent more than 50% of their time on research (Table 3). Forty-two percent of those engaged in research were M.D./Ph.D. graduates; they reported spending 55% of their time on research, as compared to 42% for their M.D. colleagues. Fifty (60%) of M.D./Ph.D. graduates reported spending more than 50% of their time doing research; the corresponding figure for M.D. graduates was 29%. The 204 (72%) respondents who included teaching among their activities reported that an average of 12.4% of their time was so spent (12.7% of M.D.s and 11.7% of M.D./Ph.D.s).

The question "Which accomplishment are you most proud of?" was answered by 127 respondents. Each respondee was assigned to one of eleven categories. Table 4 presents the distribution. It will be noted that "Teaching and Mentoring" led the responses, followed closely by leadership in organizations, committee work, research and practice, in that order.

The first survey also inquired about publications.[7] Over 80% of the 211 respondents had published at least one research paper in a peer-

Table 3.   Research Activity of 200 (75% of 272) Respondents

Any	>50% of Time
All (N=272) 200 (74%)	104 (38%)
MD (N=189) 129 (68%)	54 (29%)
MD-PhD (N=83) 71 (86%)	50 (60%)

Table 4.   Which Accomplishment Are You Most Proud Of? N=127

Teaching/mentoring (both formal and informal teaching)	22
Leadership (in a varity of organizational settings)	22
Creating or founding new entities	24
Committee work (Local, state, national, academic, practice)	13
Research	10
Practice	8
Publishing (author, editor, ed. Board, books, chapters, articles)	10
Family	6
Awards, Honors	4
Business (pharmacology, insurance co., CEO of group practice)	4
Community service	2
Inventions patented	1
Clinical studies	1
Political activism in health care reform	0

reviewed journal after graduation. The majority described their publication(s) as basic research.

Of the 254 graduates surveyed, 214, or 83%, indicated that, if they had to make the choice again, they would choose HST. Of these, 130, or 67%, attributed this to the quantitative, scientific approach of the curriculum. Over one-third of the respondents also mentioned the small class size as a reason.

Here are some typical comments on the positive influence of the quantitative/scientific approach upon choice of career:

"I chose pulmonary, one of the more quantitative fields, as my specialty."

"One of the reasons I was attracted to pathology was the bridge that pathology represents between basic science and clinical medicine."

" . . . the quantitative approach of HST was considerably more stimulating than the conventional medical curriculum."

"The thesis requirement was probably more influential in exposing me to 'hands-on' research."

"It definitely provided a background to critically evaluate patient care and research literature and practice."

"Creating testable hypotheses, testing them, measuring outcomes are an indispensable habit of mind for anything I've done since."

"I enjoyed the closer contact with professors and was given a perspective on physiology which I could not have gotten in the regular program. Also, the supportive attitude toward basic research was a major plus."

"I think that the benefits of HST are a small group of people who are bright and interested in basic science research, flexible scheduling of courses and research activites, and close interaction among students and faculty."

"I approach problems in a very quantitative way. My lectures detailing calculations and statistics demonstrate this."

"I think the quantitative approach made little difference. But, learning to break issues down analytically did help me in my career in research."

"The experience instilled me with a strong desire to apply basic science tools to solving clincally relevant questions."

"Although I feared that a quantitative emphasis would make me a poor MD, I quickly found out that I could solve complex physiological problems that left others stumped."

"The quantitative/scientific approach emphasized in HST enabled me to make the transition from basic scientist/graduate student to research clinician. However, my training in pediatrics and present pediatric practice do not satisfy me intellectually, as did my studies at Harvard/HST. Therefore, I have decided to pursue further training in genetics."

"The quantitative approach, in my case, provided a framework to base all my research, whether clinical or basic science, in a rigorous manner. In addition, the teaching methods used (small groups, hands-on, etc.) greatly influence my work."

"It's given me a better understanding of the knowledge which underlies medical practice and it allows me to read the literature better."

"I have attempted to approach clinical medicine from a rational/scientific point of view."

Summary

It is evident that the majority of the graduates of the first fourteen classes of the HST-M.D. program have chosen academic careers. Almost three-quarters hold faculty appointments, three-quarters are engaged in research, and more than a third reported devoting more than half their time to research. Seventy-five percent of respondents are active in teaching.

Geographic Distribution of Graduates of the HST-M.D. Program

The geographic distribution of graduates of the HST-M.D. program may be of interest inasmuch as it represents the dissemination and possible impact of HST's educational principles and curriculum. The whereabouts in 1995 of 457 of 465 graduates of the twenty-one classes from 1975 through 1995 were known. The HST-M.D. alumni were distributed among thirty-five states and seven foreign countries. Table 5 indicates the sixteen states with five or more graduates.

The Follow-up Studies as Outcome Evaluation

The question that must be addressed when evaluating the outcome of the HST-M.D. program is: has the program accomplished its mission? The earliest mission statement was enunciated by the founder and first director of the program, Dr. Irving M. London, in 1973:[9] "To educate physicians with a deep and quantitative understanding of the sciences of medicine . . . to prepare students for leadership roles in medicine and biomedical science." Even though no actual criteria for success of the program had been delineated at its inception, the results of the follow-up study would seem to indicate that the goal of educating physician-scientists has been achieved.

The question must be asked, however, how does this program compare to other programs with similar goals? Comparable groups of students with which this program could be compared either do not exist or have not been studied/reported. An ideal group of students for comparative analyses would be the group of students who were accepted by the program but declined. Unfortunately, the number of students who declined in favor of the regular curriculum of the Harvard Medical School is too small to serve as a control group, and the entire HMS group could not be analyzed within the confines of per-

Table 5.   Geographic Distribution of 457 Graduates of 1975–1995 (States with 5 or more graduates)

Massachusetts	160	Washington	9
California	83	Illinois	8
New York	43	Florida	7
Maryland	28	Minnesota	7
Pennsylvania	17	North Carolina	7
Mississippi	10	Colorado	6
Missouri	10	Connecticut	5
Georgia	9	Texas	5

sonnel and finances. Furthermore, some of these students may not have accepted the goals of this program.

However, several evaluations of other programs designed to educate physician/scientists have been reported in the literature. Thus, of seventy-five M.D.-Ph.D. graduates from the Medical Scientist Training Program (MSTP) at Duke University 1970–1979, 76% were in academic medicine or research and 24% in practice.[10] This figure is the same as that for the entire HST-M.D. program, of which only 30.5% held both M.D. and Ph.D. degrees. Of seventy-two M.D.-Ph.D. graduates from the MSTP program at Washington University in St. Louis, who had completed their traing, 86% were in academic positions and two others were investigators at NIH.[11] Of forty-two M.D.-Ph.D. graduates from Johns Hopkins University who had completed their training, 81% held full-time academic posts and 14% were active in research institutes.[12] An analysis of 471 graduates of MSTP programs at eight medical schools who were in career positions, reported that 90% had academic or other research positions.[13]

If we look at our M.D.-Ph.D. graduates (N=71) 91.7% held full-time faculty positions (Table 2), 86% were engaged in research, and 60% devoted more than 50% of their time to research (Table 3). These results compare quite favorably with the above-cited reports in the literature.

Notes

1. The Harvard University-Massachusetts Institute of Technology Division of Health Sciences and Technology 1969–1984. Report to the HST Review Committee, Howard W. Johnson, Chairman, June 1984.
2. Report of the Committee to Review the Harvard University-Massachusetts Institute of Technology Division of Health Sciences and Technology, September 10, 1984.

3. Report of the Harvard-Massachusetts Institute of Technology Health Sciences and Technology Advisory Committee, Richard J. Johns, M.D., Chairman, March 1988. (For membership of this committee, see Note 1 to Chapter 11.)

4. Report of the Harvard-Massachusetts Institute of Technology Health Sciences and Technology Advisory Committee, Richard J. Johns, M.D., Chairman, March 1990.

5. Report of the Harvard-Massachusetts Institute of Technology Health Sciences and Technology Advisory Committee, Richard J. Johns, M.D., Chairman, May 1992.

6. Report of the Harvard-Massachusetts Institute of Technology Health Sciences and Technology Advisory Committee, Samuel O. Thier, M.D., Chairman, March 1994. (For membership of this committee, see Note 3 to Chapter 11).

7. L. Wilkerson and W.H. Abelmann, "Producing Physician-Scientists: A Survey of Graduates from the Harvard-MIT Program in Health Sciences and Technology," *Academic Medicine* 68 (1993): 214–218.

8. W.H. Abelmann, B.D. Nave and L. Wilkerson, "Generation of Physician-Scientists Manpower: A Follow-Up Study of the First 294 Graduates of the Harvard-MIT Program of Health Sciences and Technology," *Journal of Investigative Medicine* 45 (1997): 272–275.

9. I.M. London, "The College and University in Medical Education," in W.G. Anlyan, et al., eds., *The Future of Medical Education* (Durham, North Carolina: Duke University Press, 1973), pp. 43–51.

10. W.D. Bradford, D. Anthony, C.T. Chu and S.V. Pizzo, "Career Characteristics of Graduates of a Medical Scientist Training Program, 1970–1990," *Academic Medicine* 71 (1996): 484–487.

11. C. Frieden and B.J. Fox, "Career Choices of Graduates from Washington University's Medical Scientist Training Program," *Academic Medicine* 66 (1991): 162–164.

12. D.A. McClellan and P.Talalay, "MD-PhD Training at the Johns Hopkins University School of Medicine, 1962–1991," *Academic Medicine* 67 (1992): 36–41.

13. J.B. Martin, "Training Physician-Scientists for the 1990s," *Academic Medicine* 66 (1991): 123–129.

Chapter 11

EVALUATION OF THE MEDICAL ENGINEERING AND MEDICAL PHYSICS DOCTORAL PROGRAM

Roger G. Mark, M.D., Ph.D.

As noted in Chapter 9, MIT President Jerome Wiesner envisioned the educational objective of the MEMP program as early as 1970. He felt that Harvard and MIT should collaborate in producing a new breed of physical scientists so that they could function as independent investigators of important problems at the interface of technology and clinical medicine.

To what extent has the MEMP program achieved this objective? We are now in a good position to assess both the education process and its outcome. Process may be evaluated by taking advantage of the periodic reports of the HST Advisory Committee which visited HST regularly between 1988 and 1994. Outcome evaluation is based on an analysis of the career paths and opinions of MEMP graduates through 1996.

External Advisory Committee Reviews

In 1986, an external Advisory Committee was established by MIT Provost John Deutch and HMS Dean Daniel Tosteson to periodically review the programs of the Harvard-MIT Division of Health Sciences and Technology. The Committee was to function much like a departmental visiting committee but report directly to the Provost and Dean rather than to the university corporations. The membership of the Advisory Committee was selected to include strong representation from both medical and physical sciences.[1] The Advisory Committee was to visit the HST Division approximately every two years and to focus its attention on different aspects of the Division's activities guided by specific charges prepared by the university administrations. Visits would typically include detailed meetings with HST administrators, faculty, and students.

1988

The Committee's initial visit was held in March, 1988. Its charge included some topics which related to the MEMP program:

1. Given the objectives of the Medical Engineering and Medical Physics (MEMP) Program, what is the proper balance in the curriculum between the physical/engineering sciences and the medical/clinical sciences?
2. Does it take too long to complete the Ph.D. in the MEMP program?

The Committee's report was submitted on July 13, 1988, and contained the following responses:

1. "We believe we understand the objectives of the MEMP program and the ways in which they differ from those of the Biomedical Sciences (MD) Program. The balance between the physical/engineering sciences and the medical/clinical sciences seems to be appropriate." The Committee went on, however, to suggest that HST might well consider additional tracks in the MEMP curriculum for individuals interested in the interface of the physical/engineering sciences and such areas as molecular biology, biomedical imaging science and technology, speech and hearing science, and clinical neuroscience.
2. The Advisory Committee concluded that the mean tenure of MEMP doctoral students was a little less than six years and that the program duration was not too long. The Committee stated: "Rigor in the physical sciences as well as in the biomedical sciences is required. We see no way to shorten the average duration below 6 years without compromising rigor."

The Committee's recommendations and encouragement added momentum to the subsequent development of new HST programs: a speech and hearing sciences graduate program, increased visibility of research activities for students in imaging, the inclusion of more molecular biology in the curriculum, and planning for a formal Ph.D. track at the interface of engineering and biology.

1990

The second visit of the Advisory Committee was in March 1990, and its charge was to examine the quality of research being conducted by the students in both the M.D. and MEMP programs. The Committee visited twenty-five students and faculty advisors in their research laboratories. This represented approximately 25% of those students whose research programs were mature enough for critical review. The Committee concluded that "these research projects were of excellent quality. Two of the projects were brilliant in the sense that they represented important scientific advances and at the same time reflected the student's own research initiative. Two projects were not of high quality . . . they in no sense reflect a systematic or programmatic shortcoming."

During the 1990 visit, the Committee provided additional valuable input to the administration:

• The Committee appealed to the Division to broaden the institutional representation among the entering students to HST programs and to recruit more broadly.
• The Committee felt that some MEMP students needed more mentoring from life scientists early in the process of selecting a thesis research topic, particularly if they were working in a laboratory in the mainstream of engineering or physical science. The concept of a biomedical co-advisor requirement was suggested.[2]
• The Advisory Committee indicated it was interested in investigating the clinical training component of the MEMP curriculum at a future visit.

1992

The 1992 Advisory Committee visitors were charged, among other things, to "assess the value, impact, and relevance of the clinical experience in the MEMP program." The Committee met at length with faculty, MEMP students, and MEMP alumni in order to investigate the subject. The Committee's report states:

At our last visit we questioned this aspect of the program. Our interviews with MEMP students and alumni promptly dispelled any concerns. The required clinical experience is a structured training program in the teaching hospitals that provides students with the unique opportunity to participate in patient care, to understand the issues involved in clinical decision-making, and to appreciate the needs and limitations of technology. These courses develop:

- Skills in patient interviewing and physical examinations.
- Skills in organizing and communicating clinical information, written and orally.
- Skills in integrating histories, physical examinations, and laboratory data with pathophysiologic principles, and in formulating therapeutic plans.
- Cognizance of 'real medicine' and the ethical, economic, scientific, and sociologic issues involved in patient care.

The value of the MEMP clinical experience is inestimable. For engineers, medicine is demystified, and the interface between engineering and the health sciences is erased. In the process, the intimidation of the clinical arena is dispelled. Every student interviewed had based, or planned to base, his or her future work on some aspect of their exposure during this initial clinical experience. There was resounding positive endorsement from students, alumni, and faculty alike.

1994

The make-up of the Advisory Committee changed somewhat in 1994 with rotation of some members and the addition of several new members.[3] The visit in 1994 focused heavily on serious organizational problems with the structure of HST and its governance. The Committee praised the quality of HST educational programs and its superb students. However, the Committee pointed out that if the HST Division were to include a strong research focus as part of its mission, then a stronger core faculty with a coordinated research agenda was required. The Committee viewed this issue as quite fundamental and urged the institutional leadership at MIT and HMS to address it clearly and urgently.

In assessing the MEMP program, the Committee noted that the students were of outstanding quality, the program was demanding, and the student morale was high and relatively unaffected by faculty politics. However, the Committee commented on the small size of the MEMP program and encouraged its growth. The Committee also noted the relatively small fraction of MEMP graduates entering industry and questioned whether students were given sufficient opportunities to consider industrial careers.

In summary, during its four visits from 1988 - 1994 the Advisory Committee was quite consistent in recognizing the high quality of the MEMP students, the rigor of the program's requirements in both the physical and medical sciences, the high quality of student research, and the value of the clinical experience. The Committee's suggestions regarding increased biology content in the curriculum were accepted and implemented. HST did go on to develop several new programs to increase the breadth of educational opportunity for students. The class size, however, was not enlarged significantly, primarily because of limitations in funds.

MEMP Alumni Survey

There have been a total of eighty-three graduates of the MEMP program through September, 1996. In an effort to assess the effectiveness of the doctoral program, and to provide guidance to the further development of the curriculum, the graduates were polled using a simple questionnaire. It requested current demographic information, other graduate degrees earned, current position, and percent time commitment to teaching, research/development, management, or "other." The alumni were also asked two important questions relating to the design of the MEMP doctoral program:

1. "Do you believe the MEMP program should continue its policy of requiring students to be credentialed in a standard MIT department? If so, why, based on your own subsequent career development?"
2. "Please assess the value to your own career of the heavy medical and clinical component of the MEMP program, and advise whether it should be maintained."

Of the total eighty-three alumni, replies were received from seventy-two (87%) graduates. Demographic and career information were available for all graduates, however, on the basis of mail and telephone contacts. The following sections summarize the results.

Career Choices of MEMP Graduates

It is impressive to note that of the eighty-three MEMP graduates, thirty-nine (47%) opted for an M.D. as well. Three students had the M.D. before starting MEMP, twenty were enrolled simultaneously in a dual degree program, and sixteen others went to medical school after completing the MEMP programs.[4] It is thus quite clear that MEMP attracts individuals with a strong interest in clinical medicine as well as excellent credentials in engineering and physical science. Student interest in combining MEMP with medicine has been quite consistent over the duration of the program. As shown in Figure 1, the percent of MEMP graduates choosing to go on for an M.D. degree has hovered close to 50% ever since 1982. It is of interest to note that dual degree programs are common in the M.D. program of the HST Division as well; approximately 40% of each M.D. class enrolls in an M.D./Ph.D. program.

Where are the MEMP graduates now?

Figure 2 answers this question diagrammatically. Of the thirty-nine MEMP graduates going on for an M.D. degree, twenty-one are still in training status, ranging from medical school to subspecialty fellowships. Eighteen are now employed. Of the forty-four graduates not going into medicine, five are currently post-doctoral fellows and thirty-nine are employed.

The majority (60%) of the fifty-seven MEMP graduates who have completed their training are employed as faculty members either in medical schools (sixteen) or in university departments (eighteen). Table 1 lists the university positions held by this group, and Table 2 lists the medical school appointments. As of July 1998, thirty-two MEMP graduates hold faculty positions ranging in rank from assistant to full professor (See Table 3).

Eight graduates hold non-faculty research positions: two in government laboratories (NIH), four in teaching hospitals, and two in research laboratories (one university based and one independent). Twelve Ph.D. graduates hold positions in industry, generally in senior research and development positions (See Table 4). Three Ph.D./M.D. graduates are engaged primarily in clinical care of patients.

Based on the positions held by the MEMP alumni, it is clear that virtually all have chosen career paths which are perfectly consistent with the goals of the MEMP program. Furthermore, they are filling

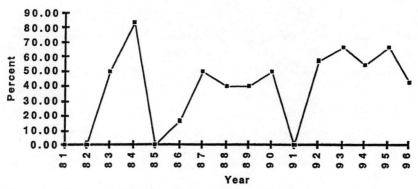

Figure 1. Percent of MEMP graduates obtaining the MD degree.

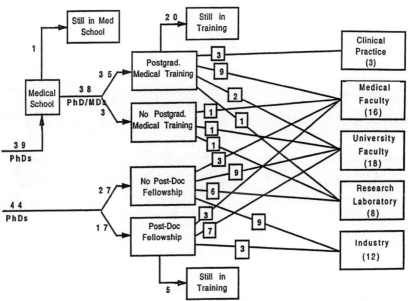

Figure 2. Flow Chart Documenting the Career Paths of the First 83 MEMP Alumni (as of 7/1/98).

Table 1: MEMP ALUMNI IN UNIVERSITY FACULTY POSITIONS

University	Faculty Appointment
1. Carnegie-Mellon University	Assistant Professor of Computer Science
2. Columbia University	Assistant Professor of Mechanical Engineering
3. Cornell University	Professor of Chemical Engineering
4. Ecole Polytechnique, Univ. of Montreal	Assistant Professor of Biomedical Engineering
5. MIT	Professor of HST and EE; Co-Director HST
6. MIT and HMS	Associate Professor of HST, MIT; Assoc Prof Medicine, HMS
7. Northwestern University	Associate Professor of Biomedical Engineering
8. Purdue University	Associate Professor of Electrical & Computer Engineering
9. Rennselaer Polytech.	Assistant Professor of Biomedical Engineering
10. University of British Columbia	Assistant Professor of Mechanical Engineering
11. University of California at Santa Barbara	Associate Professor of Chemical and Electrical & Computer Engineering
12. University of California, San Diego	Associate Professor of Bionengineering
13. University of Navarra / I.E.S.E., Spain	Professor of Management Information Systems
14. University of Texas at Austin	Associate Prof. of Electrical and Computer Engineering & BME
15. University of Texas at Austin	Professor of Electrical & Computer Engineering
16. University of Vermont	Assistant Professor of Mechnical Engineering
17. Weizmann Institute of Science	Associate Professor—Computer Science
18. Wright State University	Assitant Professor of Physics

Table 2: MEMP ALUMNI ON MEDICAL FACULTIES

Institution	Current Position
1. Harvard Medical School	Assistant Professor Medicine, Director of Pulmonary Function Lab
2. Harvard Medical School	Assistant Professor of Anesthesia (BME)
3. Harvard Medical School	Assistant Professor of Surgery
4. Harvard Medical School	Assistant Professor of Surgery (Bioengineering)
5. Harvard Medical School	Assistant Professor of Radiology
6. Harvard Medical School	Assistant Professor of Radiology
7. Harvard Medical School	Associate Professor Surgery
8. Harvard Medical School	Instructor of Medicine
9. Johns Hopkins Hospital	Cardiac Anesthesiologist
10. Medical College of Wisconsin	Assitant Professor, Biophysics
11. San Francisco General Hospital	Assistant Professor in Residence
12. University of California at Irvine	Assistant Professor of Physiology and Biophysics
13. University of California at San Francisco	Assistant Professor of Orthopedics
14. University of Michigan Medical Center	Asst Prof Radiology, Co-Director of MRI
15. University of Pennsylvania	Chief Resident in Neurosurger, HUP
16. Washington Univeristy	Assistant Professor of Medicine

Table 3. Faculty Ranks of MEMP Alumni

Rank	Number
Instructor	2
Assistant Professor	16
Associate Professor	11
Professor	3

Table 4. MEMP Positions in Industry

Manager, Clinical Applications Development	Picker International St. Davids, PA
Vice President for Engineering	Cambridge Heart, Inc. Bedford, MA
Senior Development Scientist	Ascent Technology, Inc. Pullman, WA
Director of Research and Development, Implants	Johnson & Johnson Professional, Inc. Raynham, MA
Director of Research	Aspect Medical System, Inc. Natick, MA
Senior Physicist	GE Medical Systems Applied Science Laboratory Milwaukee, WI
Research & Development Scientist	Thermo Cardiosystems Woburn, MA
Senior Engineer	Exponent, Inc. Philadelphia, PA
Research Engineer	Orthogene, Inc. Sausalito, CA
VP Clinical Applications and Regulatory Affairs	ESC Medical Systems Yokneam, Israel
Senior Scientist	Medtronic, Inc. Minneapolis, MN
Management Consultant	

influential and leadership roles nationally and internationally in the application of physical science to biomedical problems, and many are active also in clinical medicine.

Time Allocation of Graduates

The survey instrument asked alumni to estimate how their time was divided among research/development, teaching, administration, clinical work, and other activities. The data were analyzed separately in the different career categories.

Ph.D. Graduates

Of the forty-four MEMP graduates who did not pursue medical studies, five are still in post-doctoral training. The other thirty-nine individuals are working in a number of settings, including research institutions (six), academia (twenty-one), and industry (twelve). Survey responses were obtained from forty-one (93%) of the graduates. Taken as an entire group, the alumni are allocating an impressive

65% of their time to research, while teaching accounts for 16%, and administration for 17% of their time (See Table 5). It is of considerable interest to note that the high percentage of time allocation to research was seen in virtually all job classifications. Alumni in academia report that they spend about 55% of their time in research while those in industry report that 65% of their time is in R&D. Academicians teach on average 28% of their time, while spending 15% in administration/management. Alumni in industry spend about one third (34%) of their time in management.

Ph.D.—M.D. Graduates

The overwhelming majority (92%) of the thirty-eight Ph.D./ M.D. graduates went on to post-graduate clinical training. As of July 1998, twenty of them were still in training, while eighteen individuals (including the three who omitted residency training) were employed full-time (See Figure 2). Three went into full-time clinical practice, two took full-time research positions, and the remaining thirteen entered academia as faculty members at medical schools or in university departments.

Analysis of the time allocation of the employed Ph.D./M.D.s was done based on data from seventeen individuals (94%). The results (Figure 3) demonstrate that the graduates are spending the largest fraction of their time in research (44%), followed by clinical work (34%), teaching (14%), and administration (8%). The data indicate that although these Ph.D./M.D. graduates were highly motivated to become practicing physicians, they maintained a major research involvement in their eventual career patterns.

Survey Questions

Table 5. Time allocations for Ph.D.—only graduates in different types of positions

Position Type	n	Research %	Teaching %	Admin.%	Clinical %
Research Labs	6	77	6	10	6
Industry	12	65	1	34	0
Academic	21	55	28	15	0
Post-doc	5	97.5	2.5	0	0
TOTAL GROUP	44	65	16	17	2

Time Allocation for MEMP Grads in Academic Medicine

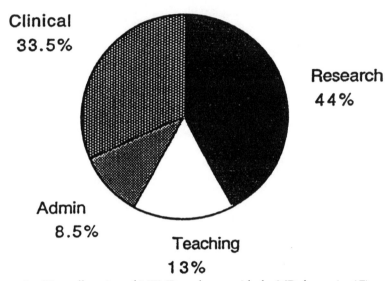

Clinical
33.5%

Research
44%

Admin
8.5%

Teaching
13%

Figure 3. Time allocation of MEMP graduates with the MD degree (n=17)

The alumni were asked to provide assessments of some MEMP program features based on their own "real world" experiences.

Question 1:

MEMP requires students to be credentialed in a standard MIT department (admission, courses, master's thesis in some cases, and doctoral qualifying exams). Do you believe this policy should be maintained? Why?

Number of responses	42
Strongly affirmative	36
Conditionally in favor	3
Opposed	3

Those in favor (93%) felt that the department-based credentialing had the following advantages:

- Maintained rigorous engineering/physics standards, which would be likely to slip if an inter-departmental or HST-based qualification process were used.
- Guaranteed that students would obtain a strong foundation in an identifiable discipline rather than end up with a shallower, broader background which they think characterizes many BME programs.
- Identifies graduates as qualified for faculty positions in traditional engineering departments. This made the difference in many cases in landing a job.
- Departmental-based credentialing tended to maintain connections between HST and departments, which is a good thing (from the point of view of thesis opportunities, teaching assistantships, faculty communication, etc.)

Three alumni were luke-warm about departmental-based qualification. Their comments include the following points:

- As more universities start undergraduate programs in BME, some excellent and highly motivated students will apply to HST but may not be competitive to gain admission to traditional departments. Unless HST admits and qualifies its own students these candidates might be lost.
- Qualifying exams might ultimately be given in HST and not require other departments . . . But this decision would be guided heavily by student and alumni feedback.
- HST-based qualifying exams would strengthen HST as an academic department . . . (But the departmental-based credentials had been critical in this individual's getting a job!)

The three individuals opposed to the department-based qualification procedure felt that:

- HST should administer its own exams and admissions because this would help to strengthen MEMP student identity.
- The master's thesis adds too much time and should be dropped. Hence, in some departments such as EECS it would no longer be possible to qualify for doctoral study.
- Preparation for doctoral study should offer several depth areas or

tracks, but not necessarily in a single department. HST should consider its own core bioengineering curriculum in selected areas.

The sentiment that HST should maintain department-based credentialing was, on the whole, extremely strong from alumni in all career areas. They seemed to feel great pride in having qualified fully as engineers or physicists, and clearly felt that this credential had stood them in very good stead in their careers. Many felt it was a critical qualification in landing their faculty or research jobs!

Question 2:

"MEMP requires a particularly heavy dose of medical courses, including a substantial clinical experience. The latter is unique in BME doctoral programs. Should this aspect of the MEMP curriculum be maintained? Has it been relevant in your own career?"

Number of responses	41
Strongly positive	38
Positive & suggestions:	3

The universal feeling was that the medical/clinical experience was a cornerstone of the MEMP program and was a major reason they had chosen it at the outset. All felt that the clinical program provided them with unique insight and knowledge of medicine which has been highly beneficial in their subsequent careers.

Typical comments:

- "Yes, it should be maintained to aid in effective interdisciplinary research and administration since the medical world (both physical constraints and way of thinking) is so different from the engineering world."
- "Yes. Clinics are very different than courses. The experience makes it much easier to interact with clinical faculty."
- "Yes, to both questions. I work with clinicians on a regular basis, and my experience helps me to communicate and to understand the clinical issues and realities."
- "I chose the MEMP program over several others because of this opportunity. I enjoyed the courses immensely, but beyond that, that knowledge and skill set give me an edge in my current position at a research/medical/educational institution. I collaborate with physicians, work with patients in clinical research, and prepare grant applications to medically oriented sponsors. (The perception

that I am familiar with medicine helps me get a little respect from physicians, too!)"
- "Absolutely yes to both questions."
- "As a scientist developing monitoring equipment for the OR environment, this aspect of the MEMP training has been invaluable. I can 'speak' the medical language (i.e., converse intelligently with my MD peers), I am familiar with the hospital environment and procedures (i.e., what is acceptable in devices and what is unacceptable), etc."
- "Yes—it has often helped me in my relationships with doctors (establishes my medical credentials) and several interviewers have said that it made my application more attractive than those of otherwise similarly-trained applicants."
- "Keep it! That's what makes the MEMP program special, and it was part of why I wanted to enter MEMP and no other program in the country. It has been useful for me to know physiology and to know how things are run in a hospital."
- "Yes! Particularly being in a clinical department the background developed from the clinical years is very important."
- "Yes—this is what 'makes MEMP MEMP.' It has been relevant by providing me (1) the vocabulary and (2) some understanding of the thought processes of clinicians. I frequently think back to my final externship (MRI imaging at MGH-east) as my reference frame for how radiologists view/deal with images, and I try to incorporate this information in my suggestions for system designs."
- "Yes. It has been a tremendously valuable part of my training. It has set me apart from most of the other BMEs in being able to converse more fluently with the biological and clinical researchers at NIH. I frequently refer to my textbooks from pathophysiology courses in my job."
- "Essential! It has been the key to understanding the pressures and feelings of practitioners. I believe that anybody working in health management (as I do) should go through this."

There were three respondents who voiced additional thoughts:

- One Ph.D./M.D. voiced the concern that the medical content might be excessively burdensome for those who do not go into medicine. (Not a single Ph.D. voiced such a concern, however!)
- One graduate urged that more molecular biology should be added—perhaps as a separate track. (Such a track has recently been approved by the HST faculty.)

- One respondent urged that students be permitted more flexibility in medical course selection. He felt that "the clinical experience was an exciting part of my tenure at HST, I'd like to see it continue at a reasonable level (?6 weeks)."

Summary and Conclusion

The MEMP doctoral program is a unique educational paradigm because of its inter-institutional character and the degree to which its students are immersed in the biomedical and clinical sciences. The program calls upon the resources of both MIT and Harvard's Faculty of Arts and Sciences to guarantee that students acquire rigorous credentials in engineering or physical science. MEMP also links the resources of the Harvard Medical School and its teaching hospitals to the education of graduate students who are equipped with an extensive knowledge base of human biology, pathophysiology, and clinical medicine.

The high caliber of the educational program, the quality of the students, and the thesis research have been consistently recognized by the external Advisory Committee. MEMP alumni have been virtually unanimous in supporting the basic design of the curriculum—particularly the departmental-based doctoral qualifying examinations and the clinical training.

MEMP graduates now occupy a wide spectrum of influential positions in academia, medicine, industry and government research laboratories. A significant number have earned M.D. degrees as well. Alumni in all career categories report that they continue to devote a major portion of their effort to research and development.

We conclude that the MEMP doctoral program has been remarkably successful in meeting the original vision of President Wiesner in 1970. It has succeeded in melding the educational resources of two great institutions to produce outstanding graduates who are well equipped to focus the power of the physical sciences and technology on important health-related problems. We would argue that it has contributed in a very central way to recognition of the Harvard-MIT community as an outstanding environment to train in Biomedical Engineering and to the increasing contributions of this community to health care. MEMP is today one of the most, perhaps the most, competitive graduate program to gain admission to in the country and its graduates represent the next generation of leaders in Biomedical Engineering education and research.

Notes

1. The 1988 HST Advisory Committee Membership:
   James B. Bassingthwaite, M.D., Ph.D.
   Director, National Simulation Resource Facility for Circulatory Mass
     Transport and Exchange
   University of Washington
   Center for Bioengineering
   Seattle, Washington

   Thomas F. Budinger, M.D., Ph.D.
   Professor, Department of Electrical Engineering and Computer Science
   Department of Radiology
   University of California
   Lawrence Berkeley Laboratory
   Berkeley, California

   Gilbert Chu, M.D., Ph.D.
   Assistant Professor, Department of Medicine
   Stanford University Medical Center
   Stanford, California

   Jerome R. Cox, Sc.D.
   Professor and Chairman
   Department of Computer Science
   School of Engineering and Applied Science
   Washington University
   St. Louis, Missouri

   Robert L. Dedrick, Ph.D.
   Chief, Chemical Engineering Section
   Biomedical Engineering and Instrumentation Branch
   Division of Research Services
   National Institutes of Health
   Bethesda, Maryland

   Richard J. Johns, M.D. (Chairman)
   Massey Professor and Director
   Department of Biomedical Engineering
   The Johns Hopkins University School of Medicine
   Baltimore, Maryland

   Peter G. Katona, Sc.D.
   Professor, Biomedical Engineering Department
   Case Western Reserve University
   Cleveland, Ohio

   John S. Lloyd, Ph.D.
   Glenville, Illinois

William F. Murphy, Jr., M.D.
Miami, Florida

John Norman, M.D.
Professor and Chairman
Department of Surgery
Marshall University School of Medicine
Huntington, West Virginia

John A. Quinn, Ph.D.
Robert D. Bent Professor of Chemical Engineering
University of Pennsylvania
Philadelphia, Pennsylvania

Helen Ranney, M.D.
Professor of Medicine
Department of Medicine
Veteran's Administration Medical Center
San Diego, California

Louis Sullivan, M.D.
President, Morehouse School of Medicine
Atlanta, Georgia

John F. Taplin
Consulting Engineer
Boston, Massachusetts

George W. Thorn, M.D.
Chairman of the Board of Trustees
Howard Hughes Medical Institute
Boston, Massachusetts

Thomas A. Waldmann, M.D.
Chief Metabolism Branch
National Cancer Institute
National Institutes of Health
Bethesda, Maryland

2. While a formal requirement for a biomedical co-advisor was never implemented, thesis committees were required to have a minimum of three members, one of whom was expected to be a life scientist.
3. The 1994 HST Advisory Committee Membership:
   William R. Brody, M.D., Ph.D.
   Director and Martin Donner Professor
   The Russell H. Morgan Department of Radiology and Radiological Science
   The Johns Hopkins University School of Medicine
   600 North Wolfe Street
   Baltimore, Maryland

Thomas F. Budinger, M.D., Ph.D.
Professor, Department of Electrical Engineering and Computer Science
Department of Radiology
University of California
Lawrence Berkeley Laboratory
Berkeley, California

Gilbert Chu, M.D., Ph.D.
Assistant Professor, Department of Medicine
Stanford University Medical Center
Stanford, California

Bernard Forget, M.D.
Professor of Medicine and Human Genetics
Department of Medicine
Yale University, School of Medicine
New Haven, Connecticut

Lee L. Huntsman, Ph.D.
Professor and Director of the Center for Bioengineering, WD12
University of Washington
Seattle, Washington

Marvin E. Jaffe, M.D.
President
The R.W. Johnson Pharmaceutical Research Institute
Route 202
Raritan, New Jersey

Stephen Malawista, M.D.
Professor of Internal Medicine
Department of Internal Medicine
Section of Rheumatology
Yale University, School of Medicine
New Haven, Connecticut

John A. Quinn, Ph.D.
Robert D. Bent Professor of Chemical Engineering
University of Pennsylvania
Philadelphia, Pennsylvania

Helen Ranney, M.D.
Professor of Medicine
Department of Medicine
Veteran's Administration Medical Center
San Diego, California

Bennett M. Shapiro, M.D.
Executive Vice President
Worldwide Basic Research
Merck Sharp & Dohme Research Laboratories
Rahway, New Jersey

John F. Taplin
Consulting Engineer
Wellesley Hills, Massachusetts

Samuel O. Thier, M.D. (Chairman)
President
Brandeis University
Waltham, Massachusetts

George W. Thorn, M.D.
Chairman of the Board of Trustees
Howard Hughes Medical Institute
Boston, Massachusetts

Thomas A. Waldmann, M.D.
Chief Metabolism Branch
National Cancer Institute
National Institutes of Health
Bethesda, Maryland

4. Fourteen of the sixteen went to HMS, one to Tufts, and one to the University of Massachusetts.

CONCLUSIONS/PERSPECTIVE

Walter H. Abelmann, M.D.

This volume has presented an overview of the conceptualization, planning, development, evolution, operation and evaluation of the Harvard-MIT Division of Health Sciences and Technology during its first twenty-five years, 1970–1995. This program constitutes a unique inter-university, interdepartmental academic venture.

We have seen how the concept of HST evolved in the 1960's. It was anchored in some of the characteristics of those years: the unfettered optimism that any scientific research or medical development could be accomplished, and that, in addition to the biological sciences, the quantitative sciences—mathematics, physics, computer science and engineering—provided untold underdeveloped opportunities for the better understanding of health and disease and hence for the betterment of human life. Governmental support—usually federal—was available for almost any well-conceived, creative and novel project, whether in basic or applied research. There was also a commitment to education, to strengthening of our universities.

In the 1940's and 1950's, much research supported by the Department of Defense and NASA had resulted in fall-out contributions to biomedical sciences and to health care. In due time, however, these sources of funds for research declined. At the same time, it had become clear that the physical and engineering sciences had much to contribute to biomedical research, both basic and applied, and the interest of many members of the faculty at MIT—as well as of students—increasingly turned to these fields. On the other side of the river, at the Harvard Medical School, the increased participation of quantitative sciences in biomedical research made the absence of a division or department of medical engineering felt. At the same time, it did not seem opportune to add such an entity.

It was against this background that HST was planned and established. As key prerequisites for this new venture, the following may be cited:

1. Strong motivation on the part of members of the faculty and students of both universities, initially mainly directed toward collaborative research.
2. Personal interest and strong support on the part of the top leadership of the two universities.
3. The perception of the need to train more physician-scientists and biomedical scientists.
4. The commitment to a rigorous curriculum.
5. The availability of funding from governmental, industrial and private sources.
6. The availability of an experienced academic leader for the directorship.

Thus the time was right, both locally and nationally. The continued success of the program relied upon the recruitment and selection of outstanding students and the enthusiasm of the combined faculty in teaching these highly motivated and capable students and in accepting them into their laboratories. At the same time, collaborative research programs expanded.

By the 1990's, however, times had changed; the HST program had to face major challenges. These included the national perception by many that biomedical scientists are in ample supply, that opportunities for new entrants are limited, and that the priority of medical education is the production of physicians to deliver primary care. Also, the institutional leaders had other priorities and less personal interest in HST. Furthermore, funds for biomedical research—especially for major collaborative projects—had become more scarce.

What can be learned from the HST experience that may benefit other, novel inter-university, interdepartmental educational and research programs? The time must be right, the importance of the goals must be visible to and accepted by both faculty and students, financial support must be available, and—most importantly—the top leadership of both institutions must have a strong personal interest in the success of the venture.

These principles were well expressed by Walter A. Rosenblith, provost of MIT in 1973:

> Thus, the period since World War II has seen the emergence of many variably successful interdepartmental or interdisciplinary ventures. When an area was ripe for such an effort—an essential complementarity of skills, a real need for jointly operable facilities, powerful motivation by an external client, and coupling of the venture to educational programs—universities have found such "inter"-units desirable and successful (at least for a time!)."[1]

Note, however, the final *caveat*. Indeed, for the continued success of an inter-institutional program, it must be well integrated into the respective organizations; i.e., institutionalized. Clearly, delineated space, funding—preferably endowment—and strong leadership are necessary ingredients in addition to basic justification and acceptance of goals and objectives.

It is our hope that this volume has provided some general information and perspectives of the HST Program of interest to those who were part of the program, a record of its founding, operation and results for those interested in the education of physician-scientists and biomedical engineering scientists, and material of interest to those who may be contemplating novel inter-institutional programs.

Note

1. W.A. Rosenblith, *Science, Technology and the University* (New York: The Rockefeller University Press, 1973) p. 79.

Appendices

APPENDIX A

Milestones in the History of HST

1966   Dr. James Shannon of the National Institutes of Health and Dr. Colin M. MacLeod of the Office of Science and Technology urge MIT to develop a new medical school and offer 50 million dollars of government support.

        After extensive review, President Howard W. Johnson and Provost Jerome B. Wiesner decide not to establish a new medical school.

        Harvard Faculty of Medicine explores the possibility of establishing a major biomedical engineering program within the Medical School.

        Dean Robert H. Ebert and Provost Jerome B. Wiesner consider possible collaboration of MIT and Harvard Medical School.

1967   Presidents Howard W. Johnson of MIT and Nathan Pusey of Harvard appoint special faculty committee which begins to explore the possibilities of collaborative efforts in health and medicine.

1968   Special faculty committee engages 150 faculty members of both universities in intensive summer study of eighteen specific areas of interaction of the life sciences and medicine with the physical sciences and engineering.

1969   Special faculty committee recommends the formation of Planning Committee to prepare detailed design of a Joint Program.

Planning Committee formed with Dr. Irving M. London of Albert Einstein College of Medicine as Chairman. Planning effort supported by Commonwealth Fund.

1970   Planning Committee recommends that "A new inter-institutional framework should be established to provide identity, coherence, and structure for the joint enterprise, a framework in which engineers, social scientists, physical scientists, physicians, and biologists may contribute as equal partners." Corporations and faculties of MIT and Harvard formally establish the Harvard-MIT Program in Health Sciences and Technology. Dr. London appointed as Director of the Program.

1971   First group of twenty-five HST students admitted into the Program as candidates for the M.D. degree.

1972   Biomaterials Science Research Program initiated.

1973   Joint Faculty Committee established to serve as senior faculty body of HST Program.

Rehabilitation Engineering Center established.

1974   Nuclear Medicine Research Program initiated.

1975   First class of HST medical students graduated.

Cancer Radiation Therapy Research Program initiated.

Biomedical Engineering Center for Clinical Instrumentation established.

Medical Radiological Physics Research Training Program established.

1976   Curriculum leading to the Ph.D. in Medical Engineering and Medical Physics developed.

Radiopharmaceutical Research Program initiated.

Research Program on Health Effects of Energy Production developed.

Institutionalization of HST Program as the Harvard-MIT Division of Health Sciences and Technology has the approval of Presidents Jerome B. Wiesner of MIT and Derek C. Bok of Harvard.

1977   Establishment of the Harvard-MIT Division of Health Sciences and Technology by vote of the corporation of MIT and Harvard University.

1978   Establishment of the Whitaker College of Health Sciences, Technology and Management at MIT.

Inauguration of the Ph.D. Program in Medical Engineering and Medical Physics (MEMP).

1981   A doctoral Program in Radiological Sciences is developed.

1984   Report of HST Review Committee (Howard W. Johnson, Chairman).

1985   Irving London, M.D., Director of the HST Division since its inception, is succeeded by Co-Directors Richard J. Kitz, M.D., and Roger G. Mark, M.D., Ph.D.

1986   Class size of HST-MD students expanded from twenty-five to thirty.

1987   Creation of five "Academic Societies" at the Harvard Medical School; HST is constituted as one of these.

The external "Advisory Committee" is appointed.

MIT's Clinical Research Center becomes part of HST.

1990   Richard J. Kitz, M.D., is succeeded by Walter H. Abelmann, M.D., as Co-Director, pro tem.

1991   Joseph V. Bonventre, M.D., Ph.D., Class of 1976, appointed as Associate Director and Associate Master in HST.

1992   Michael Rosenblatt, M.D., appointed Co-Director of HST.

Establishment of the Speech and Hearing Doctoral Program.

1994   The "Clinical Investigator Training Program" is established. HST sponsors Clinical Core Clerkships in Medicine.

1996   Martha L. Gray, Ph.D., Class of 1986, appointed Co-Director of HST.

APPENDIX B

HST COURSES OFFERED
(J= Offered jointly with another department at MIT)

010	Functional Anatomy of Man
020	Bone and Connective Tissue
021	Biology of the Skin
030	Human Pathology
040	Mechanisms of Microbial Pathogenesis
050	Topics in Quantitative Physiology
060	Endocrinology
070	Human Reproductive Biology
080	Hematology
090	Cardiovascular Pathophysiology
100	Respiratory Pathophysiology
110	Renal Pathophysiology
120	Gastroenterology
130	Introduction to Neuroscience
131	Pathophysiology of the Nervous System
140	Molecular Basis of Some Clinical Disorders
142	Molecular and Cellular Biology and Immunology
150	Principles of Pharmacology
160	Human Genetics
170	Immunology

175   Cellular and Molecular Immunology
180   Genetics and Molecular Medicine
190   Statistical Planning and Analysis of Biomedical Investigations
196   Teaching Health Sciences and Technology
198   Special Topics in Health Sciences and Technology
199   Research in Health Sciences and Technology
200   Physical Diagnosis and Introductory Clinical Experience
201   Introduction to Clinical Medicine and Medical Engineering I
202   Introduction to Clinical Medicine and Medical Engineering II
203   Clinical Experience in Medical Engineering and Medical Physics
204   Diagnostic Techniques in the Medical Specialties
205   Diagnostic Medicine/Technology Interface
210   Innovation and Conceptual Design for the Solution of Technical Problems in Clinical Medicine
220   Introduction to Patient Care and the Profession that Cares
230   Real Medicine
300   Clinical Management and Physiology of Surgical Intensive Care Patients
303   Ethics and Decision Making in Medicine
304   Five Views of Medicine
310   Advanced Cardiology
500J   Physics I
501J   Physics II
505J   Statistical and Biological Physics
510   Medical Engineering Practice
520   Artificial Internal Organs
521   Biomedical Transport Phenomena
530   Biological Effects and Medical Applications of Ultrasound and other Non-Radiation
531J   Lasers, Microwaves, Ultraviolet, Magnetic Fields and Ultrasound in Biomedical Sciences
532J   Hyperthermia: Biology, Technology, and Cancer Therapy
541J   Quantitative Physiology: Cells and Tissues
542J   Quantitative Physiology: Organ Transport Systems
543J   Quantitative Physiology: Sensory and Motor Systems
544J   Fields, Forces and Flows: Background for Physiology
550J   Computers and Patient Care

900	Topics in Economics of Health Care
901J	Health Economics
902	Current Economic and Regulatory Problems in Toxicology
903J	Health Economics Seminar
910	Medicine and Society: Historical and Sociological Perspectives
920J	Health Technology
S-11	The Art and Science of Medicine

APPENDIX C

TYPICAL FOUR- AND FIVE-YEAR HST/MD CURRICULA

Curricula for individual students are flexible, both with regard to sequence of individual courses and the number of years in residence. Representative four-year (A) and five-year (B) curricula are given here, reprinted from the 1994/5 HST Catalog.

A.   Typical Four-Year HST/M.D. Program

Year I

Fall Term
HST   010   Human Functional Anatomy
HST   030   Human Pathology
HST   160   Molecular Biology and Genetics in Modern Medicine
HST   175   Cellular and Molecular Immunology
Elective

January
Electives

Spring Term
HST   060   Endocrinology
HST   090   Cardiovascular Pathophysiology
HST   100   Respiratory Pathophysiology
HST   110   Renal Pathophysiology

Year II

Fall Term
HST   040   Mechanisms of Microbial Pathogenesis
HST   070   Human Reproductive Biology
HST   120   Gastroenterology
HST   130   Introduction to Neuroscience

January
Electives

Spring Term
HST   080   Hematology
HST   150   Principles of Pharmacology
PS-700MJ   Psychiatry
HST   200   Introduction to Clinical Medicine (ICM)

Electives
A number of elective courses at Harvard and MIT are available to
HST students. Many students elect to work as Teaching Assistants
(HST 196) or Research Assistants (HST 199) in lieu of taking a for-
mal elective subject.

Fall Term Electives
HST   220   Introduction to the Care of Patients
HST   230   Real Medicine (2nd year students only)

January Electives
HST   020   Musculoskeletal Pathophysiology
HST   140   The Molecular and Biochemical Basis of Some Clini-
cal Disorders
HST   190   Statistical Planning and Analysis of Biomedical Inves-
tigations
HST   230   Real Medicine (2nd year students only)

Spring Term Electives
HST   220   Introduction to the Care of Patients
HST   230   Real Medicine (2nd year students only)
HST   572   Future Medical Technologies
HST   920J   Health Technology

Years III and IV

Required Courses
Medicine (3 months)
Neurology
Women's and Children's Health (3 months)
Psychiatry
Surgery (2 months)
HST   240   Physician/Scientist Preceptorship (2 months)

Electives
Ambulatory Care
Radiology
Patient Doctor III

B.   Sample Five-Year Research-Oriented Program

Year I

Fall Term
HST   010   Human Functional Anatomy
HST   030   Human Pathology
HST   160   Molecular Biology and Genetics
HST   175   Cellular and Molecular Immunology
Elective

January
Elective or Research

Spring Term
HST   090   Cardiovascular Pathophysiology
HST   100   Respiratory Pathophysiology
HST   110   Renal Pathophysiology
HST   199   Research

Summer
Research

Year II

Fall Term
HST   040   Mechanisms of Microbial Pathogenesis
HST   130   Introduction to Neuroscience
HST   199   Research

January
HST   190   Statistical Planning and Analysis of Biomedical Investigations

Spring Term
HST   060   Endocrinology
HST   080   Hematology
HST   150   Principles of Pharmacology
HST   199   Research

Summer
Research

Year III

Fall Term
HST   070   Human Reproductive Biology
HST   120   Gastroenterology
HST   199   Research

January
Elective or Research

Spring Term
HST   200   Introduction to Clinical Medicine
HST   199   Research
PS-700MJ   Psychiatry

Years IV and V

Arranged as in the four-year program, allocating available elective time to research.

Credit Requirements for Graduation
The HST M.D. curriculum requires a minimum of 142 units of credit for graduation. Distribution of units is as follows:

Category	Units Required
Basic Science (B)	28
Pathophysiology (P)	20
Behavioral Medicine,	6
Health Care Policy and	52
Social Medicine	8
(SBQS)	10
Clinical (C)	18
Total	142 units

Elective
Clinical (C or CE)
Nonclinical (NCE, B, P, SBQS)

APPENDIX D

HST FACULTY
(As of 1995)

Note: Titles are listed as of the last year of service.

List of abbreviations:

HMS   Harvard Medical School

MIT   Massachusetts Institute of Technology

HST   Harvard-MIT Division of Health Sciences and Technology

HSPH Harvard School of Public Health

HU   Harvard University

*Course Head

†Core Faculty

A. FACULTY AND OFFICERS OF INSTRUCTION

Abul Khair Abbas, M.D.*
Professor of Pathology, HMS
'79–'95

Walter H. Abelmann, M.D.*
Professor of Medicine, HMS
'73–'95

Israel F. Abroms, M.D.
Assistant Professor of Neurology,
HMS
'74–'75

Joe C. Adams, Ph.D.
Associate Professor of Otology and
Laryngology, HMS
'92–'95

S. James Adelstein, M.D., Ph.D.
Executive Dean for Academic Programs in the Faculty of Medicine
Paul C. Cabot Professor of Medical
Biophysics, HMS
'73–'95

Richard B. Adler, Ph.D.
Professor of Electrical Engineering
and Computer Science, MIT
'74–'86

Paul Albrecht, Ph.D.
Lecturer, HST
'87–'93

Harold Amos, Ph.D.
Professor of Microbiology and Molecular Genetics, HMS
'73–'74

James R. Anderson, Ph.D.
Associate Professor of Biostatistics,
HSPH
'86–'89

R. Rox Anderson, M.D.
Associate Professor of Dermatology,
HMS
'88–'95

Donald Antonioli, M.D.
Associate Professor of Pathology,
HMS
'79–93

Ronald A. Arky, M.D.*
Professor of Medicine, HMS
'79–'93

Saul Aronow, Ph.D.
Lecturer in Electrical Engineering
and Computer Science, MIT
'74–'82

G. Octo Barnett, M.D.*
Professor of Medicine, HMS
'74–'91

William S. Beck, M.D.*
Professor of Medicine, HMS
'74–'95

Richard E. Belsey, M.D.
Assistant Professor of Medicine,
HMS
'74–'78

Baruj B. Benacerraf, M.D.
George Fabyan Professor of Comparative Pathology, HMS
'74–'91

George B. Benedek, Ph.D.*
Alfred H. Caspary Professor of Physics and Biological Physics, MIT
'73–'95

William Berenberg, M.D.
Professor of Pediatrics, HMS
'74–'91

Bryan P. Bergeron, M.D.
Assistant Professor of Radiology,
HMS
'90–'94

Bradford C. Berk, M.D., Ph.D.
Lecturer, HST
'87–'88

William F. Bernhard, M.D.
Professor of Surgery, HMS
'74–'78

Bruce J. Biller, M.D.
Lecturer, HST
Staff Physician, Medical Department,
MIT
'87–'94

Paul R. Billings, M.D., Ph.D.
Instructor in Medicine, HMS
'89–'92

Reginald Birngruber, Dipl. Phys.,
Ph.D., M.D.H.
Visiting Professor, HMS, HST
'90–'93

Emilio Bizzi, M.D.
Eugene McDermott Professor in the
Brain Sciences and Human Behavior
Head, Department of Brain and Cog-
nitive Sciences, MIT
'74–'90

Bengt E. Bjarngard, D.Sc.*
Professor of Radiation Therapy, HMS
'74–'89

Sissela Bok, Ph.D.*
Lecturer in Medical Ethics, HMS
'74–'82

H. Frederick Bowman, Ph.D.*
Senior Academic Administrator, HST
Lecturer in Radiation Therapy, HMS
Associate Professor of Biomedical En-
gineering, Northeastern Univ.
'74–'95

Louis D. Braida, Ph.D.*
Henry Ellis Warren Professor of Electrical Engineering, MIT
'92–'95

Eugene Braunwald, M.D.*
Hersey Professor on the Theory and
Practice of Physics, HMS
'74–'95

David C. Brooks, M.D.
Assistant Professor of Surgery, HMS
'86–'95

John R. Brooks, M.D.
Professor of Surgery, HMS
'74–'78

Gene M. Brown, Ph.D.
Whitehead Professor of Biochemistry
Department of Biology, MIT
'93–'94

M. Christian Brown, Ph.D.
Assistant Professor of Physiology,
HMS
'92–'95

Gordon L. Brownell, Ph.D.*
Professor of Nuclear Engineering,
MIT
'74–'95

David J. Bryan, M.D., Ph.D.
Instructor in Surgery, HMS
Director, Tissue and Cell Culture
Laboratory, Lahey Clinic Medical
Center
'92–'95

Stephen K. Burns, Ph.D.*
Senior Research Scientist, HST
Technical Director, Harvard-MIT
Center for Biomedical Engineering,
MIT
'74–'95

John F. Burke, M.D.
Professor of Surgery, HMS
'74–'75

Deborah Burstein, Ph.D.
Associate Professor of Radiology,
HMS
'86–'95

John B. Cadigan, Jr., B.A., M.D.*
Clinical Instructor in Medicine, HMS
'83–'90

Martin C. Carey, M.D., D.Sc.*
Professor of Medicine, HMS
'74–'95

Dennis R. Carter, Ph.D.
Assistant Professor of Orthopedic
Surgery, HMS
'82–'83

Victoria Chan-Palay, Ph.D., M.D.
Associate Professor of Neurobiology,
HMS
'79–'89

Edward J. Cheal, Ph.D.
Lecturer, HST
Manager of Applied Research, Johnson & Johnson Orthopedics
'86–'95

Roger L. Christian, M.D.
Instructor in Surgery, HMS
'79–'86

Suzanne E. Churchill, Ph.D.*
Lecturer, HST
'91–'94

W. Hallowell Churchill, Jr., M.D.*
Associate Professor of Medicine,
HMS
'74–'95

Leo T. Chylack, Jr., M.D.
Associate Professor of Ophthalmology, HMS
'86–'92

Linda G. Cima, Ph.D.*
Doherty Assistant Professor of Chemical Engineering and Health Sciences
and Technology, MIT, HST
'91–'95

John I. Clark, Ph.D.
Visiting Assistant Professor of Anat-
omy, HMS
Research Associate, Department of
Physics, MIT
'80–'82

Judy Meyers Clark, Ph.D.
Visiting Instructor of Anatomy, HST
'82–'83

Cecil H. Coggins, M.D.*
Associate Professor of Medicine,
HMS
'74–'95

Richard J. Cohen, M.D., Ph.D.*†
Professor of Health Sciences and
Technology
Director, Harvard-MIT Center for
Biomedical Engineering, HST
'78–'95

H. Steven Colburn
Associate Professor of Electrical Engineering and Computer Science,
MIT
'74–'78

Clark K. Colton, Ph.D.*
Professor of Chemical Engineering,
MIT
'80–'94

Charles E. Cook, M.D.
Instructor in Anesthesia, HMS
'87–'88

Jeffrey B. Cooper, Ph.D.
Associate Professor of Anesthesia,
HMS
'80–'94

Ramzi Cotran, M.D.
Professor of Pathology, HMS
'74–'86

Nathan Couch
Associate Professor of Surgery, HMS
'74–'78

Ernest G. Cravalho, Ph.D.*
Edward Hood Taplin Professor of
Medical Engineering, HST
'74–'95

James M. Crawford, M.D., Ph.D.
Assistant Professor of Pathology,
HMS
'91–'95

Alfred W. Crompton, D.Sc., Dr.
Phil.
Professor of Biology, HU
'73–'74

Clyde S. Crumpacker, II, M.D.*
Professor of Medicine, HMS
'93–'95

Jozef Cywinski, M.Sc., Dr.Phil.
Principal Associate in Anesthesia,
HMS
'74–'81

Alan D. D'Andrea, M.D.*
Assistant Professor of Medicine, HMS
'93–'95

Charles S. Davidson, M.D.
Senior Lecturer, HST
William Bosworth Castle Professor of
Medicine, Emeritus, HMS
'87–'95

Richard Davidson, Ph.D.
Associate Professor of Microbiology
and Genetics, HMS
'79–'82

I. John Davies, M.D.
Associate Professor of Obstetrics and
Gynecology, HMS
'79–'84

William M. Deen, Ph.D.*
Professor of Chemical Engineering,
MIT
'75–'95

Bertrand DelGutte, Ph.D.*
Associate Professor of Otology and
Laryngology, HMS
'86–'95

Allan S. Detsky, M.D., Ph.D.*
Visiting Assistant Professor, HST
'82–'88

Thomas F. Deutsch, Ph.D.
Associate Professor of Dermatology
(Applied Physics), HMS
'86–'95

C. Forbes Dewey, Ph.D.
Professor of Mechanical Engineering,
MIT
'74–'95

Peter B. Dews, Ph.D.*
Stanley Cobb Professor of Psychiatry
and Psychobiology, HMS
Professor, HST
'90–'94

G. Richard Dickersin, M.D.
Associate Professor of Pathology,
HMS
'78–'95

Jeffrey M. Drazen, M.D.*
Parker B. Francis Professor of Medicine, HMS
Chief, Combined Pulmonary Division, Brigham and Women's Hospital and Beth Israel Hospital
'91–'95

Herbert Dreyer, M.D.
Instructor, HST
'91–'93

Philip A. Drinker, Ph.D.*
Senior Associate in Surgery (Bioengi-
neering), HMS
Lecturer in Mechanical Engineering,
MIT
'74–'91

Shirley G. Driscoll, M.D.*
Professor of Pathology, HMS
'73–'91

Martin Dym, Ph.D.
Associate Professor of Anatomy,
HMS
'79–'81

Elazer R. Edelman, M.D., Ph.D.†
Hermann von Helmholtz Assistant
Professor of Health Sciences and
Technology, HST
Assistant Professor in Medicine,
HMS
'90–'95

Murray Eden, Ph.D.
Professor of Electrical Engineering
and Computer Science, MIT
'74–'78

Michael G. Ehrlich, M.D.
Instructor in Orthopedic Surgery,
HMS
'74–'78

Herman N. Eisen, M.D.*
Professor of Biology, MIT
'73–'91

Alvin Essig, M.D.
Professor of Physiology, Boston University
'74–'78

John T. Fallon, M.D., Ph.D.*
Associate Professor of Pathology, HMS
'78–'94

Leslie Shu-tung Fang, M.D., Ph.D.
Assistant Professor of Medicine, HMS
'86–'95

Don W. Fawcett, M.D.
Professor of Anatomy, HMS
'74–'78

Henry A. Feldman, Ph.D.
Associate Professor of Applied Mathematics, HSPH

Dianne M. Finkelstein, Ph.D.*
Associate Professor in the Department of Biostatistics, HSPH
Associate Professor of Biostatistics, HMS
'89–'95

Stan N. Finkelstein, M.D.*
Senior Lecturer, Health Policy and Management, Sloan School of Management, MIT
'84–'95

Gerald D. Fischbach, M.D.*
Nathan Marsh Pusey Professor and Chairman, Department of Neurobiology, HMS
Chief of Neurobiology, MGH
'92–'95

Michael C. Fishbein, M.D.
Assistant Professor of Pathology, HMS
'74–'78

Mary B. Fishman, M.D.
Instructor in Medicine, HMS
'94–'95

Thomas B. Fitzpatrick, M.D.
Professor of Dermatology, HMS
'74–'78

Jeffrey S. Flier, M.D.*
Professor of Medicine, HMS
'73–'95

M. Judah Folkman, M.D.
Julia Dyckman Andrus Professor of Pediatric Surgery, HMS
Professor of Anatomy and Cellular Biology, HMS
'74–'95

David G. Freiman, M.D.
Professor of Pathology, HMS
'74–'78

Charles Fried
Lecturer in Medical Ethics, HMS
'74–'78

Emanuel A. Friedman, M.D., Sc.D.
Professor of Obstetrics and Gynecology, HMS
'87–'88

Lawrence S. Frishkopf, Ph.D.*
Professor of Electrical and Bioengineering,
Department of Electrical Engineering and Computer Science, MIT
'74–'95

Naomi Fukagawa, M.D., Ph.D.
Assistant Professor, HST
Associate Director, Clinical Research Center, MIT
'91–'93

Barbara Fullerton, Ph.D.
Instructor, Department of Anatomy and Cellular Biology, HMS
'93–'95

Paul M. Gallop, Ph.D.*
Chairman, Department of Oral Biology and Pathophysiology, HSDM
Professor of Biological Chemistry, HMS
'74–'95

Walter J. Gamble, M.D.
Associate Clinical Professor of Pediatrics, HMS
Senior Associate in Cardiology, Children's Hospital
'84–'95

Malcolm L. Gefter, Ph.D.
Professor of Biochemistry, Department of Biology, MIT
'86–'91

Lee Gehrke, Ph.D.†
Lawrence J. Henderson Associate Professor of Health Sciences and Technology, HST
Associate Professor of Anatomy and Cellular Biology, HMS
'82–'95

Norman Geschwind, M.D.*
Professor of Neurology, HMS
'74–'85

Lorna J. Gibson, Ph.D.
Associate Professor of Civil and Environmental Engineering
Associate Professor of Mechanical Engineering, MIT
'92–'95

Edwin Hussa Gilland, Ph.D.
Lecturer, HST
Associate Research Scientist, Department of Physiology and Biophysics, New York University Medical Center
'94–'95

Leo C. Ginns, M.D.
Assistant Professor of Medicine, HMS
'84–'95

Robert M. Glickman, M.D.
Herrman L. Blumgart Professor of Medicine, HMS
'91–'95

Edward J. Goetzel, M.D.
Assistant Professor of Medicine, HMS
'74–'78

Harvey Goldman, M.D.*
Professor of Pathology, HMS
'73–'91

George E. Goslow, Ph.D.
Visiting Professor of Biology, HMS
Professor of Biology, Northern Arizona University
'86–'88

Martha L. Gray, Ph.D.†
J.W. Kieckhefer Associate Professor of Electrical and Medical Engineering, HST
Associate Professor of Electrical Engineering and Computer Science, Department of Electrical Engineering and Computer Science, MIT
'86–'95

Ann Graybiel, Ph.D.*
Associate Professor of Psychology, MIT
'79–'89

Robert A. Greenes, M.D., Ph.D.
Associate Professor of Radiology, HMS
Associate Professor, Department of Biostatistics, HSPH
'90–'95

Robert G. Griffin, Ph.D.
Professor of Chemistry, Department of Chemistry, MIT
'93–'95

Alan J. Grodzinsky, Sc.D.*
Professor of Electrical, Mechanical, and Bioengineering, Department of Electrical Engineering and Computer Science and Department of Mechanical Engineering, MIT
'80–'95

Leonard Groopman, M.D., Ph.D.
Assistant Professor of History, HU
'87–'88

John J. Guinan, Jr., Ph.D.*
Associate Professor of Otology and Laryngology, HMS
Principal Research Scientist, Research Laboratory of Electronics, MIT

Judith K. Gwathmey, V.M.D., Ph.D.
Associate Professor of Cellular and
Molecular Physiology, HMS
'94–'95

Elias P. Gyftopoulos, Sc.D.
Professor of Engineering, Chairman
of the Faculty, MIT
'73–'78

Joel F. Habener, M.D.*
Professor of Medicine, HMS
'79–'92

Edgar Haber, M.D.
Professor of Medicine, HMS
'74–'75

Charles A. Hales, M.D.
Associate Professor of Medicine,
HMS
'74–'95

David W. Hamilton, Ph.D.
Associate Professor of Anatomy, HMS
'73–'78

Michael M. Hammer, Ph.D.
Assistant Professor of Electrical Engineering and Computer Science, MIT
'74–'78

William P. Hansen, Jr., Ph.D.
Lecturer, Department of Mechanical
Engineering, MIT
'87–'90

Jeffrey E. Harris, M.D., Ph.D.*
Associate Professor of Economics and
Health Sciences and Technology, MIT
'79–'95

Tayyaba Hasan, Ph.D.
Associate Professor of Dermatology
(Biochemistry), HMS
'92–'95

Charles J. Hatem, M.D.*
Assistant Professor of Medicine, HMS
'80–'95

Wilson C. Hayes, Ph.D.
Maurice E. Mueller Professor of
Biomechanics, HMS
'79–'95

Harley A. Haynes, M.D.
Associate Professor of Dermatology,
HMS
Chief, Dermatology Division,
Brigham and Women's Hospital
'86–'95

Herbert B. Hechtman, M.D.
Professor of Surgery, HMS
Associate Surgeon, Brigham and
Women's Hospital
'83–'95

Samuel Hellman, M.D.
Professor of Radiation Therapy,
HMS
'74–'75

Lewis B. Holmes, M.D.
Professor of Pediatrics, HMS
'90–'95

Bernard Hoop, Jr., Ph.D.
Associate Professor of Medicine
(Physics), HMS
'78–'95

Nancy H.D. Hopkins, Ph.D.
Associate Professor of Biology and
Center for Cancer Research, MIT
'81–'86

David E. Housman, Ph.D.*
Professor in Biology, Department of
Biology, MIT
'90–'95

Alice Huang, Ph.D.
Professor of Microbiology and Molecular Genetics, HMS
'79–'86

Sidney H. Ingbar, M.D.*
William B. Castle Professor of Medicine, HMS
'78–'89

Donald Ingber, M.D., Ph.D.
Associate Professor of Pathology,
HMS
Visiting Scientist, Department of
Chemical Engineering, MIT
'94–'95

Edward P. Ingenito, M.D., Ph.D.
Instructor in Medicine, HMS
Instructor, HST
'84–'95

Seigo Izumo, M.D.
Associate Professor of Medicine,
HMS
'92–'94

George A. Jacoby, M.D.
Associate Professor of Medicine,
HMS
'74–'95

Rakesh K. Jain, Ph.D.*
Andrew Werk Cook Professor of Tumor Biology, HMS
'91–'95

John Jainchill, M.D.
Clinical Instructor in Medicine, HMS
'91–'95

Parviz Janfaza, M.D.
Assistant Professor, Department of
Otology and Laryngology, HMS
'93–'95

Farish A. Jenkins, Jr., Ph.D.*
Alexander Agassiz Professor of Zoology, HU
Professor of Anatomy, HST, HU
'74–'95

Philip F. Judy, Ph.D.*
Associate Professor of Radiology,
HMS
'79–'95

Roger D. Kamm, Ph.D.
Professor of Mechanical Engineering,
MIT
'83–'95

Krishna Kandarpa, M.D., Ph.D.
Assistant Professor of Radiology,
HMS
'88–'95

Michael A. Kane, M.D.
Associate Medical Director, Medical
Department, MIT
Clinical Instructor in Medicine, HMS
'86–'95

Jeffrey L. Kang, M.D., M.P.H.
Clinical Instructor in Medicine, HMS
'91–'94

Manfred L. Karnovsky
Professor of Biological Chemistry,
HMS
'74–'75

Elizabeth Kass, M.D.
Clinical Instructor in Medicine, HMS
Associate Physician in Medicine,
Beth Israel Hospital
'91–'95

Roger E. Kaufman, Ph.D.
Associate Professor of Mechanical
Engineering, MIT
'74–'78

Homayoun Kazemi, M.D.*
Professor of Medicine, HMS
'74–'95

Tony M. Keaveny, Ph.D.
Instructor, Orthopedic Surgery, HMS
'93–'95

Samuel W. Kennedy, Ph.D.*
Lecturer on Cell Biology, HMS
Lecturer, HST
'91–'95

Robert V. Kenyon, Ph.D.
Assistant Professor of Aeronautics
and Astronautics, MIT
'80–'86

William M. Kettyle, M.D.*
Assistant Clinical Professor of Medicine, HMS
'78–'95

Sherwin V. Kevy, M.D.
Associate Professor of Pediatrics,
HMS
'74–'78

Nelson Y-S Kiang, Ph.D.*
Eaton Peabody Professor of Health
Sciences and Technology, HST
Professor of Physiology, Department
of Otology and Laryngology, HMS
'87–'95

John G. King
Professor of Physics, MIT
'74–'78

Thomas V. King, M.D.
Clinical Instructor in Orthopedic Surgery, HMS
'86–'92

Richard J. Kitz, M.D.
Henry Isaiah Dorr Professor of Research and Teaching in Anesthetics
and Anaesthesia, HMS
Co-Director, HST
'86–'94

John L. Kitzmiller, M.D.
Assistant Professor of Obstetrics and
Gynecology, HMS
'79–'82

Henry Klapholz, M.D.*
Associate Professor of Obstetrics, Gynecology and Reproductive Biology,
HMS
'85–'95

James Bradley Kobler, Ph.D.
Assistant Professor of Otology and
Laryngology, HMS
Director, Mosher Laryngology Research Laboratory, Massachusetts Eye
and Ear Infirmary
'93–'95

Irene E. Kochevar, Ph.D.*
Associate Professor of Dermatology,
HMS
'88–'95

Richard E. Kronauer, Ph.D.*
Gordon McKay Professor of Mechanical Engineering, HU
'74–'95

John C. Kryder, M.D.
Lecturer, HST
Physician/Administrator, Medical
Department, MIT
'87–'95

David J. Kuter, M.D., D.Phil.*
Assistant Professor, HMS
Visiting Scientist, Department of Biology, MIT
'91–'95

C. Grant C. LaFarge, M.D.
Assistant Clinical Professor of Pediatrics, HMS
'74–'78

Thomas J. Lamont, M.D.
Assistant Professor of Medicine,
HMS
'74–'78

Robert S. Langer, Jr., Sc.D.
Kenneth J. Germeshausen Professor
of Chemical and Biomedical Engineering, Department of Chemical
Engineering, MIT
'81–'95

Samuel Latt, M.D., Ph.D.*
Associate Professor of Pediatrics,
HMS
'74–'88

Cato T. Laurencin, M.D., Ph.D.
Instructor, HST
'88–'94

Alexander Leaf, M.D.
Jackson Professor of Clinical Medicine, Emeritus, HMS
'73–'91

Raphael C. Lee, M.D., Sc.D.
Karl R. Van Tassel Assistant Professor of Electrical and Bioengineering,
Department of Electrical Engineering and Computer Science, MIT
Assistant Professor of Surgery (Plastic), HMS
'84–'89

Richard T. Lee, M.D., Ph.D.
Assistant Professor of Medicine, HMS
'92–'95

Robert S. Lees, M.D.†
Professor of Health Sciences and
Technology, HST
'88–'95

Padmakar P. Lele, M.D., Ph.D.*
Professor of Mechanical Engineering,
MIT
'74–'94

George E. Lewinnek, M.D.
Instructor in Orthopedic Surgery,
HMS
'79–'86

M. Charles Liberman, Ph.D.
Associate Professor of Physiology,
Department of Otology and
Laryngology, HMS
'92–'95

Norman S. Lichtenstein, M.D.
Assistant Professor of Medicine, HMS
'74–'80

Andrew H. Lichtman, M.D., Ph.D.*
Assistant Professor in Pathology,
HMS
'92–'95

J. David Litster, Ph.D.
Professor of Physics
Associate Provost
Vice President for Research
Director, Whitaker College
Director, Francis Bitter National Magnet Lab, MIT
'74–'95

Steven E. Locke, M.D.
Assistant Professor of Psychiatry,
HMS
'93–'95

Irving M. London, M.D.*†
Grover M. Hermann Professor of
Health Sciences and Technology,
Emeritus, HST
Professor of Medicine, Emeritus,
HMS
Professor of Biology, Emeritus, MIT
Director, HST
'73–'95

Michael C. Long, M.D.
Instructor in Anesthesia, HMS
'81–'86

Edmund G. Lowrie, M.D.
Assistant Professor of Medicine,
HMS
'74–'86

Kilmer S. McCully, M.D.
Assistant Professor of Pathology,
HMS
'74–'78

Deedra McClearn, B.A., M.A.
Instructor in Anatomy, HST
'82–'85

E. Regis McFadden, M.D.
Associate Professor of Medicine,
HMS
'77–'84

Thomas A. McMahon, Ph.D.*
Gordon McKay Professor of Applied
Mechanics and Professor of Biology,
HU
'73–'95

Barbara J. McNeil, M.D., Ph.D.
Ridley Watts Professor of Health
Care Policy
Head, Department of Health Care
Policy
Professor of Radiology, HMS
Kieckhefer Lecturer, HST
'79–'95

James L. Madara, M.D.
Professor of Pathology, HMS
'83–'95

Boris Magasanik, Ph.D.
Professor of Biology, MIT
'73–'88

Harvey J. Makadon, M.D.*
Assistant Professor of Medicine, HMS
Assistant Professor of Health Policy
and Management, HSPH
'93–'95

Robert W. Mann, Sc.D.
Whitaker Professor of Biomedical Engineering, Department of Mechanical
Engineering, MIT
'73–'94

Eugene J. Mark, M.D.
Associate Professor of Pathology,
HMS
'79–'95

Roger G. Mark, M.D., Ph.D.*†
Co-Director, Harvard-MIT Division of
Health Sciences and Technology
Grover M. Hermann Professor of
Health Sciences and Technology and
Professor of Electrical Engineering,
MIT
Assistant Professor of Medicine, HMS
'73–'95

Katherine M. Martien, M.D.
Instructor, HST
'92–'95

Donald B. Martin, M.D.
Associate Professor of Medicine,
HMS
'73–'78

John J. Mekalanos, M.D., Ph.D.
Professor of Microbiology and Molecular Genetics, HMS
'84–'95

Edward W. Merrill, Sc.D.
Carbon P. Dubbs Professor of Chemical Engineering, MIT
'74–'94

Martin C. Mihm, Jr., M.D.
Assistant Professor of Pathology and
Dermatology, HMS
'74–'78

Borivoje B. Mikic, Sc.D.*
Professor of Mechanical Engineering, MIT
'74–'86

Clarke F. Millette, Ph.D.
Assistant Professor of Anatomy,
HMS
'83–'88

John W. Mills, Ph.D.
Assistant Professor of Anatomy, Department of Medicine, HMS
'74–'82

Richard N. Mitchell, M.D., Ph.D.
Assistant Professor of Pathology,
HMS
'93–'95

Frederic R. Morgenthaler, Ph.D.
Professor of Electrical Engineering
and Computer Science, MIT
'79–'95

Joseph F. Mortola, M.D.
Associate Professor of Obstetrics,
Gynecology, and Psychiatry, HMS
'92–'95

John M. Moses, M.D.
Lecturer, HST
Assistant Clinical Professor of Medicine, HMS
'91–'95

Michael A. Moskowitz, M.D.*
Professor of Neurology, HMS
'80–'95

James E. Muller, M.D.
Associate Professor of Medicine,
HMS
'86–'93

Richard C. Mulligan, Ph.D.
Assistant Professor of Biology, MIT
'83–'86

John R. Murphy, Ph.D.
Associate Professor of Microbiology
and Molecular Genetics, HMS
'79–'85

Brian W. Murray
Research Associate in Nuclear Engineering, MIT
'74–'75

Elizabeth R. Myers, Ph.D.
Instructor, Department of Orthopedic Surgery, HMS
Senior Research Associate, Department of Orthopedic Surgery, Beth Israel Hospital
'93–'94

Joseph B. Nadol, Jr., M.D.*
Walter Augustus LaCompte Professor and Chairman, Department of Ontology and Laryngology, HMS
'92–'95

Alan Natapoff, Ph.D.*
Research Associate in Aeronautics and Astronautics, MIT
'73–'78

Walle J.H. Nauta, M.D., Ph.D.*
Professor of Psychology, MIT
'74–'88

Alan C. Nelson, Ph.D.*
Assistant Professor of Nuclear Engineering, MIT
Assistant Professor of Health Sciences and Technology
'80–'87

Ronald S. Newbower, Ph.D.
Associate Professor of Anesthesia, HMS
'74–'95

Norman S. Nishioka, M.D.
Assistant Professor of Medicine, HMS
'90–'95

R. Alan North, Ph.D.
Professor of Applied Biological Sciences, MIT
'86–'87

Walter H. Olson, Ph.D.*
Associate Professor of Health Sciences and Technology, HST
Associate Professor of Electrical Engineering and Computer Sciences, MIT
'79–'86

Charles M. Oman, Ph.D.
Senior Research Engineering, Department of Aeronautics and Astronautics, MIT
'74–'95

David C. Page, M.D.
Associate Professor of Biology, Department of Biology, MIT
'90–'95

Sanford Palay, M.D.
Bullard Professor of Neuroanatomy, HMS
'79–'91

J. Anthony Parker, M.D., Ph.D.*
Associate Professor of Radiology, HMS
'85–'93

John Albert Parrish, M.D.
Professor and Chairman, Department of Dermatology, HMS
'88–'95

Madhukar Anant Pathak, M.D., Ph.D.
Instructor, HST
'86–'95

Igor Paul
Associate Professor of Mechanical Engineering, MIT
'74–'78

William T. Peake, Sc.D.*
Professor of Electrical Engineering and Computer Science, MIT
'74–'95

Justin D. Pearlman, M.D., Ph.D.*
Assistant Professor of Medicine and Assistant Professor of Radiology, HMS
'90–'95

James E. Pennington, M.D.
Assistant Professor of Medicine, HMS
'79–'86

James H. Philip, M.D.
Associate Professor of Anesthesia,
HMS
'80–'94

Mark Phillippe, M.D.
Instructor in Obstetrics and Gynecology, HMS
'81–'85

Daniel A. Pollen, Ph.D.
Associate Professor of Physiology,
HMS
'74–'78

John T. Potts, Jr., M.D.
Jackson Professor of Clinical Medicine, HMS
'74–'95

Carmen A. Puliafito, M.D.
Associate Professor of Ophthalmology, HMS
Assistant in Ophthalmology, Massachusetts Eye and Ear Infirmary
'87–'92

Steven D. Rauch, M.D.
Assistant Professor in Otolaryngology, HMS
'86–'95

Stephen A. Raymond, Ph.D.
Lecturer, HST
'79–'82

Peter Reich, M.D.
Chief of Psychiatry, Medical Department, MIT
Professor of Psychiatry, HMS
'74–'95

Stanley J. Reiser, M.D., Ph.D.*
Associate Professor of History of
Medicine in the Faculty of Medicine,
HMS
'79–'82

Glenn D. Rennels, M.D., Ph.D.†
Thomas Cabot Assistant Professor of
Artificial Intelligence in Medicine,
Department of Electrical Engineering and Computer Science, MIT
and HST
'89–'90

Helmut G. Rennke, M.D.
Associate Professor of Pathology,
HMS
'86–'95

Paul O. Roberts
Professor of Civil Engineering, MIT
'74–'78

Dwight R. Robinson, M.D.*
Professor of Medicine, HMS
'74–'95

Kenneth L. Rock, M.D.
Associate Professor of Pathology,
HMS
'94–'95

Robert M. Rose, Sc.D.*
Professor of Materials Science and
Engineering, MIT
'74–'86

Bruce R. Rosen, M.D., Ph.D.*
Associate Professor of Radiology,
HMS
Director of Radiological Sciences,
Department of Nuclear Engineering,
MIT
'84–'95

Robert D. Rosenberg, M.D., Ph.D.
Professor of Biology, Department of
Biology, MIT
Professor of Medicine, HMS
'78–'95

Michael Rosenblatt, M.D.†
Co-Director, HST
Robert H. Ebert Professor of Molecular Medicine, HMS
'92–'95

John J. Rosowski, Ph.D.
Associate Professor of Otology and
Laryngology, HMS
Research Scientist, Research Labora-
tory of Electronics, MIT
'93–'95

John L. Rowbotham, M.D.
Assistant Clinical Professor Surgery,
HMS
'74–'86

Robert H. Rubin, M.D.*
Associate Professor of Medicine,
HMS
'93–'95

Robert C. Rustigian, Ph.D.
Associate Professor of Microbiology,
HSDM
'74–'80

William A. Ruth, M.D., M.P.H.
Clinical Instructor in Medicine, HMS
Chief of Medicine, Medical Department, MIT
'86–'95

Kenneth J. Ryan, M.D.
Professor of Obstetrics and Gynecology, HMS
'74–'75

Harvey M. Sapolsky
Associate Professor of Political Science, MIT
'74–'78

J. Philip Saul, M.D.
Assistant Professor of Pediatrics,
HMS
'89–'95

Priscilla A. Schaffer, Ph.D.
Professor of Microbiology and Molecular Genetics, HMS
'86–'95

Robert H. Schapiro, M.D., Ph.D.
Clinical Associate Professor of Medicine, HMS
'74–'95

Robert J. Scheuplein
Principal Associate in Dermatology
(Biophysics), HMS
'74–'78

Isaac Schiff, M.D.
Associate Professor of Obstetrics and
Gynecology, HMS
'83–'90

Alan L. Schiller, M.D.
Lecturer on Pathology, HMS
Irene Heinz Given and John Laporte
Given Professor and Chairman of
Pathology, Mt. Sinai Medical Center
'74–'95

Peter H. Schiller, Ph.D.
Professor of Neuroscience, Department of Cognitive and Brain Sciences, MIT
'86–'91

Frederick J. Schoen, M.D., Ph.D.*
Lawrence J. Henderson Associate
Professor of Health Sciences and
Technology, HST
Associate Professor of Pathology,
HMS
'83–'95

William C. Schoene, M.D.
Associate Professor of Pathology,
HMS
'82–'95

Martin Schultz
Director, Hearing and Speech Division, Children's Hospital Medical
Center
'74–'78

Nevin S. Scrimshaw, M.D., Ph.D.
Professor of Nutrition, MIT
'73–'74

Daniel C. Shannon, M.D.*
Professor of Pediatrics, HMS
Professor of Health Sciences, HST
'74–'95

Ascher H. Shapiro, Ph.D.
Professor of Mechanical Engineering,
MIT
'74–'75

Debra S. Shapiro, M.D.
Instructor, HST
'90–'92

Phillip A. Sharp, Ph.D.
Salvador E. Luria Professor
Center for Cancer Research
Head, Department of Biology, MIT
'82–'95

Herbert Sherman
Principal Associate in Medicine (Engineering), HSPH
'74–'75

Elaine Li Shiang, M.D.
Clinical Instructor, HMS
Physician, Medical Department, MIT
Assistant Director, Clinical Research
Center, MIT
'84–'95

Robert L. Siddon, Ph.D.
Associate Professor of Radiation
Therapy, HMS
'86–'89

Richard S, Sidell
Assistant Professor of Mechanical Engineering, MIT
'74–'78

Richard L. Sidman, M.D.*
Bullard Professor of Neuropathology,
HMS
Chief, Division of Neurogenetics,
New England Regional Primate Research Center
'90–'92

William M. Siebert, Sc.D.
Ford Professor of Engineering, Department of Electrical Engineering
and Computer Science, MIT
'74–'92

William Silen, M.D.
Professor of Surgery, HMS
'74–'75

Patricio Silva, M.D.
Associate Professor of Medicine,
HMS
'86–'92

Harvey B. Simon, M.D.
Assistant Professor of Medicine,
HMS
Physician, Massachusetts General
Hospital
'94–'95

Clement B. Sledge, M.D., Sc.D.
Chairman, and John B. and
Buckminster Brown Professor of Orthopedic Surgery, Department of Orthopedic Surgery, HMS
Brigham and Women's Hospital
'81–'95

Arthur A. Smith, Ph.D.
Lecturer in Electrical Engineering,
MIT
'74–'78

Kenneth A. Smith, Sc.D.
Associate Provost, MIT
Vice President for Research, MIT
'86–'92

Thomas W. Smith, M.D.
Professor of Medicine, HMS
'83–'95

Louis D. Smullin, S.M.
Dugald Caleb Jackson Professor of
Electrical Engineering, MIT
'74–'74

Michael T. Snider, M.D., Ph.D.
Assistant Professor of Anesthesia,
HMS
'79–'82

Aziza H. Soliman-Fam
Lecturer on Anatomy, HMS
'74–'78

Daniel Souder, M.D.
Instructor in Medicine at the Massachusetts General Hospital, HMS
'79–'86

Ellen Spar, M.D.*
Clinical Instructor, HMS
'92–'95

Richard F. Spark, M.D.
Associate Clinical Professor of Medicine, HMS
'86–'94

Myron Spector, Ph.D.
Professor of Orthopedic Surgery (Biomaterials), HMS
'91–'95

Reynold Spector, M.D.
Assistant Professor of Medicine, HMS
'74–'78

John B. Stanbury, M.D.
Professor of Nutrition and Food Science, MIT
'73–'89

H. Eugene Stanley, Ph.D.
Associate Professor of Physics, MIT
'74–'78

Kenneth N. Stevens, D.Sc.*
Professor, Department of Electrical Engineering and Computer Science, MIT
'94–'95

Gary R. Strichartz, Ph.D.
Professor of Anesthesia (Pharmacology), HMS
'89–'95

Denise J. Strieder, M.D.
Associate Professor of Pediatrics, HMS
'74–'81

Maryrose P. Sullivan, Ph.D.
Lecturer, HST
'93–'95

Lloyd V. Sutfin
Research Associate in Orthopedic Surgery, HMS
'74–'78

David Swann, Ph.D.
Associate Professor of Biological Chemistry, HMS
'74–'78

George Szabo
Principal Research Associate in Oral Surgery, HSDM
'74–'78

Peter Szolovits, Ph.D.
Associate Professor of Computer Science and Engineering, Department of Electrical Engineering and Computer Science, MIT
'86–'95

Clifford J. Tabin, Ph.D.*
Associate Professor of Genetics, HMS
'92–'95

Melvin L. Taymor, M.D.
Clinical Professor of Obstetrics and Gynecology, Emeritus, HMS
'86–'95

Jonathan Teich, M.D., Ph.D.
Lecturer, HST
'84–'86

Richard S. Teplick, M.D.
Associate Professor of Anesthesia, HMS
'81–'95

Carol Tereszkiewicz, M.D.
Lecturer, HST
'91–'92

Edwin D. Trautman, Ph.D.
Instructor in Anesthesia (Biomedical Engineering), HMS
'81–'84

John T. Truman, M.D.
Assistant Professor of Pediatrics, HMS
'74–'87

Ruth E. Tuomala, M.D.
Assistant Professor in Obstetrics, Gynecology, and Reproductive Biology, HMS
'94–'95

H. Richard Tyler, M.D.
Professor of Neurology, HMS
'74–'91

Jose G. Venegas, Ph.D.
Assistant Professor of Anesthesia (Bioengineering), HMS
'86–'95

Manjeri A. Venkatachalam
Assistant Professor of Pathology, HMS
'74–'78

Felix M.H. Villars, D.Sc. Nat.*
Professor of Physics, Emeritus, MIT
Lecturer in Physics, HMS
'74–'95

Arthur R. vonHippel
Professor of Electrical Engineering and Computer Science, Emeritus, MIT
'74–'78

Thomas Waggener, Ph.D.
Lecturer, HST
'85–'86

Alan C. Walker, MD
Associate Professor of Anatomy, HMS
'74–'78

Conrad Wall, III, Ph.D.
Associate Professor of Otolaryngology, HMS
Research Affiliate, Man-Vehicle Lab, MIT
'87–'95

Christopher T. Walsh, Ph.D.
Professor of Chemistry and Biology, MIT
'80–'85

Jack R. Wands, M.D.
Associate Professor of Medicine, HMS
'78–'95

Steven Christopher Ward, Ph.D.
Visiting Assistant Professor of Anthropology, HU
Visiting Assistant Professor of Health Sciences and Technology, HST
'81–'82

James Ware, Ph.D.
Associate Professor of Biostatistics, HSPH
'82–'89

Paul Wassarman
Assistant Professor of Biological Chemistry, HMS
'74–'78

David F. Waugh, Ph.D.
Professor of Biology, HMS
'74–'75

Stephen Waxman, M.D.
Assistant Professor of Neurology, HMS
'74–'78

James C. Weaver, Ph.D.*
Senior Research Scientist, HST
Associate Director, Harvard-MIT Division of Health Science and Technology Center for Biomedical Engineering, MIT
'74–'95

Edward William Webster, Ph.D.
Professor of Radiology (Physics), HMS
'78–'86

Arnold N. Weinberg, M.D.*
Professor of Medicine, HMS
Medical Director and Head, Medical Department, MIT
Physician, Massachusetts General Hospital
'89–'95

Steven E. Weinberger, M.D.*
Associate Professor of Medicine, HMS
Beth Israel Hospital
'93–'95

Milton M. Weiser, M.D.
Assistant Professor of Medicine, HMS
'74–'78

Charles Weiss, M.D.
Instructor in Orthopedic Surgery,
HMS
'74–'78

Michael Weiss, M.D., Ph.D.
Assistant Professor of Biological
Chemistry and Molecular Pharmacology, HMS
Assistant Professor, HST
'91–'92

Thomas F. Weiss, Ph.D.*
Thomas A. Gerd Perkins Professor of
Electrical Engineering, Department of
Electrical Engineering and Computer
Science, MIT
'74–'95

Robert M. Weisskoff, Ph.D.
Assistant Professor of Radiology, HU
Physician, Department of Obstetrics
and Gynecology, Brigham and
Women's Hospital
'94–'95

Carol Whitbeck, Ph.D.
Lecturer, HST
Senior Lecturer, Mechanical Engineering, MIT
'91–'92

Augustus A. White, III, M.D.
Professor of Orthopedic Surgery,
HMS
'79–'95

James L. Whittenberger, M.D.
James Stevens Simmons Professor of
Public Health and Professor of Physiology, HSPH
'73–'82

Sheila E. Widnall, Ph.D.
Chairman of Faculty, MIT
'79–81

Allen W. Wiegner, Ph.D.
Lecturer, HST
'87–'88

Luann Wilkerson, Ed.D.
Lecturer on Medical Education,
HMS
'91–'92

Thomas Willemain
Assistant Professor of Urban Studies,
MIT
'74–'78

Gordon H. Williams, M.D.
Professor of Medicine, HMS
'86–'94

Kenneth Wright
Office of Sponsored Programs, MIT
'74–'75

Richard J. Wurtman, M.D.
Professor of Neuroscience, Department of Brain and Cognitive Sciences
Director, Clinical Research Center,
MIT
'74–'95

Ioannis V. Yannas, Ph.D.*
Professor of Mechanical Engineering, Department of Mechanical
Engineering
Professor of Polymer Science and
Engineering, Department of Material
Science and Engineering, MIT
'74–'95

Martin L. Yarmush, M.D., Ph.D.*
Visiting Scientist, Department of
Chemical Engineering, MIT
'84–'95

Lawrence R. Young, Sc.D.
Professor of Aeronautics and Astronautics, Department of Aeronautics
and Astronautics, MIT
'73–'95

Geraldine Zagarella, M.D.
Clinical Instructor of Medicine, HMS
Physician, Urban Medical Group
'91–'95

Warren M. Zapol, M.D.
Reginald Jenney Professor of Anesthesia, HMS
Massachusetts General Hospital
Lecturer, Department of Chemical Engineering, MIT
'73–'95

Marvin Zelen, Ph.D.*
Professor of Statistical Science, HSPH
'80–'91

RESEARCH MEMBERS

Robert E. Zimmerman, M.S.E.E.
Principal Associate in Radiology, HMS
Research Affiliate, Laboratory for Nuclear Science, MIT
'78–'95

Dan Adam, Ph.D.
Visiting Assistant Professor, HST
'80–'83

Mary Amdur, Ph.D.
Associate Professor of Toxicology, HSPH
'77–'86

Karen S.H. Antman, M.D.
Assistant Professor of Medicine, HMS
'82–'86

Philip E. Auron, Ph.D.
Visiting Assistant Professor, HST
'83–'88

Paul J. Axelrod, M.D.
Instructor in Medicine, HMS
'77–'86

William H. Barry, M.D.
Associate Professor of Medicine, HMS
'82–'84

Kenneth A. Bauer, M.D.
Associate Professor of Medicine, HMS
'90–'94

János M. Beér, D.Sc.
Professor of Chemical Engineering, MIT
'77–'85

Irving A. Berstein, Ph.D.
Assistant Director for Research Program Development, HST
'74–'86

Tushar Bhattacharjee, Ph.D.
Research Associate, MIT
'82–'85

Klaus Biemann, Ph.D.
Professor of Chemistry, MIT
'82–'85

Ernesto E. Blanco, B.M.E., R.P.E.
Lecturer, Department of Mechanical Engineering, MIT
'82–'86

William D. Bloomer, Ph.D.
Associate Professor of Radiation Therapy, HMS
'77–'84

Jeffrey B. Blumberg, Ph.D.
Associate Professor of Pharmacology, Northeastern University
'81–'86

Bertrand A. Brill, M.D., Ph.D.
Professor, Nuclear Medicine, University of Massachusetts
'93–'95

William F. Busby, Jr., Ph.D.
Research Associate, Department of
Nutrition and Food Science, MIT
'77–'85

Resy Cavallesco, Ph.D.
Visiting Scientist, HST
'89–'95

John T. Chaffey, M.D.
Associate Professor of Radiation
Therapy, HMS
'74–'85

Jane-Jane Chen, Ph.D.
Principal Research Scientist, HST
'86–'95

Michael Chorev, Ph.D.
Research Affiliate, HST
Associate Professor in Pharmaceutical
Chemistry, The Hebrew University of
Jerusalem
'93–'95

John R. Clark, M.D.
Instructor in Medicine, HMS
'85–'93

Catherine E. Costello, Ph.D.
Senior Research Scientist, Department
of Chemistry, MIT
'80–'94

George F. Dalrymple, Ph.D.
Research Affiliate, Department of Mechanical Engineering, MIT
'74–'90

Michael A. Davis, Sc.D.
Assistant Professor of Radiology,
HMS
'77–'81

Alan Davison, Ph.D.
Professor of Chemistry, MIT
'77–'92

Carlo DeLuca, M.D.
Principal Research Associate in Or-
thopedic Surgery (Anatomy), HMS
Lecturer in Mechanical Engineering,
MIT
'77–'86

William Dietz, M.D., Ph.D.
Research Scientist, HST
'93–'95

William K. Durfee, Ph.D.
Associate Professor of Mechanical
Engineering, MIT
'89–'93

David J. Edell, Ph.D.
Principal Research Scientist, HST
'82–'95

Gideon Eden, Ph.D.
Research Associate in Health Sciences and Technology, HST
'77–'82

John F. Elliot, Ph.D.
Professor of Metallurgy, Department
of Materials Science and Engineering, MIT
'77–'82

David R. Elmaleh, Ph.D.
Associate Professor in Radiology,
HMS
'77–'95

Thomas J. Ervin, M.D.
Assistant Professor of Medicine,
HMS
'82–'85

Merrill I. Feldman, M.D., D.M.D.
Director, Radiation Medicine, Boston
University Medical Center
'82–'83

Woodie C. Flowers, Ph.D.
Professor of Mechanical Engineering, MIT
'77–'94

James G. Fox, D.V.M.
Professor and Director, Division of
Comparative Medicine, MIT
'83–'95

Leslie R. Fox, Ph.D.
Research Associate in Health Sciences and Technology, HST
'77–'82

Lisa Freed, M.D., Ph.D.
Research Scientist, HST
'90–'95

Emil Frei, III, M.D.
Richard and Susan Smith Professor of Medicine, HMS
'82–'91

Joseph M. Furman, M.D., Ph.D.
Research Associate, HST
'80–'81

Melvin J. Glimcher, M.D.
Harriet M. Peabody Professor of Orthopedic Surgery, HMS
'74–'90

John J. Godleski, M.D.
Assistant Professor of Pathology, HMS
'81–'83

John E. Hall, M.D.
Professor of Orthopedic Surgery, HMS
'74–'86

Robert I. Handin, M.D.
Associate Professor of Medicine, HMS
'87–'94

Robert N. Hanson, Ph.D.
Associate in Radiology, HMS
Assistant Professor of Medical Chemistry, Northeastern University
'77–'91

Jack J. Hawiger, M.D., Ph.D.
Associate Professor of Medicine, HMS
'86–'90

Bin He, Ph.D.
Research Scientist, HST
'91–'93

Terence S. Herman, M.D.
Associate Professor of Radiation Therapy, HMS
'87–'93

W. Andrew Hodge, M.D.
Director of Clinical Research, Harvard-MIT Rehabilitation Engineering Center
'89–'93

Neville Hogan, Ph.D.
Professor of Mechanical Engineering, MIT
'89–'94

B. Leonard Holman, M.D.
Philip H. Cook Professor of Radiology, HMS
'77–'93

George B. Horvorka, M.A.
Visiting Scientist, HST
'83–'86

Jack B. Howard, Ph.D.
Professor of Chemical Engineering, MIT
'77–'86

Charles E. Huggins, M.D.
Associate Professor of Surgery, HMS
Senior Lecturer, Department of Mechanical Engineering, MIT
'74–'86

John Idoine, Sc.D.
Instructor in Radiology, HMS
Research Affiliate, Laboratory for Nuclear Science, MIT
'81–'83

David Israel, Ph.D.
Instructor in Medicine, HMS
Research Affiliate, HST
'94–'95

Maxine Jochelson, M.D.
Assistant Professor in Radiology, HMS
'89–'93

Alun G. Jones, Ph.D.
Associate Professor of Radiology, HMS
Research Affiliate, HST
'77–'95

C. William Kaiser, M.D.
Chief of Surgery, Veterans Administration Hospital, Manchester, New Hampshire
'82–'83

Michael L. Kaplan, M.D.
Research Associate in Radiology, HMS
'84–'86

Kenneth R. Kase, Ph.D.
Associate Professor of Radiation Therapy, HMS
'77–'85

Amin I Kassis, Ph.D.
Associate Professor in Radiology, HMS
'80–'94

Peter K. Kijewski, Ph.D.
Assistant Professor of Radiation Therapy, HMS
'77–'86

Jonathan A. King, Ph.D.
Professor of Biology, MIT
'77–'86

Christoph R. Körber, Ph.D.
Visiting Assistant Professor and Max Kade Fellow, HST
'83–'85

Robert J. Krane, M.D.
Associate Professor and Chairman, Department of Urology, Boston University Medical Center
'82–'83

Arthur L. LaFleur, Ph.D.
Research Scientist, Energy Laboratory, MIT
'82–'85

Richard C. Lanza, Ph.D.
Principal Research Scientist, Laboratory for Nuclear Science (Physics), MIT
Associate in Radiology (Nuclear Medicine), HMS
'81–'91

Ronald D. Larsen, Ph.D.
Instructor in Radiation Therapy, HMS
'77–'81

Ann M. Lees, M.D.
Assistant Professor of Medicine, HMS
'89–'95

Martin B. Levene, M.D.
Associate Professor of Radiation Therapy, HMS
'74–'80

Daniel H. Levin, Ph.D.
Senior Research Scientist, HST
'82–'92

Jack N. Lindon, Ph.D.
Instructor in Surgery, HMS
Visiting Scientist, Department of Chemistry, MIT
'77–'88

Elijahu Livni, Ph.D.
Assistant Radiochemist, Massachusetts General Hospital
'84–'86

Jacob J. Lokich, M.D.
Assistant Professor of Medicine, HMS
'82–85

John P. Longwell, Sc.D.
Professor of Chemical Engineering, MIT
'77–'85

Jean F. Louis, Ph.D.
Professor of Aeronautics and Astronautics, MIT
'77–'85

Denni C. Lynch, M.D., Ph.D.
Assistant Professor of Medicine, HMS
'89–'94

Hywel Medoc-Jone, M.D.
Radiologist-in-Chief, New England Medical Center
'82–'86

Edward W. Merrill, Ph.D.
Carbon P. Dubbs Professor of Chemical Engineering, MIT
'74–'94

George B. Moody
Research Engineer, HST
'90–'92

James C. Murphy, D.V.M., Ph.D.
Director, Research Animal Diagnostic Laboratory, Division of Comparative Medicine, MIT
'82–'86

William V. McDermott, M.D.
David W. and David Cheever Professor of Surgery, HMS
'73–'86

Jan McDonagh, Ph.D.
Associate Professor of Pathology, HMS
'86–'94

Rudi D. Neirinckx, Ph.D.
Associate in Radiology, HMS
'77–'80

Christian E. Newcome, D.V.M.
Clinical Veterinarian, Division of Comparative Medicine, MIT
'82–'86

William H. Newman, D.Ing.
Visiting Scientist, HST
'89–'93

Matthew A. Nugent, Ph.D.
Research Affiliate, HST
'94–'95

Bjorn R. Olsen, M.D., Ph.D.
Professor of Anatomy, HMS
'89–'94

Kohei Ono, B.S.
Visiting Scientist, HST
'92–'93

Louis S. Osborne, Ph.D.
Professor of Physics, MIT
'77–'88

Alan B. Packard, Ph.D.
Assistant Professor of Radiology, HMS
'89–'93

Anthony T. Patera, Ph.D.
Associate Professor, Department of Mechanical Engineering, MIT
'83–'86

Henry M. Paynter, Sc.D.
Professor of Mechanical Engineering, MIT
'74–'83

William A. Peters, Ph.D.
Principal Research Engineer, Energy Laboratory, MIT
'81–'85

Chi-Sang Poon, Ph.D.
Principal Research Scientist, HST
'89–'95

William M. Rand, Ph.D.
Lecturer, Department of Nutrition and Food Science, MIT
'82–'86

Joe M. Rife, Ph.D.
Lecturer, Energy Laboratory, MIT
'77–'85

David R. Rigney, Ph.D.
Research Affiliate, HST
Assistant Professor of Medicine, HMS
'87–'95

Patrick Riley, Ph.D.
Assistant Biomedical Engineer, Massachusetts General Hospital
'89–'94

Mary F. Roberts, Ph.D.
Associate Professor, Department of Chemistry, MIT
'82–'86

Michael J. Rosen, Ph.D.
Principal Research Scientist and Lecturer, Department of Mechanical Engineering, MIT
'77–'94

Robert D. Rosenberg, M.D.
Assistant Professor of Medicine, HMS
'78–'83

Robert Rosenthal, Ph.D.
Instructor in Orthopedic Surgery,
HMS
'74–'86

Derek Rowell, Ph.D.
Professor of Mechanical Engineering,
MIT
'74–'95

Andrew L. Salner, M.D.
Clinical Instructor in Radiation Therapy, HMS
'82–'83

Edwin S. Salzman, M.D.
Professor of Surgery, HMS
'74–'94

Adel F. Sarofim, Sc.D.
Professor of Mechanical Engineering,
MIT
'77–'84

Marc B. Schenker, M.D.
Instructor in Medicine, HMS
'81–'86

Paul S. Schluter, Ph.D.
Research Affiliate, HST
'82–'84

Kevin Schomacker, Ph.D.
Research Associate, Northeaster University
Research Affiliate, HST
'93–'95

Kenneth L. Schunk, D.V.M.
Assistant Professor, Department of
Medicine, Tufts University School of
Veterinary Medicine
'82–'88

Sheldon Roy Simon, M.D.
Instructor in Orthopedic Surgery,
HMS
Lecturer in Mechanical Engineering,
MIT
'74–'93

Henry S. Slayter, Ph.D.
Principal Associate, Department of
Cellular and Molecular Physiology,
HMS
'86–'94

Joseph M. Smith, M.D., Ph.D.
Research Scientist, HST
'88–'90

Thomas J. Smith, Ph.D.
Associate Professor of Industrial Hygiene, HSPH
'81–'84

Frank D. Speizer, M.D.
Professor of Environmental Science
in the Faculty of Public Health
Edward H. Kass Professor of Medicine, HMS
'81–'86

Jeffrey I. Steinfeld, Ph.D.
Professor of Chemistry, MIT
'77–'88

Malcolm W.P. Strandberg, Ph.D.
Professor of Physics, MIT
'77–'88

H. William Strauss, M.D.
Professor of Radiology, HMS
'90–'94

Herman D. Suit, M.D.
Professor of Radiation Therapy,
HMS
'79–'93

Göran K. Svensson, D.Sc.
Associate Professor of Radiation
Therapy, HMS
'79–'93

Huyhn Van Tan, Ph.D.
Visiting Scientist, HST
'82–'85

Rebekah A. Taube
Associate in Radiology, HMS
'85–'86

William G. Thilly, Sc.D.
Associate Professor of Toxicology,
MIT
'77–'83

John R. Tole, Ph.D.
Research Associate, HST
'77–'83

S. Ted Treves, M.D.
Professor of Radiology, HMS
'77–'95

Dorothy Tuan, Ph.D.
Principal Research Scientist, MIT
'82–'91

Lucia Vaina, Ph.D., D.Sc.
Research Scientist, HST
'87–'95

David F. Waugh, Ph.D.
Professor of Biophysics in Biology,
MIT
'77–'85

Ralph R. Weicheselbaum, M.D.
Instructor in the Joint Center for Radiation Therapy, HMS
'77–'86

Alfred D. Weiss, M.D.
Assistant Professor of Neurology,
Massachusetts General Hospital,
HMS
Research Associate in Aeronautics
and Astronautics, MIT
'73–'86

W. Keasley Welch, M.D.
Franc D. Ingraham Professor of Neu-
rosurgery, HMS
'74–'82

Gerald N. Wogan, Ph.D.
Professor of Toxicology
Chairman, Department of Nutrition
and Food Science, MIT
'77–'85

Monty Woods, III, M.D.
Research Affiliate, HST
'77–'86

Kazuo Yana, Ph.D.
Research Affiliate, HST
'94–'95

Michael R. Zalutsky, Ph.D.
Principal Associate in Radiology
(Nuclear Medicine), HMS
'81–'86

Appendix E
HST Graduates and Their Thesis Topics

Part 1—List of HST M.D. and M.D.- Ph.D. Thesis Titles by Year of Graduation

1978

Student	Degree	Thesis Title	Thesis Supervisor
Adams, David H.	MD	Dynamics of Center of Mass Applicability to Gait Analysis	Dr. Sheldon Simon
Berdine, Gilbert	MD	Properties of Gas Flow in A Central Airway Cast	Dr. Jeffrey Drazen
Blum, Richard	MD	Propranolol, Beta-Adrenergic Blockade, and the Limitation of Myocardial Infarct Size	Dr. Peter Maroko
Bockenstedt, Paula	MD	The Role of Prostaglandin Synthetase in Thrombin Induced Platelet Aggregation	Dr. Robert Handin
Camazine, Scott	MD	Native Zuni Indian Medical Practices with Special Reference to the Pharmacological and Physiological Bases of Plant Remedies	Dr. George Lamb
Cassel, Douglas	MD	8-Methoxypsoralen and Ultraviolet Light: A Probe of Chromosome Structure	Dr. Samuel Latt
Cheung, Nai Kong	MD, PhD	Genetic Control of Immune Tolerance	Dr. Baruj Benacerraf
Choi, Dennis	MD, PhD	Pharmacological Evidence for GABA as a Neurotransmitter in Dissociated Spinal Cord Cell Cultures	Dr. Gerald Fischbach
Detsky, Allan	MD, PhD	An Economic Analysis of Policy Issues in the Supply of Medical Services	Dr. Jerome Rothenberg
Fifer, Michael	MD	Myocardial Contractility in Aortic Stenosis as Determined from the Rate of Stress Development During Isovolumic Systole	Dr. William Grossman
Freedman, Roger	MD	Calcium Metabolism in the Small Bowel	Dr. Milton Weiser

Student	Degree	Thesis Title	Thesis Supervisor
Ho, David	MD	Thrombolytic Therapy in Pulmonary Embolism and Deep Vein Thrombosis	Dr. Arthur A. Sasahara
Knirk, Jerry	MD	Dynamics of Center of Mass and Applicability to Gait Analysis	Dr. Sheldon Simon
Mazer, Norman	MD	Size and Shape of Bile Salt, BS-Licithin and BS-L-Cholesterol Micelles Using Quasi-Elastic Light Scattering Spectroscopy	Dr. Martin Carey
Newman, Ronald	MD	The Effect of Patient Noncompliance with Oral Penicillin Regimens on the Incidence of Rheumatic Fever	Dr. Reynold Spector
Pinkston, Paula	MD	A Method of Isolation of Juxtaglomerular Cells	Dr. A. Clifford Barger
Silverberg, Alan	MD	Spectrum of and Resistance to Mecillinam—a Novel Penicillin Antibiotic	Dr. Louis Weinstein
Smith, William	MD, PhD	The Biochemical Basis of Wound Healing and Pathologic Scar Formation	Dr. Jerome Gross
Solway, Julian	MD	A Monkey Model for Investigation of the Minor Components of Hemoglobin	Dr. H. Franklin Bunn
Swartz, Mitchell	MD	Reduction of Methemoglobin and Oxygen Using Methylene Blue, Light, and Electricity	Dr. Stephen Senturia
Weigle, David Scott	MD	The Modification of Neuronal Protein Metabolism by Neural Activity	Dr. Michael Moskowitz
Wise, Elizabeth	MD	Epidemiology of Multiple Sclerosis	Dr. David Poskanzer

Student	Degree	Thesis Title	Thesis Supervisor
		1979	
Barnett, Marguerite	MD	A Method of Determination of Folylpolyglutamate Biosynthesis in Stimulated Human Lymphocyte Cultures	Dr. William Beck
Bogen, Daniel	MD, PhD	The Mechanical Disadvantage of Myocardial Infarction: A Model of the Infarcted Ventricle	Prof. Thomas McMahon
Brenkus, Lawrence	MD	Mathematical Modeling of Lead Kinetics in Humans in Health and Disease	Dr. John Graef and Dr. Robert Strong
Brodie, Howard	MD	A Non-invasive Method for Evaluating Relative Glottal Aperture	Dr. Denise Strieder
Deckelbaum, Lawrence	MD	Systemic Vasodilators in the Treatment of Congestive Heart Failure	Dr. J.A. Markis
Faller, Douglas	MD, PhD	Mapping of the Genome of the Murine Leukemia Virus	Dr. N. Hopkins
Fintel, Dan	MD	Angiotensin II and Renal Function in Normal Man	Dr. Richard Re
Flicker, Wayne	MD, PhD	Carbon Monoxide Poisoning and a Proposed Treatment: Photodissociation of Carboxyhemoglobin	Dr. J.A. Parrish
Jaski, Brian	MD	Sodium Permeability and the Atrial Resistance to Cell Swelling during Metabolic Blockade	Dr. Michael Pine
Murphy, Alma	MD	(Section I) The Kinetics of Morphological Head Damage Process in Hela Cells: (Section II) Hyperthemia: Review of the Potential Use of Heat in Cancer Therapy	Dr. Ernest Cravalho

Student	Degree	Thesis Title	Thesis Supervisor
Numata, Tetsuto	MD	Effect of Hydrostatic Press on Proteoglycan Synthesis by Calf Articular Cartilage	Dr. Henry Mankin and Prof. Robert Mann
Pober, Joseph	MD	Effects of Hypoxia on Contraction of Cultured Myocardial Cells	Dr. William Barry
Resnick, Arthur	MD	Exercise-Induced Asthma: Heat Exchange Hypotheses and Critical Assessment of the Effects of Hyperoxia	Dr. E.R. McFadden
Safranek, Louis	MD, PhD	Endocrine Regulation in the Tobacco Hornworm *Manduca sexta*	Dr. Carroll M. Williams Dr. S. Leeman
Samoszuk, Michael	MD	Anamnestic Acceptance as a New Model for Tumor Immunology	Dr. Herman Eisen
Shields, Anthony	MD, PhD	Defectiveness in Murine Leukemia Viruses	Dr. David Baltimore
Sorge, Joseph	MD	Immunogenetics of the Male Antigen and Its Role in Sex Determination	Dr. Herman Eisen
Sukhatme, Vikas	MD, PhD	Varying Cell Shape in Tissue Culture by Changing Substrate Surface Charge	Dr. J. Folkman and Dr. A. Grodzinsky
Swerdlow, Barry	MD	Malignant Characteristics of Ventricular Premature Beats in a Population with Ventricular Tachycardia in the Absence of Acute Myocardial Infarction	Dr. Roger Mark Dr. Paul Axelrod
Walters, Bradford	MD, PhD	The Effects of Cyclic AMP on the Phosphorylation of Synaptosomal Plasma Membrane and Postsynaptic Junctional Lattices	Dr. M.L. Shelanski

Student	Degree	Thesis Title	Thesis Supervisor
		1980	
Bridges, Maria Alexander	MD, PhD	Protein Phosphorylation	Dr. Robert Perlman and Dr. Joseph Avruch
Chu, Gilbert	MD, PhD	The Kinetics of Target Cell Lysis by Cytotoxic T Lymphocytes: A Description by Poisson Statistics	Dr. Herman Eisen
Clark, Sharon	MD	Temperature Regulation in the Pediatric Patient After Trauma: An Analysis of Hematoma as the Cause of Fever	Dr. Michael Ehrlich
Hawryluk, Ann	MD	A Critical Analysis of the Literature Pertaining to the Development of Gait in Children	Dr. Sheldon Simon
Mercando, Anthony	MD	A Mircoprocessor-based System for Measuring Pulmonary Function Using a Full-Body Plethysmograph	Dr. E.R. McFadden
Moskowitz, David	MD	The Effect of Vitamin D Metabolites on the Bovine Parathyroid Gland	Dr. Joel Habener
Pettiford, Herman	MD	Culture of Enzymatically Dispersed Anterior Pituitary Cells: Use in the Investigation of Prolactin Regulation	Dr. David Cooper and Dr. William Chin
Redner, Robert	MD	Regulation of the In Vitro T Cell Response to Azo-Benzenearsonate Coupled Cells	Dr. Mark Greene
Scally, Michael	MD	The Role of Tyrosine in Catecholamine Synthesis	Dr. Richard Wurtman

Student	Degree	Thesis Title	Thesis Supervisor
Sell, Jeffrey	MD	Chemical Antroneurolysis With and Without Highly Selective Vagotomy	Dr. William Silen
Spitzer, Peter	MD	Nonparametric Computer-aided Diagnosis: Bahadur's Technique	Dr. G.O. Barnett
Star, Robert	MD	Acid-Base Physiology: Quantitative Models of Blood and Extracellular Fluid	Dr. Reinier Beeuwkes, III
Turner, Joan	MD	The Role of Edema in Myocardial Stiffness	Prof. Thomas McMahon
von Schulthess, Gustav	MD, PhD	N-Particle Distributions in Aggregating Systems: Aggregation of Antigen Coated Latex Spheres by Antibody	Prof. George Benedek
Walicke, Patricia	MD, PhD	Neurobiology Transmitter Metabolism in Cultured SCG Neurons	Dr. Paul Patterson
Weinberger, Judah	MD, PhD	Genetic Analysis of T Lymphocyte Specificity	Dr. Benacerraf and Dr. Dorf
Wolf, Robert	MD	Biochemical Studies of Bovine Testicular Hyaluronidase in Dog with Coronary Artery Occlusion	Dr. James Muller Dr. Eugene Braunwald

Student	Degree	Thesis Title	Thesis Supervisor
		1981	
Alleyne, Claudia	MD	Induction of Desaturated Phosphatidylcholine Synthesis in Cultured Fetal Lung Cells by Dexamethasone: Role of Protein and RNA Synthesis	Dr. J. Torday
Bessman, Edward	MD	A Mathematical Technique for Enhancing the Accuracy of *In Vivo* Bone Strain Measurements	Dr. D. Carter
Bridges, Charles	MD, PhD	Binary Decision Trees and the Diagnosis of Acute Myocardial Infarction	Dr. Octo Barnett
Cataldo, Nicholas	MD	Cultural Bovine Anterior Pituitary Cells: I. Thyroid Hormones Stimulate and Cortisol Inhibits Prolactin Secretion II. Dopaminergic Ligand Binding to Intact Cells in Culture	Dr. David Cooper
Chiu, Y. Christopher	MD	Mechanical Properties of CAT Papillary Muscle	Dr. L.E. Ford
Eidelberg, David	MD	Symmetry and Asymmetry in the Human Posterior Thalamus: A Cytoarchitectonic Analysis in Normals and in One Case of Developmental Dyslexia	Dr. Albert Galaburda
Fong, Chin-to	MD	Depletion of Alloreative Cytotoxic T-Lymphocytes Using Liposomes Prepared From Plasma Membranes of P815 Mastocytoma Cells	Dr. Herman Eisen
Goldberg, Mark	MD	The Effect of Erythrocyte Membrane Preparations on the Polymerization of Sickle Hemoglobin	Dr. H. Franklin Bunn
Groopman, Leonard	MD, PhD	Doctors' Dilemmas: The French Medical Profession, 1803–1845	Dr. Stanley Reiser

Student	Degree	Thesis Title	Thesis Supervisor
Hahn, Peter	MD, PhD	Procoagulant from the Guinea Pig Line 10 Carcinoma: A Mediator of Trousseau's Syndrome?	Dr. Harold Dvorak
Jaffe, Joshua	MD	The Effect of Early Exercise on Myocardial Infarct Size Following Coronary Artery Occlusion in the Rat	Dr. Paulo Radvany Dr. Walter Abelmann
Kelsick, Cavalle	MD	Immuosuppression and Infectious Disease: Effect of Cyclophosphamide and Cortisone Acetate Immuno-suppressive Therapy on the Biosynthesis of C3 and C5 by Bronchoalveolar Macrophages	Dr. James Pennington
Koh, Edward	MD, PhD	The Paraventricular Nucleus of the Hypothalmus and Visceral Control	Prof. Walle Nauta
Lee, Hon-Chi	MD, PhD	Biosynthesis, Metabolism and the Role of Carnitine in Health and Disease	Dr. Paul Gallop
Lieberman, Judy	MD, PhD	Gentamicin Bolus or Continuous Infusion?	Dr. Peter Goldman
Ling, Alexander	MD	Volume Determination of Lesions in Cranial Computed Tomographic Images Using Boundary Detection	Dr. John Correia
Lisak, James	MD	Calcium Action Potentials in Mammalian Cortical Neurons in Cell Culture	Dr. Marc Dichter
Madsen, Joseph	MD	Effects of Prenatal Treatment of Rats with HALO Peridol: Possible Consequences of Retained Drug	Dr. Ross Baldessarini

Student	Degree	Thesis Title	Thesis Supervisor
Mazzei, William	MD	Correlation of Maximum Expiratory Flow and Airway Area	Dr. Mary Ellen Wohl
Neubig, Richard	MD, PhD	Agonist and Antagonist Interactions with Nicotinic Acetylcholine Receptors from *TORPEDO*: A Comparison of Binding and Function	Dr. Jonathan Cohen
Pastan, Steven	MD	A Quantitative Analysis of the Use of the Sputum Culture and Sputum Gram Stain in the Diagnosis of Community-acquired Pneumococcal Pneumonia	Dr. Mark Aronson Dr. Anthony Komaroff
Pincus, David	MD, PhD	Gentamicin Bolus or Continuous Infusion?	Dr. Peter Goldman
Slater, Cecelia	MD	Neutrophil Actin Dysfunction: Studies on the Role of Actin in Cellular Motility	Dr. Thomas Stossel
Susman, Pia	MD	Macrophage-Lymphocyte Interations *In Vitro*. A *Scanning Electron Microscopy Study*	Dr. John Caulfield
Verkman, Alan	MD, PhD	Physical Perturbation Studies of Biological Membrane Systems	Dr. Arthur Solomon
Vuckovic, Alexander	MD	Blood Levels of S-Adenosylmethionine in a Psychiatric Inpatient Population	Dr. Bruce Cohen
Wax, Amy	MD	Studies on the Anatomy of Substance P Neurons in the Sympathetic Nervous System	Dr. Richard Zigmond and Dr. Susan Leeman

1982

Student	Degree	Thesis Title	Thesis Supervisor
Cook, Charles	MD	COMED, A Generalized, Table-Driven System for Computerized Medical Education	Dr. Octo Barnett
Coughlin, Shaun	MD, PhD	Regulation of Vascular Prostacyclin Synthesis	Dr. Michael Moskowitz
Dushane, Theodore	MD	Application of the Suga-Sugawa and Windkessel Models to the Analysis of the Aortic Blood Pressure Waveform	Dr. Richard Cohen
Farhi, Eli	MD, PhD	Interactions Between the Renal Baroreceptor, Circulating Epinephrine, Salt Intake, and Cardiopulmonary Receptors in the Control of Plasma Renin Activity in the Conscious Dog	Dr. Clifford Barger
Fung, Kaihi	MD	Dose-Response Effects of Atropine on Thermal Stimulus-Response Relationships in Asthma	Dr. E. Regis McFadden
Hahn, Jin	MD	Effects of Disulfide Reduction on Ligand Binding Properties of Acetylcholine Receptor from TORPEDO	Dr. Jonathan Cohen
Hsaio, Karen	MD, PhD	Bilaterally Projecting Retinal Ganglion Cells to the Optic Tracts in Normal and Monocular Hamsters	Dr. Gerald Schneider
Ingenito, Edward	MD, PhD	Respiratory Fluid Mechanics and Heat Transfer	Dr. E. Regis McFadden
Karlan, Beth	MD	The Order of Events Leading to Surface Immunoglobulin Capping: Analysis of a Transmembrane Signal	Dr. Robert Ashman (Dr. Herman Eisen)
Khosla, Sundeep	MD	Effect of Adrenocorticotrophic Hormone (ACTH) and Prostaglandins on Renal Concentrating Ability	Dr. Reinier Beeuwkes, III Dr. Randall Zusman
Narrett, Matthew	MD	Alterations in Thyroid Hormone Economy in Non-Thyroid Illness	Dr. Sidney Ingbar
Okunieff, Paul	MD	Toxicity, Radiation Sensitivity Modification and Combined Drug Effects of Ascorbic Acid with Minsonidazole In Vivo on FS aII C3H Murine Tumors	Dr. Herman Suit

Student	Degree	Thesis Title	Thesis Supervisor
Plisko, Andrew	MD	Effect of Tissue Donor Age on Responsiveness to Specific Growth Factors of Cultured Human Fibroblasts and Keratinocytes	Dr. Barbara Gilchrest
Relman, David	MD	The Characterization of Vibriophages and Their Uses in the Study of *Vibrio Cholerae* Genetics	Dr. John Murphy
Sarris, George	MD	Identification of an Apolipoprotein E Receptor on a Human Hepatoma Cell Line	Dr. Jan Breslow / Dr. Vassilis Zannis
Schwartz, Joseph	MD	The Influence of Dietary Fat on the Sympathetic Nervous System	Dr. Lewis Landsberg
Scott, Neal	MD, PhD	The Cardiovascular Effects of Tyrosine	Dr. Richard Wurtman / Dr. Bernard Lown
Shinnar, Meir	MD, PhD	Spectral Analysis of Surface Electromyography	Dr. Mark Hallett
Singer, Samuel	MD	Chloride Ion Exchange Between Blood, Brain and CSF	Dr. Homayoun Kazemi
Spindel, Eliot	MD, PhD	Extrahypothalamic TRH: Identification, Metabolism, and Interaction with Amphetamine	Dr. Richard Wurtman
Taylor, Pamela	MD	A Method for Preparation of Placental Chorionic Villi and Development of an Affinity Chromatography System for the Separation of Glycosylated Amino Acids	Dr. Michael Brownlee
Trepman, Elly	MD	The Role of Cell Shape in Growth and Phenotypic Expression of Human Chondrocytes	Dr. Judah Folkman
Villarreal, Victor	MD	Serotonin Receptor in Rabbit Corneal Epithelium	Dr. Arthur Neufeld
Wage, Michael	MD, PhD	A Method for Deconvolution of DNA Flow Histograms Incorporating Biological Constraints; Application to the Analysis of DNA Replication Kinetics	Dr. Samuel Latt

1983

Student	Degree	Thesis Title	Thesis Supervisor
Anderson, Warren	MD	Binding Studies with High Affinity Antidigoxin Monoclonal Antibodies: A Model System for Antigen-Antibody Interaction	Dr. Michael Margolies
Balk, Stephen	MD, PhD	Cytolytic T Lymphocyte Recognition of Allogeneic Target Cells and Purified Plasma Membranes	Dr. Matthew Mescher
Baron, Margaret	MD, PhD	Initiation of Poliovirus Replication In Vitro	Dr. David Baltimore
Bedrosian, Camille	MD	Molecular Mechanism of Aminoacyl-tRNA Recognition of tRNA	Dr. Paul Schimmel
D'Andrea, Alan	MD	High Resolution Analysis of the Timing of Replication of Specific DNA Sequences During the S Phase of Mammalian Cells	Dr. Samuel Latt
Drews, Reed	MD	Transport of a Renin Inhibitor Across Rabbit Jejunum In Vitro	Dr. James Burton
Dunham, Jeffrey	MD, PhD	Affinity Maturation and Antibody Diversity	Dr. Herman Eisen
Edelman, Elazer	MD, PhD	Regulation of Drug Delivery From Porous Polymers by Oscillating Magnetic Fields	Dr. Robert Langer
Erny, Raymond	MD, PhD	Regulation of Adenylate Cyclase and Catecholamine Synthesis by Adenosine in Pheochromocytoma Cells	Dr. John Wagner
Feldmann, Edward	MD	Non-Invasive Assessment of the Progression of Carotid Artery Disease and the Risk of Focal Cerebal Ischemia	Dr. Robert Ackerman
Friedman, Alan	MD	Erythropoiesis: Molecular Studies on Hemoglobin Switching, Commitment, and Globin Gene Induction	Dr. David Housman
Geller, Robert	MD	The Structure of Crystallized N-Acetyl-Phenylalany1-tRNA^{Phe}	Dr. Alex Rich

Student	Degree	Thesis Title	Thesis Supervisor
Golub, Howard	MD, PhD	A Physioacoustic Model of the Infant Cry and Its Use for Medical Diagnosis and Prognosis	Dr. Kenneth N. Stevens
Gordon, Gilad	MD	Intranasal Administration of Insulin Via Insulin-Bile Salt Aerosols	Dr. Jeffrey Flier
Martin, David	MD	Design Considerations for a Microcomputer-Based Learning, Recall, and Secretarial Aid for the Physician	Dr. Octo Barnett
Massaquoi, Steve	MD	Refinement and Extension of the McCarley-Hobson Reciprocal-Interaction Model of REM Sleep Control	Dr. R.W. McCarley
Naini, Ali	MD	Modulation of Vascular Prostacyclin Synthesis: Parameters of the Thrombin Effect	Dr. Michael Moskowitz
Schnitzer, Jay	MD, PhD	Transport of Macromolecules Across the Aortic Wall with Special Attention to Low Density Lipoproteins	Drs. Clark Colton, Kenneth Smith, Robert Lees, and Michael Stemerman
Semigran, Marc	MD	Nucleotide Metabolism in Ataxia Telangiectasis, Fanconi's Anemia and Bloom's Syndrome Cells	Dr. Lorraine Gudas
Shaknovich, Alex	MD	Aspects of Regulation of Glomerular Filtration During Maturation	Dr. Norman Hollenberg
Shapiro, Craig	MD	A Case-Control Study of the Effectiveness of BCG Vacine Against Childhood Tuberculosis in Cali, Colombia	Dr. Charles Hennekens
Siegel, Lawrence	MD	Endorphins and Alveolar Hypoxic Pulmonary Vasoconstriction	Dr. Charles Hales
Smith, Barbara	MD, PhD	Studies on the Multistep Origin of Tumor-Forming Ability in CHEF Chinese Hamster Embryo Fibroblasts	Dr. Ruth Sager
Teich, Jonathan	MD, PhD	An Integrated Image Analysis and Program-Development System for a Computer-Controlled Microscope	Dr. William Siebert

1984

Student	Degree	Thesis Title	Thesis Supervisor
Anderson, Richard	MD	Selective Thermal Damage from Pulsed Laser Sources	Dr. John A. Parrish
Bailin, Michael	MD	The Effect of Topical Anaesthetic Spray on the Gait and Posture of Parkinsonian Subjects	Profs. Mohamed Sabbahi, William Abend, Carlo Deluca
Baker, Richard	MD	Intraocular Pressure Regulation in Insulin Dependent Diabetics	Dr. Alec Walker
Canning, Michael	MD	Studies of Reovirus Persistent Infections	Dr. Bernard Fields
Donovan, Joanne	MD, PhD	Quasielastic Light Scattering Studies of the Formation of Micelles of Human Apolipoproteins A-I and A-II Lichthins and Bile Salts	Dr. George Benedek
Doupe, Allison	MD, PhD	Effects of Glucocorticoids on Development of Sympathetic Nervous System	Dr. Paul Patterson
Dreyer, Evan	MD, PhD	Affinity Labelling Studies of the Acetylcholine Receptor	Dr. John Cohen
Grad, Oren	MD	Fuzzy Set Theory: A New Approach to Clinical Decision Analysis	Dr. Milton Weinstein
Ivashkiv, Lionel	MD	A Genetic Analysis of Parathyroid Hormone Secretion and Signal Sequence Function	Dr. Henry Kronenberg
Lee, Angel	MD, PhD	Structure-Function Relations in HGB, and Atomic Mechanisms for High Cooperativity	Dr. Arthur Solomon, Dr. Martin Karplus
Liang, Tsanyang	MD	Resolving the Roles of Plyoma HR-T Gene Products in Cell Transformation and Lytic Infection: Using the Technique of Oligonucleotide-Directed Mutagenesis	Prof. Thomas Benjamin

Student	Degree	Thesis Title	Thesis Supervisor
Macklis, Jeffrey	MD	Noninvasive Laser Lesioning of Dye-Targeted Mammalian Neurons	Dr. Richard Sidman
Nash, Ira	MD	The Search for a Novel Mutant of *Corynebacterium Diptheriae*	Dr. John Murphy
Negrin, Robert	MD	Characterization of 185,000 Dalton Protein Specifically Associated Transfectants Transformed with a Rat Neuroblastoma Oncogene	Dr. Robert Weinberg
Pacella, Bernard	MD	Production of Fibrin-Specific Antibodies by Using Synthetic Peptide Immunogens Corresponding to Newly Exposed Fibrin Amino Termini of Thrombin Cleavage Sites	Dr. Gary Matsueda
Page, David	MD	Homologous Single-Copy Sequences on the Human X and Y Chromosomes	Dr. David Botstein
Pegg, William	MD	Studies on a General Method for Somatic Cell Hybridization	Dr. Herbert Lazarus
Picus, Joel	MD	The Immune System of a Naturally Occurring Hemato-poietic Chimeric Primate: *Saguinus Oedipus*	Dr. Norman L. Letvin
Samuelson, John	MD, PhD	Surface Characteristics of Cercariae & Schistosomula *S. mansoni*	Dr. John Caulfield
Shuldiner, Alan	MD	Synthesis and Biological Properties of N-Cyclo-(LEU^5) Enkephalin	Dr. Michael Rosenblatt
Stecker, Mark	MD	A New Theoretical Approach to Micellar Systems	Dr. George Benedek
Yodlowski, Marilyn	MD, PhD	Evidence for Neurotransmitter Plasticity *In Vivo*: Effects of 6-OHDA on Cholinergic Innervation in Rats	Dr. Story Landis
Zelenetz, Andrew	MD, PhD	The Cloning of Rous Sarcoma Virus and the Characterization of Transformation by the *src* Gene via Transfection	Dr. Geoffrey Cooper

1985

Student	Degree	Thesis Title	Thesis Supervisor
Block, Bethany	MD	Ultrastructural Studies of Immunolabelled Alzheimer Paired Helical Filaments	Dr. Dennis Selkoe
Bradley, Scott	MD	Increased Expression vs. Altered Protein Product in the Activation of a Human Oncogene	Prof. Robert Weinberg
Bueno, Raphael	MD	The Role of the glnB, glnD, and glnL Products in the Regulation of Glutamine Synthetase and Nitrogen Metabolism in Escherichia coli	Prof. Boris Magasanik
Duerr, Ann	MD, PhD	Malaria: Mechanisms of Invasion into and Release from Erthrocytes	Dr. John David
Huang, Paul	MD, PhD	Cloning of Genes for Surface Antigens of *Leishmania Tropica* and *Donovani*	Dr. John David
Imanishi, Yuri	MD	Photo-Correlation Spectroscopy of Intracellular Hemoglobin S Aggregation at Physiological Oxygen Pressures	Prof. Toyoichi Tanaka
Ivarsson, Bengt	MD	In Vitro Construction of an Endothelialized Smooth Muscle Cell Tube with Potential as a Small Vessel Prosthesis	Dr. Anthony Whittemore
Joseph, David	MD	Can Peripheral Measurements of Venous Pressure Provide Clinically Useful Information?	Dr. James Philip
Konner, Melvin	MD, PhD	Universals of Behavioral Development in Relation to Brain Myelination	Dr. Irven DeVore
Koren, Michael	MD	Prophylaxis Against the Acid Aspiration Syndrome in Obstetric Patients: A Decision Analysis	Dr. Harvey Fineberg

Student	Degree	Thesis Title	Thesis Supervisor
Laks, Mitchell	MD, PhD	Group Representation Theory	Dr. David Kazhdan
Leifer, Dana	MD	Applications of Monoclonal Antibodies and Tissue Culture Methods to Neurobiology	Dr. Colin Barnstable
Lo, Steve	MD	Growth-Dependent Polyadenylation at the SV40 Late Poly(a) Site in DHFR Modular Genes	Dr. Phillip Sharp
Monitto, Constance	MD	O Lasers and Liposomes: A Description of an Attempt to Use Liposomes as Temperature Sensitive Probes in *In Vitro* Studies of Selective Photothermolysis	Dr. John Parrish / Dr. Steven Jacques
Nuchtern, Jed	MD	The Effect of Exercise Conditioning on Cardiovascular Control in Hypertensive Patients	Dr. Daniel Shannon
Oates, Dale	MD, PhD	Effect of Chronic Prostacyclin Infusion on Platelet Function and Smooth Muscle Cell Proliferation	Dr. Michael Stemerman
Prince, Martin	MD, PhD	Selective Photo-Removal of Atheromatous Arterial Obstructious	Dr. John Parrish
Roberts, Drucilla	MD	Mechanism of Cardiac Tissue Desensitization to Catecholamine Exposure	Dr. James Marsh
Show, Joyce	MD	Traditional Eskimo Illness Beliefs and Cross-Cultural Doctor-Patient Communication	Dr. Arthur Kleinman
Van Wesep, Robert	MD, PhD	The Analysis of Geographical Clustering of Disease	Dr. Marvin Zelen
Weiss, Michael	MD, PhD	NMR Studies of Repressor and Operator	Dr. Martin Karplus
Wiggs, Janey	MD	Characterization of Murine Suppressor T Lymphocyte Generation in Vitro	Dr. Steven Burakoff

1986

Student	Degree	Thesis Title	Thesis Supervisor
Becker, Pamela	MD, PhD	The Spectrin-Actin-Protein 4.1 Interaction in Normal and Abnormal Erythrocyte Membranes	Prof. Samuel Lux
Benaron, David	MD	Improving Outpatient Compliance with Medication Regimes Utilizing Electronic Dose Response Priming	Dr. Jerome Avorn
Bodenstein, Lawrence	MD, PhD	Developmental Neurobiology	Dr. R.L. Sidman
Brown, Nancy	MD	Mechanism of Bile Salt-Mediated Transport of Insulin Across the Nasal Mucosa	Dr. Alan Moses Dr. Martin Carey
Camazine, Brian	MD	Neurogenic Histaminergic Vasodilation in Skeletal Muscle: Mediation by Central Alpha 2-Adrenoceptor Stimulation	Dr. W. John Powell
Dixon, Mark	MD	Bioprosthetic Heart Valve Calcification: Studies of Mechanism and Prevention	Dr. Robert Levy
Elrick, Jean	MD	Effects of Increased Ionized Calcium on Left Ventricular Function in Neonatal Lambs	Dr. Marshall Jacobs
Farley, David	MD	Effect of Catecholomines on Aldosterone Secretion	Dr. Gordon Williams

Student	Degree	Thesis Title	Thesis Supervisor
Finkel, Toren	MD, PhD	Biochemistry of ras Gene Products Cellular Oncogenes	Dr. Geoffrey Cooper
Ierardi, Lynn	MD, PhD	Transformation of the Nuclear Matrix During Mouse Spermatogenesis	Dr. Anthony Bellvé
Ko, Bing Ho	MD, PhD	Mechanisms of Heat and Mass Transfer Across A Double-Diffusive Interface	Prof. Kenneth Smith
Liu, Alexander	MD	Isolation of Osteocalcin Fragments from Peritoneal Dialysate	Dr. Caren Gundberg
Onesti, Stephen	MD	Somatostatin-Containing Cells in the Rabbit Retina	Dr. Joseph Martin
			Dr. Stephen Sagar
Pollack, Michael	MD	Computer Tools for Medical Decision Making	Dr. Robert Greenes
Schaffer, Jean	MD	Functional Analysis of ORI$_L$, A Herpes Simplex Virus Type 1 Origin of DNA Synthesis	Dr. Priscilla Schaffer
Seldin, David	MD, PhD	Biochemistry of Mast Cell Subclasses	Dr. K.F. Austen
Smith, Joseph	MD, PhD	The Stochastic Nature of Cardiac Electrical Instability: Theory and Experiment	Dr. Richard Cohen

1987

Student	Degree	Thesis Title	Thesis Supervisor
Alter, Craig	MD	Helium Neon Laser Scattering by Human Skin	Dr. John Parrish Dr. Steven Jacques
Backer, Jonathan	MD	Reconstitution of a Phospholipid "Flippase" from Rat Liver Endoplasmic Reticulum	Dr. E.A. Dawidowicz
Berger, Ronald	MD, PhD	Analysis of Cardiovascular Control System Using Broad-Band Stimulation	Dr. Richard Cohen
Burley, Stephen	MD	X-Ray Crystallographic Studies of Some Model Therapeutic Agents for Sickle Cell Anemia and of Protein Structure Stabilization	Prof. G.A. Petsko Dr. Joel Habener
Chen, Neil	MD	Potentiation of the Antiangiogenic Activity of Heparin-Steroid Combination by Sodium 2-Hydroxy-4 Nitro-a-Toluenesulfonate, A Synthetic Inhibitor of Arylsulfate Sulfohydrolase Heparin in the Presence of Hydrocortisone	Dr. Judah Folkman
Cummings, David	MD	Characterization of Antigens Associated with Human Hepatocellular Carcinoma, Using Monoclonal Antibodies	Dr. Jack Wands
Doerschuk, Peter	MD, PhD	A Markov Chain Approach to Electrocardiogram Modeling and Analysis	Prof. Alan Willsky
Frosch, Matthew	MD, PhD	GABA Activated Currente and Channels in Cultural Rat Cortical Neurons	Dr. M.A. Dichter

Student	Degree	Thesis Title	Thesis Supervisor
Fung, Claire	MD	Stage I Testis Cancer: The Importance of Primary Testis Pathology in Predicting Metastatic Potential	Dr. Marc Ganick
Hiehle, John	MD	In Vitro Analysis of Biologic Variables Which May Affect the Outcome of Nd:YAG Laser Balloon Angioplasty	Dr. J. Richard Spears
Hsu, Frank	MD	The Characterization of Tumor a Gene Derived form Activated B Cells and Macrophages	Dr. Ellis Reinherz
Liu, Eugene	MD	Transferrin Receptor Mediated Intoxication of Target Cells by a Transferrin-CRM45 Conjugate Toxin	Dr. Terry Strom
Marcantonio, Ed	MD	The Inositol Cycle in Polyoma Virus Infected NIH3T3 Cells	Dr. Thomas Benjamin
Moore, Marcia	MD, PhD	Metabolism of Selected Barbiturate Compound by P-450 Isozyme	Prof. C.T. Walsh
Olson, Erik	MD	Effects of Milrinone on Contractile State and Cyclic Nucleotide Metabolism in Cultured Chick Embryonic Ventricular Cells	Dr. James Marsh
Reicin, Alise	MD	Deregulation of c-myc Oncogene in Virus-Induced Thymic Lymphomas AKR/J Mice	Dr. Paul O'Donnel Dr. Erwin Fleissner
Romanelli, John	MD	Metabolic and Histologic Studies of Dye Laser Retinal Photocoagulation Lesions	Dr. Carmen Puliafito
Roth, David	MD	Isolation and Characterization of a Vitamin D Responsive Gene	Dr. Henry Kronenberg
Sperber, David	MD	Magnetic Resonance Imaging of Intraocular Melanomas and Simulating Lesions	Dr. James Augsburger
Waldman, Richard	MD	Identification of Functional Regions on the I-A^b Molecule by Site-Directed Mutagenesis	Dr. Jonathan Seidman

1988

Student	Degree	Thesis Title	Thesis Supervisor
Bernstein, Paul	MD, PhD	Biochemistry and Pharmacology of Rhodopsin Regeneration in the Vertebrate Eye	Dr. Robert Rando
Brodey, Benjamin	MD	The Impact of AIDS on Large Massachusetts Corporations	Dr. Steven Gortmaker Dr. David Calkins
Cheung, Luke	MD	Sodium and Water-Suppressed Proton Nuclear Magnetic Resonance Spectroscopy of Normal and Neoplastic Tissues	Dr. Deborah Burstein Dr. Eric Fossell
Chung, Jay	MD, PhD	Regulation of the C-MYC Proto-Oncogene in Burkitt Lymphoma	Dr. Philip Leder
Cohen, David	MD, PhD	Studies of Biliary Lipid Secretion and Aggregation in Model and Native Biles	Dr. Martin Carey
Cohen, Steven	MD	Y-79 Retinoblastoma Cells Have Receptors for Vitamin D and Their Growth is Inhibited by Vitamin D *In Vitro and In Vivo*	Dr. Daniel Albert
Eagon, John	MD	Quantitative Frequency Analysis of the Electrogastrogram During Prolonged Motion Sickness	Dr. Charles Oman
Freed, Lisa	MD	An Enzymatic Bioreactor Based on Suspended Particles of Agarose-Immobilized-Heparinase	Dr. Robert Langer
Greenberg, Steven	MD	Neurokinin A in the Feline Trigeminovascular System	Dr. Michael Moskowitz
Haigh, Linda	MD	The Role of Cholesterol in Regulating Muscarinic Cholinergic and Beta Adrenergic Responsiveness in Cultured Chick Atrial Cells	Dr. Jonas Galper
Harbury, Lisa	MD	*In situ* Hybridization to Diagnose Leishmania	Dr. Dyann Wirth
Hey, Lloyd	MD	Health Status and Health Care in Greater Boston Adolescent Emergency Shelters: New Opportunities for Health Providers to Join the Team	Dr. Patricia McArdle

Student	Degree	Thesis Title	Thesis Supervisor
Lee, Raymond	MD	Efficacy and Preliminary Toxicity Testing of a New Blood Substitute	Dr. Gus Vlahakes
Leong, Rebecca	MD	The Effects of Acupuncture on the Hormonal Response to Stress	Dr. Bart Chernow
Levin, Leonard	MD, PhD	Immune Functions of Astrocytes	Dr. Howard Weiner
Lui, Eugene	MD, PhD	Transferrin Receptor Mediated Intoxication of Target Cells by a Transferrin-CRM45 Conjugate Toxin	Dr. Terry Strom
McFarland, Eric	MD, PhD	Nuclear Spin Transfer Studies of Chemical Reactions in Living Systems	Dr. Martin Kushmerick
Okada, Annabelle	MD	The Contribution of Mitochondria to Calcium Homeostasis in Cultured Heart Cells	Dr. Thomas Smith
Rogers, William	MD, PhD	Sequence Heterogeneity in the Kinetoplast DNA Mini-circle of *Leishmania* and Its Application to the Detection and Identification of *Leishmania*	Dr. Dyann Wirth
Saxberg, Bo	MD, PhD	A Theoretical Model for the Electrical Activity of the Heart	Dr. Richard Cohen
Sege, Robert	MD, PhD	Genetics Analysis of IDL Endocytosis: Molecular Characterization of Mutant and Revertant Cells	Dr. Monty Krieger
Senechek, David	MD	Lymphadenopathy and Aids	Dr. Donald Abrams
Spangler, Gregory	MD, PhD	Persistence of SV40-Derived Plasmids in Mice	Dr. David Livingston Dr. Thomas Benjamin
Spencer, Richard	MD, PhD	^{31}p NMR Spectroscopy Studies of Cardiac Energetics and Function in the Perfused Rat Heart	Dr. Joanne Ingwall
Stolpen, Alan	MD, PhD	Cytokine-Mediated Regulation of Endothelial Cell Morphology and Membrane Dynamics	Dr. David Golan Dr. Jordan Pober
Tan, Swee Lian	MD	Electron Spin Echo Spectroscopy of Ethanolamine Ammonia-Lyase, A Vitamin B12-Dependent Enzyme	Dr. William Orme-Johnson, III

1989

Student	Degree	Thesis Title	Thesis Supervisor
Aronow, Michael	MD	Characterization of a Rat Osteoblast-Like Culture System	Dr. Jane Lian
Baer, Margaret	MD	Molecular Analysis of Specific mRNA-Protein Interaction	Dr. Lee Gehrke
Bernstein, Howard	MD	Extracorporeal Enzymatic Heparin Removal: Use in a Sheep Dialysis Model	Dr. Robert Langer
Bienenstock, Arielle	MD	Role of Langerhans in T Cell Activation: Effect of Ultraviolet B. Irradiation	Dr. Jeanette Thorbecke
Bishai, William	MD, PhD	Diptheria Toxin Gene	Dr. John Murphy
Chang, Chin-Yen	MD	The Development of a System to Measure Electrode Impedances and the Electrical Characteristics of Neural Tissue Surrounding a Chronically Implanted Neural Signal Transducer	Dr. David Edell
Chueh, Henry	MD	Expert Knowledge Management System and Video Base	Dr. Octo Barnett Dr. William Beck
Diamandis, Peter	MD	The Artificial Gravity Sleeper: A Deconditioning Countermeasure for Long Duration Space Habitation	Prof. Laurence Young
Forman, Stuart	MD, PhD	Mechanism of Action of Anesthetics on the Function of the Post-Synaptic Cholinergic Ion Channel from *Torpedo Membrane Vesicles and Effects of n-alkanols on Receptor Function*	Dr. Keith Miller
Iwamoto, Satori	MD	Part I. "Characterizing a Region of Differential Splicing in the Duchenne Muscular Dystrophy Gene" Part II. "A Method for Producing Radiolabeled Probes via Polymerase Chain Reaction Amplification	Prof. Louis Kunkel
Janicek, Michael	MD	Defects in the Progression of the Lytic Cycle of a Herpes Simplex Virus Type I Mutant Lacking Both Copies of the Immediate-Early Gene for ICPO	Dr. David Knipe

Student	Degree	Thesis Title	Thesis Supervisor
Klickstein, Lloyd	MD, PhD	The Human C3b/C4b Receptor (CR1): A Polymorphic Protein Containing Long Homologous Repeats	Dr. Douglas Fearon
Kujovich, Jody	MD	Mechanism of Calcification of Bioprosthetic Heart Valves: Role of Phospholipids in the Initiation of the Process	Dr. Frederick Schoen
Lara, Maria Elena	MD	Assessment of Lung Sounds Measurement Techniques	Dr. Daniel Shannon
Liccini, Paul	MD	Cyclic AMP-Dependent Regulation of Glycerol Phosphate Dehydrogenase Expression in Neonatal Rat Oligodendrocyte Cultures	Dr. Jean De Vellis
Renshaw, Andrew	MD	Development of *in vivo* Testing and Applications of a Particulate Composite Bone Cement	Dr. Wilson Hayes
Selden, Richard	MD, PhD	The Regulation of Polypeptide Hormone Gene Expression and the Development of a Model Somatic Cell Gene Therapy System	Dr. Howard Goodman
Shafman, Timothy	MD	The Effects of Tiazofurin on the Induction of Mouse Erythroleukemia Cell Differentiation	Dr. Donald Kufe
Sorensen, Gregory	MD	Biochemical Correlation of the Magnetic Resonance Appearance of Cerebral Hemorrhage in the Rat	Dr. Bruce Rosen
Starr, Philip	MD, PhD	Synaptic Transmission in the Peripheral Auditory System	Dr. William Sewell
Stein, Lincoln	MD, PhD	Cloning of Developmentally Regulated Genes Schistosoma Mansoni	Dr. John David
Tannanbaum, James	MD	The Graphical Display of Laboratory Information	Dr. Howard Bleich

1990

Student	Degree	Thesis Title	Thesis Supervisor
Barnett, Faith	MD, PhD	Molecular Aspects of the Development and Regulation of Schwann Cells	Dr. Richard Sidman
Bogenschutz, Michael	MD	Molecular Analysis of MDR-Like Genes and RNA Transcripts in Drug-Resistant and Drug-Sensitive Strains of *Plasmodium Falciparum*	Dr. Dyann Wirth
Borud, Loren	MD	A Novel Strategy for Mapping Cytotoxic T Cell Epitopes of the gp160 Glycoprotein of the Human Immunodeficiency Virus	Dr. Malcolm Gefter
Canning, Susan	MD	Fine Mapping and Sequence Analysis of Deletions of the Retinoblastoma Gene	Dr. Thaddeus Dryja
Chen, Catherine	MD	Selective Degradation of T Cell Antigen Receptor Chains Retained in a Pre-Golgi Compartment	Dr. Richard Klausner
Chen, Diane	MD	Genetic Linkage Study of Two Neurodegenerative Motor-Sensory Diseases	Dr. Guy Rouleau
Chernoff, Daniel	MD, PhD	Kinetic Analysis of Local Anesthetic Binding to Sodium Channels	Dr. Gary Strichartz
Cudkowicz, Merit	MD	Neuropathological and Neurochemical Changes in the Cerebral Cortex in Huntington Disease Patients	Dr. Neil Rowall
Davis, Benjamin	MD	Construction of a CD4+ T Cell Line That Inducibly Expresses the HIV Transactivator Protein, TAT	Dr. William Haseltine
Doering, Elana	MD	Osmosis: Theories of Neutral Solvent Flow	Prof. Thomas Weiss
Francis, Howard	MD	Patterns of Innervation of Outer Hair Cells in the Chimpanzee	Dr. Nelson Kiang

Student	Degree	Thesis Title	Thesis Supervisor
Freese, Andrew	MD, PhD	Drug and Gene Delivery into the Central Nervous System: Implications for Neurological Diseases(MD Thesis) / Excitoxic Mechanisms in Huntington's Disease(PhD Thesis)	Dr. Robert Langer
Frohlich, Mark	MD	Enhanced Expression of the Protein-Kinase Substrate p36 in Human Hepatocellur Carcinoma	Dr. Jack Wands
Hajjar, Roger	MD	Calcium Responsiveness of Myofilaments in Cardiac Muscle: A Novel Approach of Characterizing Calcium Activation in Human Myocardium	Dr. Judith Gwathmey
Hurlbert, Anya	MD, PhD	The Computation of Color	Dr. Tomaso Poggio
Lebowitz, Howard	MD	A Comparison of Negative Impedance Ventilation with Conventional Mechanical Ventilation in a Rabbit Model	Dr. Chi-Sang Poon
Lee, Kathleen	MD	Accuracy of Computed Tomography in the Diagnosis of Abdominal Trauma: A Retrospective Evaluation	Dr. Robert Novelline
Lewin, John	MD	The Effect of Dietary Fatty Acid Composition on the Methyl and Methylene Proton NMR Line-widths in Rats	Dr. Eric T. Fossel
Lowy, Adam	MD	The Generation of Cytotoxic T Lymphocytes to the HIV-1 tat Protein	Dr. Man-Sun Sy

Student	Degree	Thesis Title	Thesis Supervisor
Mortensen, Eric	MD, PhD	Evaluation of Factors Affecting Hormone Binding (Insulin) and the Intrinsic Hormone Stimulated Tyrosine Kinase Activity Associated with the B Subunit of the Receptor	Dr. Guido Guidotti
Nastelin, Jennifer Green	MD	Pancreatic Islet Cell Transplantation: Optimization of Islet Cell Adhesion by Altering Polymer Surface Characteristics	Dr. Joseph Vacanti
Pierce, Eric	MD, PhD	Antibodies to and Studies of the X-Linked Chronic Granulomatous Disease Protein	Dr. Stuart Orkin
Powell, David	MD	NMR Studies of Sodium-Calcium Exchange in Perfused, Beating Frog Hearts	Dr. Eric Fossel
Saxberg, Bror	MD, PhD	A Modern Differential Geometric Approach to Shape from Shading	Dr. Tomaso Poggio
Sleckman, Barry	MD, PhD	Role of the CD4 Molecule in T Cell Activation	Dr. Steven Burakoff
Taratuta, Elena	MD	Statistical Properties of the Long-term Heart Rate Time Series	Dr. Richard Cohen
Wilson, Byron	MD	Antigenic Changes of Neoplastic Transformation	Dr. Jack Wands
Wolf, Nancy	MD	Hyperostosis and Bone Metabolism in Fishes	Dr. Julie Glowicki
Wu, Benson	MD	Oral Enzyme Treatment for Hyperbilirubinemia	Dr. Robert Langer
Yu, John	MD	Studies in the Molecular Pathogenesis: Linkage Analysis of Candidate Susceptibility Genes and RNA Accumulation Studies in Postmortem MS Brain Tissue	Dr. Stephen Hauser

Student	Degree	Thesis Title	Thesis Supervisor
		1991	
Appel, Marvin	MD, PhD	Closed-Loop Identification of Cardiovascular Regulatory Mechanisms	Dr. Richard Cohen
Blacklow, Stephen	MD, PhD	The Evolution of Improvements in Catalytic Efficiency: Mutants of the Enzyme Triosephosphate Isomerase	Dr. Jeremy Knowles
Chaudhry, Hina	MD	Laser-Induced Relaxation of Vascular Smooth Muscle	Dr. Irene Kochevar
Chen, Chinfei	MD, PhD	Voltage Dependent Calcium Channels in 3T3 Fibroblasts	Dr. Peter Hess
Daly, George	MD, PhD	Implicating the bcr/abl Gene in the Pathogenesis of Chronic Myelogenous Leukemia	Dr. David Baltimore
Eydelman, Malvina	MD	Concentrated Amblyopia Therapy at Threshold Stimuli with Auditory Reinforcement	Dr. Shirley Wray
Glaser, Thomas	MD, PhD	Genetic Linkage Analysis of Mouse Chromosomes 2,, 12 and 19	Dr. David Housman
Grund, Stephen	MD	Demonstration of Cooperation Between Adipocytes and Endothelial Cells in the Synthesis of Prostacyclin by Human Adipose Tissue	Dr. Lloyd Axelrod
Ko, Albert	MD, PhD	Immunological Aspects of Schistosomiasis	Dr. John David
Kuhn, Duncan	MD	Block of Hippocampal NMDA Receptor Responses by Tricyclic Antidepressants	Dr. Mark Mayer

Student	Degree	Thesis Title	Thesis Supervisor
Marroquin, Edmundo	MD	Control of Respiration Under Simulated Airway Compression	Dr. Chi-Sang Poon
Paik, Leo Seung Kon	MD	Interleukin-1B: Analysis of Structural and Functional Relationships	Dr. Lee Gehrke
Pearson, Gregory	MD, PhD	The Cholera Toxin Genetic Element: A Site-Specific Transposon	Dr. John Mekalanos
Sah, Robert	MD, PhD	Biophysical Regulation of Matrix Synthesis, Assembly and Degradation in Dynamically Compressed Calf Cartilage	Dr. Alan Grodzinsky
Shaw, Albert	MD, PhD	Molecular Genetic Analysis of the Membrane Immunoglobulin Antigen Receptor	Dr. Philip Leder
Slanetz, Priscilla	MD	Hemoglobin Blood Substitutes in Preoperative Autologous Blood Donation	Dr. Gus Vlahakes
Stelling, John	MD	Statistical Analysis of Quadratic Pressure-Flow Relationships in Intravenous Therapy	Dr. James Philip
Wang, Ming Xu	MD, PhD	Screening Genomes to Identify and Characterize DNA Sequences Involved in Strong DNA-Protein Interactions	Dr. George Church

1992

Student	Degree	Thesis Title	Thesis Supervisor
Barsotti, Martitia	MD, PhD	The Source of Proteins in the Aqueous Humor of the Eye	Dr. Roger Kamm
Bogan, Jonathan	MD	Genetic Mapping and Molecular Biology of the Human Y Chromosome	Dr. David Page
Brown, Gregory	MD, PhD	Load-Bearing Role of the Human Knee Meniscus	Prof. Derek Rowell
Cameron, Scott	MD, PhD	Analysis of the Gibbon Interleukin-3 Promotor Region Using In-vivo Genomic Footprinting	Dr. Bernard Mathey-Prevot
de la Torre, Ralph	MD	Intravascular Laser Induced Cavitation: A Study of the Mechanics with Possible Detrimental and Beneficial Effects	Dr. R. Rox Anderson
Dunn, James	MD, PhD	Development of a Bioartificial Liver	Dr. Martin Yarmush Dr. Ronald Tompkins
Goradia, Tushar	MD, PhD	Stochastic Models for Human Gene Mapping	Dr. William Bassert
Graham, Scot	MD	Enzyme and Size Profiles in Chronically Inactive Cat Soleus Muscle Fibers	Dr. Roland Roy
Hartman, Audrey	MD	Diffusion Coefficient of Protons in Compressed Cartilage	Dr. Deborah Burstein Dr. Martha Gray
Huang, George	MD	Design of Retroviral Vectors Transducing the Human β-globin Gene and Hypersensitive Site 2 Derivatives of the Locus Control Region of the Human β-globin Gene Cluster	Dr. Philippe LeBoulch
Johnston, S. Claiborne	MD	Species Specificity of the Interaction of LFA-1 with Intercellular Adhesion Molecules	Dr. Timothy Springer
Lee, Lawrence	MD	Retroviral Oncogene Induced Growth Deregulation of Murine Helper T Lymphocytes	Dr. Andrew Lichtman
Lee, Vivian	MD, PhD	Visual Impairment in Diabetic Oklahoma Indians	Dr. Elisa Lee

Student	Degree	Thesis Title	Thesis Supervisor
Marciniak, Robert	MD, PhD	Human Immunodeficiency Virus 1 Tat Protein: A Eukaryotic Processivity Factor	Dr. Phillip Sharp
McClellan, Mark	MD, PhD	Appropriateness of Care: A Comparison of Global and Outcome Methods to Set Standards	Dr. Robert Brook / Dr. Barbara McNeil
McKinstry, Robert	MD, PhD	Ultrafast NMR Imaging of Brin Water Mobility	Dr. Bruce Rosen
Murakawa, George	MD	Effects of Human Insulin Gene Expression on Endogenous Glucose Homeostasis in Transgenic Mice	Dr. Richard Selden
Nguyen, Ben	MD	Mechanism of Nitric Oxide and Cyclic GMP Inhibition of Signal Transduction in Activated Human Platelets	Dr. Edwin Salzman
Rago, Oscar	MD	Dynamics of Neutrophil Accumulation During Reperfusion of the Globally Ischemic Rabbit Heart	Dr. Lawrence Cohn
Reynolds, Dale	MD, PhD	The Molecular Biology of Mast Cell Preoteases and Additions Immunology	Dr. K. Frank Austen
Rokos, Ivan	MD	The Isolation and DNA-Sequencing of the Mouse α1 (IX) Collagen Gene for Use in Transgenic Mouse Experiments	Dr. Bjorn Olsen
Salant, Evan	MD	Surface Probe for Electrokinetic Detection of Cartilage Degeneration	Dr. Alan J. Grodzinsky
Tanaka, George	MD	Nuclear Magnetic Resonance Studies of Mannose Metabolism in the Normal and Diabetic Mammalian Lens	Dr. Hong-Ming Cheng
Tong, Lucene	MD	A Study of the Biological Chromophores in Human Arterial Wall	Dr. Michael Feld
Wu, Thomas	MD, PhD	Efficient Diagnosis of Multiple Disorders	Dr. Ramesh Patil / Dr. Peter Szolovits
Yang, Jane	MD	Molecular Mechanisms in the Regulation of Heme-Regulated e1F-2α Protein Kinase	Dr. Irving London / Dr. Jane-Jane Chen

1993

Student	Degree	Thesis Title	Thesis Supervisor
Badizadegan, Kamran	MD	Development and Partial Characterization of a Perfusion Culture System for Isolated Rat Hepatocytes	Dr. Martin Yarmush
Dutta, Sanjoy	MD	Prolonged Release of Local Anesthetics from a Biodegradable Matrix: *In Vitro and In Vivo* Characteristics	Dr. Charles Berde Dr. David Masters Dr. Robert Langer
Fernandez, Harold	MD	Cloning of Band 3-Related Anion Exchanger (AE3) from Human Heart	Dr. Seth Alper
Fleming, Mark	MD	Dominant Negative Mutants of Transcription Factor mXBP1	Dr. Laurie Glimcher
Frucht, Steven	MD	Biochemical Characterization of β-Amyloid in Alzheimer's Disease	Dr. Edward Koo
Gleit, Zachary	MD	Localization of Upstream Elements Responsible for the Regulation of Transcription of the Mouse Class-II MHC E_β Gene	Dr. Laurie Glimcher
Goldstein, Allan	MD	Stretch-Induced Hypertrophy of Primary Rat Skeletal Muscle Cells *In Vitro*	Dr. Seigo Izumo
Goodman, David	MD	The Influence of Age, Diagnosis and Gender on Proper Use of Metered Dose Inhalers	Dr. Jeffrey Drazen
Guyton, Gregory	MD	Measurement of Muscle Saturation in Free-Diving Weddell Seals Using a Dual-Wavelength NIR Spectrophotometer	Dr. Warren Zapol
Hahn, Samuel	MD	The Effects of Low Density Lipoproteins on Cell Proliferation and Extracellular Matrix mRNA Expression	Dr. Robert Lees
Helman, Joshua	MD	The Pathogenesis of Parathyroid Neoplasia: Towards Cloning a Novel Putative Oncogene and the Possible Role of the Parathyroid Hormone Receptor	Dr. Andrew Arnold
Huang, David	MD, PhD	Optical Coherence Tomography	Prof. James Fujimoto

Student	Degree	Thesis Title	Thesis Supervisor
Huertas, Pedro	MD, PhD	Modulation of Signal Transduction of the Insulin Receptor by the Lipid Membrane Environment	Dr. Joel Swanson
Labow, Brian	MD	The Effect of Interleukin-1 on the Metabolic Properties of Epiphyseal Cartilage	Dr. Martha Gray / Dr. Lee Gehrke
Lai, Amy	MD	Effects of Recombinant Human Interleukin-1 Beta and Mechanical Compression on the Physical and Metabolic Properties of Calf Epiphyseal Cartilage	Dr. Lee Gehrke / Dr. Martha Gray
Leffler, Christopher	MD	Noninvasive Evaluation and Mathematical Studies of Atrioventricular Nodal Function	Dr. Richard Cohen / Dr. J. Philip Saul
Li, Peter	MD	Characterization of the LIM Motif in the Presumptive Transcription Factor *lin-11* from *Caenorhabditis Elegans*	Prof. Christopher Walsh
McCue, Michael	MD, PhD	Electrical Activation of the Medical Olivocochlear Neuron Pool	Prof. John Guinan
Meyerson, Matthew	MD	Human Protein Kinesis Which Regulates Cell Division	Dr. Edward Harlow
Morse, Nicholas	MD	Evaluating the Effectiveness of Nephromancer: A Renal Pathology Tutorial for the Macintosh Computer	Dr. Bryan Bergeron
Naqvi, H. Faraz	MD	Type Specific Characterization of Matrix Metalloproteinases Secreted by Bovine Capillary Endothelial Cells with Isolation and Cloning of an Inhibitor	Dr. Marsha Moses / Dr. Robert Langer
Priebe, Gregory	MD	Efforts Towards Rational Drug Design: Multivalent Sialosides as Potential Inhibitors of Attachment of Influenza Virus	Prof. Jeremy Knowles
Pu, William	MD	Functional Analysis of the bZIP DNA-Binding Domain of Yeast GCN4	Dr. Kevin Struhl

Student	Degree	Thesis Title	Thesis Supervisor
Reiter, Evan	MD	The Effect of Olivocochlear Efferent Stimulation on Auditory Threshold Shifts Induced by Intense Tone Exposures	Dr. Charles Liberman
Roth, Heidi	MD	Recognition Memory in Amnesia: An Examination of Underlying Processes	Dr. Mieke Verfaellie
Sanger, Terence	MD, PhD	A Neural Network Technique for Adaptive Control of Distributed Nonlinear Systems	Prof. Emilio Bizzi
Song, Lucy	MD	Characterization of a Bradykinin Binding Site in PC12 Cells and Correlation of Binding with Phosphatidy-Inositol Turnover	Dr. Patrick Hogan
Tsai, Eugene	MD	Lymphocytes as Drug Carriers for MR Contrast Agents	Dr. Ralph Weissleder
Tseng, Elaine	MD	Sequence of the Murine Lymphocyte Function-Associated Molecule-1α Subunit and Its Expression in Cos Cells	Dr. Timothy Springer
Van Nice, Faith	MD, PhD	The Effect of Ortho-Hydrogen Concentration on the Nuclear Spin-Lattice Relaxation Rate of Carbon Monoxide at 4.2K	Dr. John Waugh
Vonderheide, Robert	MD	Very Late Antigen-4-Dependent Lymphocyte Adhesion to Vascular Cell Adhesion Molecule-1	Dr. Timothy Springer
Weaver, Yaffa	MD	A Variable Repetition Rate Picosecond Neodymium: YAG photodisruptor for Precision Intraocular Microsurgery	Dr. Carmen Puliafito
Wu, George	MD	Characterizations of the *In Vitro* and *In Vivo* Biocompatibility of Galactose-Derivatized Poly (Ethyleneoxide) as a Model Material for Hepatocyte Transplantation	Prof. Linda Cima
Wu, Samuel	MD	Use of Bi-Specific Heteroconjugated Antibody "Antigen Mimics" and T Cells with a Truncated Antigen Receptor ζ Chain to Explore the Mechanism of T Cell Activation	Dr. Jonathan Ashwell
Yang, Michael	MD	Hollow Fibers as Vehicles for Hepatocyte Transplantation	Dr. Donald Ingber

1994

Student	Degree	Thesis Title	Thesis Supervisor
Baraga, Joseph	MD, PhD	*In situ* Chemical Analysis of Biological Tissue: Vibrational Raman Spectroscopy of Human Atherosclerosis	Dr. Michael Feld Dr. Richard Rava
Burstein, Harold	MD, PhD	Regulation and Functions of Interleukin-4 During *in vivo* Immune Responses	Dr. Abul Abbas
Chin, Douglas	MD	Mechanisms of Impaired Immune Function Following Thermal Trauma: *in vitro Studies in a Murine Model*	Dr. John Mannick
Chin, Richard	MD	*In vivo* Determination of DNA Protein Interaction with *E. Coli:* A Global Approach Based on Methylation Patterns	Dr. George Church
Dang, Long	MD, PhD	An Analysis of Cell-Cell Interaction and Antigen Presentation by B Lymphocytes	Dr. Baruj Benacerraf
Flaherty, Alice	MD, PhD	Contributions of Motor and Somatosensory Cortex to Movement Control in the Primate Striatum	Dr. Ann Graybiel
Gipe, Robert	MD	The Loss of Nicotonic Receptor Responsiveness in PC-12 Pheochromocytomoa Cells Exposed to Reduced Extra-cellular Sodium	Dr. Greg Koski
Gozani, Shai	MD, PhD	Sensory Information Represented by a Class of Interneurons in the Cricket Cercal Sensory System	Dr. John Miller
Hadlock, Tessa	MD	The Interaction of a Local Anesthetic, Tetracaine, with Model Membranes: Equilibrium and Kinetic Studies Using Intrinsic Drug Fluorescence	Dr. Gary Strichartz
Hahn, William	MD, PhD	The Role of the CD2 Glycoprotein in T Cell Activation and Adhesion	Dr. Steven Burakoff
Hu, Kenneth	MD	Analysis of an Erythroid-Specific Enhancer Involved in the Transcriptional Control of the Human β-Globin Gene Cluster	Dr. Philippe LeBoulch

Student	Degree	Thesis Title	Thesis Supervisor
Huang, Philip	MD	The Localization of Transduction Channels in Mechanosensory Hair Cells	Dr. David Corey
Hung, Rebecca	MD, PhD	Applications of Photoacoustic Calorimetry to the Study of Transient Organic Intermediates	Dr. George Whitesides
Kaji, Eugene	MD, PhD	Regulation of Secretary Protein Transport from the Endoplasmic Reticulum	Dr. Harvey Lodish
Karp, Seth	MD	Molecular Cloning and Chromosomal Localization on the Key Subunit of the Human N-methyl-D-aspartate Receptor	Dr. M. Flint Beal
Kerrihard, Thomas	MD	The Epidemiology of Suicidal Ideation in AIDS	Dr. Alexandra Beckett
Kim, Young-Jo	MD, PhD	Effects of Compression on Cartilage Matrix Synthesis, Structure, and Processing: Physical Stimuli and Cellular Mechanisms	Dr. Alan Grodzinsky
Lee, Betty	MD	Use of a Single Strand Conformational Polymorphism to Delineate the Potential Link Between Mullerian Inhibiting Substance and Early Onset Ovarian Cancer	Dr. Patricia Donahoe
Li, Vincent	MD	Studies of Angiogenesis in Human Cancers: Detection, Activity, and Clinical Implications of an Angiogenic Factor (bFGF) in the Body Fluids of Cancer Patients	Dr. Judah Folkman
Maggard, Melinda	MD	Activated MIS Blocks Autophosphorylation of EGF Receptor: A Protein-Tyrosine Phosphatase Dependent Action	Dr. Patricia Donahoe
Malek, Adel	MD, PhD	Molecular Regulation of the Endothelial Cell by Fluid Shear Stress	Dr. Seigo Izumo
McGovern, Terence	MD	Retinal Blood Flow Determinations in the Diabetic Animal Model Using Video Fluorescein Angiography – The Role of Various Mediators in Flow Changes	Dr. Sven Bursell

Student	Degree	Thesis Title	Thesis Supervisor
Medoff, Benjamin	MD	Expression of Endothelial-Leukocyte Adhesion Molecules in Atherogenesis	Dr. Myron Cybulsky
Murphy, Elizabeth	MD	Investigation of Homologous Recombination Efficiency in Mammalian Cells	Dr. Tyler Jacks
Nohria, Anju	MD	Expression and Controlled Release of Interleukin-1 Receptor Antagonist	Dr. Robert Langer
Oscasio, Wendell	MD	Analysis of Fluctuations in Heart Rate and Blood Pressure	Dr. David Rigney
Oliver, James	MD, PhD	Analysis of Glomerular Permselectivity in the Rat Using Theoretical Models of Hindered Transport	Dr. William Deen
Satcher, Robert	MD, PhD	A Mechanical Model of Vascular Endothelium	Dr. C. Forbes Dewey
Stufflebeam, Steven	MD	Objective Detection and Localization of Multiple Sclerosis Lesions on Magnetic Resonance Brainstem Images: Correlation with Auditory Evoked Potentials	Dr. Robert Levine
Szal, Sara	MD	[Ca^2+]I Signaling in Pregnant Human Myometrium	Dr. Ellen Seely
Wilson, John	MD	The Mechanical Basis of Respiratory-Cardiovascular Interaction	Dr. J. Philip Saul
Wu, Mary	MD	*In Vivo* Versus *In Vitro Degradation of Controlled Release Polymers for Brain Tumor Therapy*	Dr. Robert Langer
Zhu, Henry	MD	The Effects of Ovarian Sex Steroids and Growth Factors in the Regulation of Myometrial and Leiomyoma Smooth Muscle Cell Proliferation and Extracellular Matrix Production	Dr. Romana Nowak

Student	Degree	Thesis Title	Thesis Supervisor
		1995	
Albers, Mark	MD, PhD	Mechanisms of Action of Immunosuppressive Agents	Prof. Stuart Schreiber
Celi, Ann	MD	Myocardial Ultrasonic Tissue Characterization Using the Autocorrelation Function	Dr. Richard Lee
Faryniarz, Deborah	MD	The Contractile Mechanisms in the Healing Medial Ligament: An Immunohistochemical and Ultrastructural Study in Rabbits	Dr. Myron Spector
Fogaça, Marcelo	MD	Cartilage Immunology and Transplantation	Dr. Joseph Vacanti
Frangioni, John	MD, PhD	Intracellular Characterization of Protein Tyrosine Photophase 1B Tumor Biology	Dr. Benjamin Neel
Helman, David	MD	Characterizations of a Myelin PO-Like cDNA Clone in the Central Nervous System	Dr. Stuart Lipton
Hung, Albert	MD, PhD	Regulation of Expression and Processing of the β-Amyloid Precursor Protein of Alzheimer's Disease	Dr. Dennis Selkoe
Ito, Keita	MD, ScD	Movement Induced Orientation of Collagen Fibers in Cartilaginous Tissues	Prof. Robert Mann
Kosowsky, Jeffrey	MD, PhD	Optimization with Smooth Dynamical Systems	Dr. Roger Brockett

Student	Degree	Thesis Title	Thesis Supervisor
Lee, ChenWei	MD	Mutational Analysis of the Parathyroid Hormone Receptor: An Examination into the Structural Basis of the Ligand-Receptor Interaction	Dr. Henry Kronenberg
Lee, Richard	MD	Studies of Skin Graft Rejection Using MHC Class II-Deficient and MHC-Deficient Mice	Dr. Hugh Auchincloss, Jr.
Lesperance, Leann	MD, PhD	Compositional Studies of Cartilage Matrix Using NMR Spectroscopy	Dr. Martha Gray
Lin, Herbert	MD, PhD	Expression Cloning and Characterization of the Type II and Type III TGF-Beta Receptors	Dr. Harvey Lodish
Martinez, Camilo	MD, PhD	Molecular Regulation of Corticotropin-Releasing Hormone Gene Expression by the Protein Kinase-A Pathway and Glucocorticoids	Dr. Joseph Majzoub
Mazzoni, Pietro	MD, PhD	Spatial Perception and Movement Planning in the Posterior Parietal Cortex	Dr. Richard Anderson
McHugh, John	MD	Photoaffinity Derivatized Local Anesthetics Which Label the Voltage-Dependent Sodium Channel	Dr. Gary Strichartz
Povsic, Thomas	MD	Syndecans Are Regulated by a cAMP Mediated Mechanism During Wound Repair	Dr. Merton Bernfield
Raman, Chitra	MD	Proton Diffusivity in Cartilage and Cartilage Macromolecules Using Nuclear Magnetic Resonance	Dr. Deborah Burstein

Student	Degree	Thesis Title	Thesis Supervisor
Rosario, Vernon	MD, PhD	Sexual Psychopaths: Doctors, Patients, and Novelists Narrating the Erotic Imagination in 19th-Century France	Dr. Arthur Kleinman
Saito, Yoriko	MD	The Role of Erythropoietin and Erythropoietin Receptor in the Pathogenesis of Murine and Human Erythroleukemia	Dr. Alan D'Andrea
Shaw, Stanley	MD, PhD	DNA Knotting In-vitro and In-vivo	Dr. James Wang
Smith, James	MD	A Biologically Plausible Model for Transparent Motion/Computational Neuroscience	Dr. Ellen Hildreth
Strauss, Eric	MD	Molecular Mechanisms Controlling GATA-1 Gene Expression and Globin Locus Control Region Function in Erythroid Cells	Dr. Stuart Orkin
Trob, Joshua	MD	Insulin Stimulation of MAP and S6 Kinases in Liver and Muscle of Intact Rat	Dr. C. Ronald Kahn
Wald, Heidi	MD	The Retina in Diabetes: Biochemical and Physiologic Markers of Dysfunction	Dr. Sven Bursell
Zhang, Kang	MD, PhD	Genetic and Molecular Studies of Macular Degeneration	Dr. Jonathan Seidman

Part 2—HST Ph.D. Thesis Titles by Year of Graduation

Name	Degree Yr	Thesis Title	Thesis Supervisor
Jonathan Valvano Professor, Electrical and Computer Engineering, University of Texas, Austin	9/1/81	The Use of Thermal Diffusivity to Quantify Tissue Perfusion	H. Frederick Bowman, Ph.D. MIT
Tamar Flash Associate Professor—Computer Science, Weizmann Institute of Science	6/1/83	Organizing Principles Underlying the Formation of Arm Trajectories	Emilio Bizzi, M.D. MIT
Dennis Orgill Assistant Professor of Surgery, HMS	6/1/83	The Effects of an Artificial Skin on Scarring and Contraction in Open Wounds	Ionnis V. Yannas, Ph.D. MIT
Ronald Tompkins John Francis Burke Professor of Surgery, HMS, Massachusetts General Hospital	6/1/83	*In Vivo* Transport of Low-Density Lipoprote in in the Arterial Walls of the Squirrel Monkey	Clark K. Colton, Ph.D. Kenneth A. Smith, Ph.D. MIT
Jose Venegas Assistant Professor of Anesthesia, HMS, Massachusetts General Hospital	6/1/83	Efficiency and Distribution of High Frequency Ventilation	Ascher H. Shapiro, Ph.D. Charles A. Hales, Ph.D. MIT
Edward Ingenito Assistant Professor of Medicine, HMS	2/1/84	Respiratory Fluid Mechanics and Heat Transfer	E. Regis McFadden, Jr., M.D. BWH
David Sebok Manager, Clinical Applications Development Picker International, Wayne, PA	2/1/84	The Membrane, Interstitium, Lymphatic System: A Model of Lung Water Dynamics	Edwin D. Trautman, Ph.D. HMS

Name	Degree Yr	Thesis Title	Thesis Supervisor
Anthony Patriarco Physician, Children's Medical Center, Martinsville, VA	6/1/84	The Prediction of Individual Muscle Forces During Human Movement	Robert W. Mann, Sc.D. MIT
Bruce R. Rosen Associate Professor of Radiology, HMS Director of Clinical NMR, Massachusetts General Hospital	6/1/84	NMR Chemical Shift Imaging	Alan C. Nelson, Ph.D. MIT
Joanne Donovan Assistant Professor of Medicine, HMS, Veterans Administration Medical Center Boston, MA	9/1/84	Quasielastic Light Scattering Studies of the Formation of Micelles of Human Apo lipoproteins A-I and A-II, Lecithins and Bile Salts	George B. Benedek, Ph.D. MIT
Elazer Edelman Associate Professor of Health Sciences and Technology, MIT Associate Professor of Medicine, HMS	9/1/84	Regulation of Drug Delivery from Porous Polymer Matrices Using Oscillating Magnetic Fields	Robert S. Langer, Sc.D. MIT
David Carley Research Associate Professor of Medicine, University of Illinois College of Medicine and Pharmacology	9/1/85	The Stability of Respiratory Control in Man: Mathematical and Experimental Analyses	Daniel C. Shannon, M.D. MGH
Zvi Ladin Associate Professor of BME Vice President, Clinical Applications and Regulatory Affairs, ESC Medical Systems, Yokneam, Israel	9/1/85	Set-Theoretic Analysis of Multi-Link Systems with Applications to Gait	Woodie C. Flowers, Ph.D. MIT

Name	Degree Yr	Thesis Title	Thesis Supervisor
Joseph Smith Assistant Professor of Medicine, Washington University	2/1/86	The Stochastic Nature of Cardiac Electrical Instability: Theory and Experiment	Richard J. Cohen, M.D., Ph.D.MIT
Deborah Burstein Associate Professor of Radiology, HMS, Beth Israel-Deaconess Medical Center	6/1/86	NMR Studies of Intracellular Sodium in the Perfused Frog Heart	Eric T. Fossel, Ph.D. BIH and HMS
Edward Cheal Director of Research and Development, Implants, Johnson & Johnson rofessional, Inc.	6/1/86	Trabecular Bone Remodeling Around Implants	Wilson C. Hayes, Ph.D. BIH and HMS
Paul Albrecht Vice President for Engineering, Cambridge Heart, Inc.	9/1/86	Stochastic Characterization of Chronic Ventricular Ectopic Activity	Roger G. Mark, M.D., Ph.D. MIT
Martha Gray Co-Director, HST Professor of HST and Electrical Engineering, MIT	9/1/86	Response to Mechanical Loading by Ephiphyseal Plate Chondrocytes	Alan J. Grodzinsky, Sc.D. MIT
Josep Valor-Sabatier Professor of Management Information Systems, University of Navarra, Barcelona, Spain	9/1/86	Mathematical Tools and Budgetary Mechanisms for Hospital Cost Control	Barbara J. McNeil, M.D. Regina Herzlinger, Ph.D. BWH and HMS
Nancy Allbritton Assistant Professor, University of California, Irvine	6/1/87	The Role of Calcium in the Destruction of Target Cells by Cytotoxic T Cells	Herman N. Eisen, M.D. MIT

Name	Degree Yr	Thesis Title	Thesis Supervisor
Eric McFarland Associate Professor of Chemical and Nuclear Engineering, University of California, Santa Barbara	6/1/87	Nuclear Spin Transfer Studies of Chemical Reactions in Living Systems	Martin J. Kushmerick, M.D., Ph.D. BWH
W. Mark Saltzman Professor, School of Chemical Engineering, Cornell University	6/1/87	A Microstructural Approach for Modeling Diffusion of Bioactive Macromolecules in Porous Polymers	Robert S. Langer, Sc.D. MIT
Robert Cothren, Jr. Project Staff, TRW Systems and Information, Walnut Creek, CA	9/1/87	Design and Development of a Multifiber Shielded Laser Catheter for Removal of Atherosclerotic Plaque	Michael S. Feld, Ph.D. MIT
Patrick Riley Technical Director, Biomotion Laboratory, Massachusetts General Hospital	2/1/88	Modeling of the Biomechanics of Posture and Balance	Robert W. Mann, Sc.D. MIT
Richard Spencer Chief, Nuclear Magnetic Resonance Unit, National Institute on Aging, NIH	6/1/88	31P Nuclear Magnetic Resonance Spectroscopy Studies of Cardiac Energetics and Function in the Perfused Rat Heart	Joanne S. Ingwall, Ph.D. BWH and HMS
Joseph T. Walsh, Jr. Associate Professor of Biomedical Engineering, Northwestern University	6/1/88	Pulsed Laser Ablation of Tissue: Analysis of the Removal Process and Tissue Healing	John A. Parrish, M.D. MGH and HMS
Jeffrey C. Lotz Assistant Professor of Orthopedics, University of California, San Francisco, Medical School	9/1/88	Hip Fracture Risk Predictions by X-Ray Computed Tomography	Wilson C. Hayes, Ph.D. BIH and HMS

Name	Degree Yr	Thesis Title	Thesis Supervisor
Martin Prince Co-Director, Division of MRI, University of Michigan Medical Center, Ann Arbor, MI	9/1/88	Selective Laser Ablation of Diseased Tissue: Investigations on a Safe Method of Opening Occluded Arteries	John A. Parrish, M.D. MGH and HMS
Cynthia Sung Senior Staff Fellow—BME and Instrumentation Program, National Institutes of Health, BEIP/NCRR, Bethesda, MD	2/1/89	A Study of Polyethelene Oxide-Polysiloxane Networks as Biomaterials for Drug Release	Edward W. Merrill, Ph.D. MIT
Mehmet Toner Associate Professor of Surgery (Bioengineering), HMS, Massachusetts General Hospital	2/1/89	Thermodynamics and Kinetics of Ice Nucleation Inside Biological Cells During Freezing: As Applied to Mouse Oocytes	Ernest G. Cravalho, Ph.D. MIT
Daniel M. Chernoff Clinical Instructor, University of California, San Francisco	6/1/89	Frequency Analysis of Catheter Systems Used for Invasive Blood Pressure Monitoring	Roger G. Mark, M.D., Ph.D. MIT
Kevin T. Powell Carle Clinic, Urbana, IL	6/1/89	Mammalian Cell Clonal Growth and Secretion Measurements Using Gel Microdroplets and Flow Cytometry	James C. Weaver, Ph.D. MIT
George R. Wodicka Associate Professor of Electrical and Computer Engineering, Purdue University	6/1/89	Acoustic Transmission in the Respiratory System	Daniel C. Shannon, M.D. MGH and HMS
Robert L.-Y. Sah Assistant Professor of Bioengineering, University of California, San Diego	2/1/90	Biophysical Regulation of Matrix Synthesis, Assembly, and Degradation in Dynamically Compressed Calf Cartilage	Alan J. Grodzinsky, Sc.D. MIT

Name	Degree Yr	Thesis Title	Thesis Supervisor
Charles Stearns Senior Physicist, Applied Science Laboratory, GE Medical Systems	2/1/90	Accelerated Image Reconstruction for a Cylindrical Positron Tomograph Using Fourier Domain Methods	Gordon L. Brownell, Ph.D. MIT
Martitia Barsotti Internal Medicine, Sansum Medical Center, Santa Barbara, CA	6/1/90	The Source of Proteins in the Aqueous Humor of the Eye	Roger D. Kamm, Ph.D. MIT
Gregory Brown Sports Medicine Fellow, University of Western Ontario, London, Ontario, Canada	6/1/90	Load-Bearing Role of the Human Knee Meniscus	Derek Rowell, Ph.D. MIT
Scott Greenwald Director of Research, Aspect Medical Systems, Inc., Natick, MA	6/1/90	Improved Detection and Classification of Arrhythmias in Noise-Corrupted Electrocardiograms Using Contextual Information	Roger G. Mark, M.D., Ph.D. MIT
Rebecca R. Richards-Kortum Associate Professor of Electrical Engineering, University of Texas, Austin	6/1/90	Fluorescence Spectroscopy as a Technique for Diagnosis of Pathologic Conditions in Human Arterial, Urinary Bladder, and Gastro-Intestinal Tissues	Michael S. Feld, Ph.D. MIT
Jonathan Bliss Senior Development Scientist Ascent Technology, Inc., Pullman, WA	2/1/91	Rapid Determination of Antimicrobial Susceptibility Using Gel Microdroplets and Flow Cytometry	James C. Weaver, Ph.D. MIT
Natacha DePaola Assistant Professor of Biomedical Engineering, Rensselaer Polytechnic Institute	2/1/91	Focal and Regional Responses of Endothelium to Disturbed Flow In Vitro.	C. Forbes Dewey, Ph.D. MIT

Name	Degree Yr	Thesis Title	Thesis Supervisor
Brent Foy Assistant Professor, Physics Department, Wright State University, Dayton, OH	6/1/91	NMR Characterization of Interstitial Myocardial Sodium	Deborah Burstein, Ph.D. BIH and HMS
Lyle Borg-Graham Postdoctoral Fellow, Institut Alfred Fessand, France	2/1/92	On Directional Selectivity in Vertebrate Retina: An Experimental and Computational Study	Tomaso Poggio, Ph.D. MIT
Michael Buschmann Assistant Professor, Ecole Polytechnique, University of Montreal, Institute of Biomedical Engineering, Montreal, Canada	2/1/92	Chondrocytes in Agarose Culture: Development of a Mechanically Functional Matrix, Biosynthetic Response to Compression, and Molecular Model of the Modulus	Alan J. Grodzinsky, Sc.D. MIT
James Dunn Research Fellow, University of California, Department of Surgery, Los Angeles, CA	6/1/92	Development of a Bioartificial Liver	Martin Yarmush, M.D., Ph.D. MGH and HMS
Howard M. Loree, II Research and Development Scientist, Thermo Cardiosystems, Woburn, MA	6/1/92	The Mechanics of Atherosclerotic Plaque Rupture	Roger D. Kamm, Ph.D. MIT
Marvin Appel Cardiac Anesthesiologist	6/3/92	Closed Loop Identification of Cardiovascular Regulatory Mechanisms	Richard J. Cohen, M.D., Ph.D. MIT

Name	Degree Yr	Thesis Title	Thesis Supervisor
Andrew Freese Chief Resident in Neurosurgery, Hospital of University of Pennsylvania	6/3/92	Excitotoxic Mechanisms in Huntington's Disease	Joseph B. Martin, M.D., Ph.D. MGH and HMS
Joseph Baraga Transitional Medicine Internship, Department of Radiology, University of Minnesota, Minneapolis, MN	9/1/92	*In Situ* Chemical Analysis of Biological Tissue: Vibrational Raman Spectroscopy of Human Atherosclerosis	Michael S. Feld, Ph.D. MIT
David Huang Resident, Cardiac Unit, MGH	5/28/93	Optical Coherence Tomography	James G. Fujimoto, Ph.D. MIT
James Oliver Resident, Department of Medicine, Walter Reed Army Medical Center Washington, DC	6/3/93	Analysis of Glomerular Permselectivity in the Rat Using Theoretical Models of Hindered Transport	William M. Deen, Ph.D. MIT
Tai Sing Lee Assistant Professor, Carnegie Mellon University, Center for Neural Basis Cognition, Mellon Institute, Pittsburgh, PA	6/10/93	Surface Inference by Minimizing Energy Functionals: A Computational Framework for the Visual Cortex	David Mumford, Ph.D. HU

Name	Degree Yr	Thesis Title	Thesis Supervisor
Kathleen Donahue Assistant Professor of Biophysics, Biophysics Research Institute, Medical College of Wisconsin	9/15/93	Studies of Gd-DTPA Relaxivity and Proton Exchange Rates in Tissue with Implications for MR Imaging of Regional Myocardial Perfusion	Deborah Burstein, Ph.D. BIH and HMS
Leann Lesperance Resident in Pediatrics, Children's Hospital, Boston, MA	9/15/93	Compositional Studies of Cartilage Matrix Using NMR Spectroscopy	Martha L. Gray, Ph.D. Deborah Burstein, Ph.D. MIT, BIH and HMS
Michael McCue Resident in Neurosurgery	9/15/93	Acoustic Responses from Primary Vestibular Neurons	John J. Guinan, Ph.D. MEEI and HMS
Amy Corinne Courtney Project Scientist, BME, Cleveland Clinic Foundation, Cleveland, OH	5/27/94	Mechanical Properties of the Proximal Femur: Changes with Age	Thomas A. McMahon, Ph.D. HU
Bernard Fine House Staff, Division of Hematology, Stanford School of Medicine, Stanford, CA	5/27/94	Light Scattering by Aqueous Protein Solutions that Exhibit Liquid-Liquid Phase Separation	George B. Benedek, Ph.D. MIT
Edward Guo Assistant Professor, Department of Mechanical Engineering Columbia University, NY, NY	5/27/94	Fatigue of Trabecular Bone: High Cycle Microcrack Propagation Versus Low Cycle Creep	Thomas A. McMahon, Ph.D. HU

Name	Degree Yr	Thesis Title	Thesis Supervisor
Keita Ito Research Staff, AO/ASIF Research Institute Switzerland	5/27/94	Movement-Induced Orientation of Collagen Fibrils in Cartilaginous Tissues	Robert W. Mann, Sc.D. MIT
Adel M. Malek Clinical Fellow in Surgery, HMS, Brigham and Women's Hospital, Boston, MA	5/27/94	Functional and Molecular Characterization of the Vascular Endothelial Response to Fluid Shear Stress	Seigo Izumo, M.D. BIH and HMS
Teung Shen Medical Student, Mount Auburn Hospital, Cambridge, MA	5/27/94	Superparamagnetic Contrast Agents for Magnetic Resonance Imaging	Thomas J. Brady, M.D. MGH and HMS
Daniel K. Sodickson Postdoctoral Fellow, Cardiovascular Division, Beth Israel Deaconess Medical Center, Boston, MA	5/27/94	Spin-Spin Couplings in Two Limits: Experimental, Theoretical, and Computational Studies of Dipole-Coupled Nuclear Spins in Solids	John S. Waugh, Ph.D. MIT
Frank J. Rybicki, III Resident, Radiology Department, Brigham and Women's Hospital, Boston, MA	6/1/94	A Novel Encoding Technology for Magnetic Resonance Imaging (MRI)	Samuel Patz, Ph.D. BWH and HMS
Mickey Bhatia J.P. Morgan and Company, Inc., Corporate Risk Management Group, New York, NY	9/1/94	Wavelet Transform-Based Multi-Resolution Techniques for Tomographic Reconstruction and Detection	Allan S. Willsky, Ph.D. MIT

Name	Degree Yr	Thesis Title	Thesis Supervisor
Julie E. Greenberg Research Scientist, Research Lab of Electronics, Massachusetts Institute of Technology	9/1/94	Improved Design of Microphone-Array Hearing Aids	Patrick M. Zurek, Ph.D. MIT
Antony Hodgson Assistant Professor, , Department of Mechanical Engineering, University of British Columbia Vancouver, British Columbia, Canada	9/1/94	Inferring Central Motor Plans from Attractor Trajectory Measurements	Neville Hogan, Ph.D. MIT
Stephen Robinovitch Director, Biomechanics Research Laboratory, Orthopedic Surgery, San Francisco General Hospital, San Francisco, CA	9/1/94	Hip Fracture and Fall Impact Biomechanics	Wilson C. Hayes, Ph.D. BIH and HMS
Lisa Shieh Intern, Department of Medicine, Stanford University Stanford, CA	2/1/95	Erosion and Release from Biodegradable Polyanhydrides	Robert S. Langer, Sc.D. MIT
Jerrold L. Boxerman Intern, Radiology Department, Johns Hopkins Hospital, Baltimore, MD	6/8/95	Non-Invasive Measurement of Physiology Using Dynamic Susceptibility Contrast NMR Imaging	Robert M. Weisskoff, Ph.D. MGH and HMS

Appendix F

MAJOR RESEARCH PROJECTS

Harvard—MIT Division of Health Sciences and Technology
Funded Research and Principal Investigators
by Academic Years

Title	PI	Years
Metabolism of the Erythrocyte (Hemoglobin Synthesis and Hematopoiesis)	London, I.M., M.D.	1972 –
Biomaterials Science	Mann, R.W., Sc.D.	1972 – 78
Rehabilitation Engineering Center	Berenberg, W., M.D. Mann, R.W., Sc.D.	1973 – 91
Nursing Home Telemedicine	Mark, R.G., M.D., Ph.D.	1974 –
Nuclear Techniques in Medicine	Adelstein, S.J., M.D., Ph.D.	1975 – 78
Optimization of Dose Distribution in Cancer Radiation Therapy	Levine, M., M.D. Bjarngard, B.E., Ph.D.	1975 – 83
Medical Radiological Physics Training	Bjarngard, B.E., Ph.D.	1975 – 82
A Portable System for Real-Time Arrhythmia Analysis	Mark, R.G., M.D., Ph.D.	1975 – 85
Biomedical Engineering Center for Clinical Instrumentation	Mark, R.G., M.D., Ph.D.	1976 – 80
Harvard-MIT Program in Short-Lived Radiopharmaceuticals	Adelstein, S.J., M.D., Ph.D.	1977 – 92
Thromboresistant Materials	Salzman, E.W., M.D. Rosenberg, R.D., M.D., Ph.D.	1977 –
Studies on Conduction in Demyelinated Central Axons in situ	Waxman, S.G., M.D.	1977 – 80
Cryopreservation of the Isolated Rat Heart	Cravalho, E.G., Ph.D.	1977 – 80
Corneal Curvature by Electrical Heating	Olson, W.H., Ph.D. Benedek, G.B., Ph.D.	1978 – 80

Title	PI	Years
Control of Protein Synthesis	Levine, D.H., Ph.D. Gehrke, L., Ph.D.	1978 –
Environmental Health Sciences Center	Wogan, G.N., Ph.D.	1978 –
Environmental Health Sciences Program	Thilly, W.G., Ph.D.	1978 – 84
A Computer System for 2 and 3 Dimensional Imaging	Osborne, L.S., Ph.D.	1979 – 80
Mapping Hypoxic Regions of the Retina	Shapiro, A.H., Sc.D. Olson, W.H., Ph.D.	1979 – 80
Measures of Mental Workload	Tole, J.R., Sc.D.	1979 – 80
Instrumentation for Clinical Vestibular Testing	Young, L.R., Sc.D.	1979 – 82
Antigen-Antibody Agglutination	Cohen, R.J., M.D., Ph.D.	1979 – 82
CDTI Crew Function Assessment	Tole, J.R., Sc.D.	1979 – 83
Harvard-MIT Biomedical Engineering Center	Mark, R.G., M.D., Ph.D.	1979 –
Measurement of Perfusion from Tissue Thermal Properties	Bowman, H.F., Ph.D.	1979 –
Bedside Arrythmia Monitor – Evaluation	Mark, R.G., M.D., Ph.D.	1979 –
Myocardial Perfusion Scintigraphy Using the Mesh Chamber	Osborne, L.S., Ph.D.	1979 –
An Ultrasonic Phased Array for Localized Hyperthermia	Cravalho, E.G., Ph.D.	1980 – 81
Oculomotor Function in Patients	Kenyon, R.V., Ph.D.	1980 – 81
Phase Behavior of Lens Cell Cytoplasm in Cataract	Clark, J.I., Ph.D.	1980 – 81

Title	PI	Years
Treatment of Tumors by Hyperthermia	Lele, P.P., M.D., Ph.D.	1980–82
Continuous MS Monitoring of Liver Alcohol Metabolism	Brunengraber, H., M.D., Ph.D.; Weaver, J.C., Ph.D.	1980–83
A New Approach to the Analysis of Radiopharmaceuticals	Jones, A.G., Ph.D.; Davison, A., Ph.D.	1980–83
Application of Immobilized Hydrogenase for Heavy Water	Weaver, J.C., Ph.D.; Klibanov, A.M., Ph.D.	1980–83
Non-Invasive Blood Perfusion Measurements	Bowman, H.F., Ph.D.	1980–84
Fracture and Viscoelastic Characteristics of the Human Cervical Spine	Hayes, W.C., Ph.D.	1980–
Instrumentation for Clinical Vestibular Testing	Young, L.R., Sc.D.	1980–84
Beat-to-Beat Fluctuations in ECG and Hemodynamic Parameters	Cohen, R.J., M.D., Ph.D.	1980–86
Autonomic Regulation/Cardiopulmonary	Shannon, D.C., M.D.	1980–90
The Effects of 60 Hz Magnetic Fields on Bovine Embryos	Nelson, A.C., Ph.D.; Frankel, E.G., Ph.D.	1981
Development of Non-Invasive Instruments for Dark Adaptation	Soloman, N.; Tole, J.R., Sc.D.	1981
Molecular Basis of Globin Gene Expression	Tuan, D.Y., Ph.D.	1981–82
Use of Autoradiographic Methods for Physiologic Disposition	Elmaleh, D.R., Ph.D.	1981–82

Title	PI	Years
Thermal Dosimetry and Blood Flow Measurements for Hyperthermia	Bowman, H.F., Ph.D. Lele, P.P., M.D., Ph.D.	1981–82
Regulation of Protein Synthesis by Double-Stranded RNA	Levine, D.H., Ph.D.	1981–83
Effect of Hemin on Adipocyte	Chen, J.J., Ph.D.	1981–84
Interdisciplinary Research on Biophysical and Biological Mechanisms	Grodzinsky, A., Sc.D.	1981–84
A Random Process Model for Atrial Fibrillation	Cohen, R.J., M.D., Ph.D.	1981–84
Development of a Chronic Multiplexed Nerve Electrode	Edell, D.J., Ph.D.	1981–84
Quantitative Formulations of Wolff's Law in Trabecular Bone	Hayes, W.C., Ph.D.	1981–
Phase I Evaluation of Equipment for Hyperthermia Treatment of Cancer	Lele, P.P., M.D., Ph.D.	1981–
Mechanisms of Ventricular Fibrillation	Cohen, R.J., M.D., Ph.D.	1981–
Study of Diesel Exhaust Exposure in Railroad Workers	Speizer, F.E., M.D.	1981–
Gel Microdroplets for Microbiology	Weaver, J.C., Ph.D.	1981
New Approach to the Analysis of Radiopharmaceuticals	Jones, A.G., Ph.D.	1981–
Growth of Heart Cells in Tissue Culture	Mark, R.G., M.D., Ph.D.	1981–
High Resolution Track Etch Autoradiography in Neutron…	Brownell, G.L., Ph.D.	1982–83
Tissue Oxygen Flow Probe Development	Bowman, H.F., Ph.D. Weaver, J.C., Ph.D.	1982–83
256 Electrode Integrated Circuit Cell Culture Array	Edell, D.J., Ph.D.	1982–84

Title	PI	Years
Myocardial Perfusion Scintigraphy Using the Mesh Chamber (Fabrication of Equipment)	Osborne, L.S., Ph.D.	1982 – 84
Studies in Tissue Transport	Weaver, J.C., Ph.D.	1982 – 84
Research in Neural Prostheses	Edell, D.J., Ph.D.	1982 – 84
Study of N-Particle Distribution for Macromolecular Aggregates	Cohen, R.J., M.D., Ph.D.	1982 – 84
Role of Protein Phosphorylation in Regulation of Adipose Tissue	Chen, J.J., Ph.D.	1982 – 84
Neutron Capture Therapy	Brownell, G.L., Ph.D.	1982 – 85
Stress Morphology Relations for Trabecular Bone *in vivo*	Hayes, W.C., Ph.D.	1982 –
Tumor Hyperthermia: Science, Technology, and Evaluation	Bowman, H.F., Ph.D.	1982 –
Transcutaneous Blood Gas, pH and Cardiac Output	Weaver, J.C., Ph.D.	1982 –
Spatial Mapping of Enzymes	Weaver, J.C., Ph.D.	1982 –
Cryopreservation of Organs	Cravalho, E.G., Ph.D.	1982 –
Bovine Embryo Transfer Technology	Cravalho, E.G., Ph.D.	1982 –
An HMO for Nursing Home Patients	Mark, R.G., M.D., Ph.D.	1982 –
Studies in Microbiology	Weaver, J.C., Ph.D.	1983 – 84
Non-Traumatizing, Acc. Transcutaneous Blood Gas Interface	Weaver, J.C., Ph.D.	1983 – 84
Development and Evaluation of an Auditory Prosthesis Based on Thin Film Technology	Edell, D.J., Ph.D.	1983 – 84

Title	PI	Years
Stress Morphology Relations for Trabecular Bone *in vivo*	Hayes, W.C., Ph.D.	1983 – 84
Non-Invasive Assessment of Cardiorespiratory Function and Regulation by Mathematical Analysis of Periodic Waveforms	Cohen, R.J., M.D., Ph.D.	1983 – 84
Control of Protein Synthesis in Normal and Interferon-Treated Cells	London, I.M., M.D. Thomas, S., Ph.D.	1983 – 85
Modulation of mRNA Structure by mRNA Binding Proteins	Gehrke, L., Ph.D.	1983 – 86
Environmental Health Sciences Center	Wogan, G.N., Ph.D.	1983 – 88
Structural Proteins in Bioprosthetic Valve Clarification	Nelson, A.C., Ph.D.	1983 – 88
Regulating Gene Expression	Gehrke, L. Ph.D.	1983 –
Regulation of Gene Expression in Plants Structure of Messenger RNA	Gehrke, L., Ph.D.	1983 –
The Regulation of Gene Expression in Normal Cellular Differentiation and Human Leukemia Cells	London, I.M., M.D.	1983 –
Measurement of the Temporal Evaluation of Cluster Size Distributions of Latex Microspheres Undergoing Antigen Antibody Agglutination Reactions	Benedek, G.B., Ph.D. Cohen, R.J., M.D., Ph.D.	1983 –
Mathematical Analysis of Short Term Fluctuations in Cardiorespiratory Parameters: A New Clinical Diagnostic Tool	Cohen, R.J., M.D., Ph.D.	1983 –
Cancer Hyperthermia: Temperature, Perfusion, Oxygen Profilometer	Bowman, H.F., Ph.D.	1983 –
Physical Forces in Skeletal Growth and Development: Quantification	Lee, R., M.D., Ph.D.	1983 –
Development of a Centralized Consistent-Environment Base for Computerized Analysis of Nucleic Acid Sequence Data	Gehrke, L., Ph.D.	1983

Title	PI	Years
Interleukin I	Gehrke, L., Ph.D. Auron, P.E., Ph.D.	1983 – 88
Electrode Arrays Based on Thin Film Technology	Edell, D.J., Ph.D.	1983 –
Instrumental Research for Biotech. Data Acquisition from Gel Micro	Weaver, J.C., Ph.D.	1984 – 85
Cardiorespiratory Stress Physiology	Cohen, R.J., M.D., Ph.D.	1984 – 85
Harvard-MIT Rehabilitation Engineering Center	Mann, R.W., Sc.D.	1984 – 92
Measurement of Perfusion from Tissue Thermal Properties	Bowman, H.F., Ph.D.	1984 – 88
Myocardial Perfusion Scint. Using a New Technique	Osborne, L.S., Ph.D.	1984 – 87
Program Project in Thrombosis and Artherosclerosis	Rosenberg, R., Ph.D.	1984 – 92
High Level Visual Functions in the Aged: Comp. Anal.	Vaina, L.M., Ph.D., Sc.D.	1984 – 87
Cluster Size Distrib. In Polymers and Coll.	Cohen, R.J., M.D., Ph.D.	1984 – 87
Sorting Methods for More Sensitive Arrhythmia Analysis	Mark, R.G., M.D., Ph.D.	1984 – 88
Role of Physical Forces in the Control Skeletal Growth and Development	Lee, R., M.D., Ph.D.	1985 –
Implantation of the Cochlear Nerve	Edell, D.J., Ph.D.	1985 –
Analysis of Beat-to-Beat Fluctuations in Electrocardiogram	Cohen, R.J., M.D., Ph.D.	1985 – 86
Mechanical Control of Vasc. Tissue Structure-Composition	Lee, R., M.D., Ph.D.	1985 – 86
Systems Analysis of Cardiorespiratory Control	Cohen, R.J., M.D., Ph.D.	1985 – 87
The Bone Absorptiometer	Osborne, L.S., Ph.D.	1985 – 87

Title	PI	Years
Automated Screening for Hyperproduction of Amino Acids	Weaver, J.C., Ph.D.	1985 – 87
Rapid Biodetection: A New Approach	Weaver, J.C., Ph.D.	1985 – 88
Enhan. Transtat. or Engin. Plant Messenger RNA	Gehrke, L., Ph.D.	1985 – 88
Tactile Substitution Using Neural Interface	Edell, D.J., Ph.D.	1985 – 88
Analysis of Biochemical Activity in Small Volumes	Weaver, J.C., Ph.D.	1985 – 88
Thromboresistant Materials	Salzman, E.W., M.D.	1985 – 88
Ident. And Char. Of Trancription Enhancer Sequencer	Tuan, D.Y., Ph.D.	1985 – 88
Therapeutic Laser-Tissue Interaction	Parrish, J.A., M.D.	1985 –
Closed-Loop Evaluation of the Baro-Receptor Reflex	Saul, J.P., M.D.	1986 – 87
Microbial Measurement and Manipulation Gel Micro	Weaver, J.C., Ph.D.	1986 – 87
Interfragmentary Strain Hypothesis and Fract. Healing	White, A.A., Ph.D.	1986 – 88
Advanced ECG Signal Proc. and Arrhythmia Analysis	Mark, R.G., M.D., Ph.D.	1986 – 91
Stochastic Analysis of Ventricular Beat Generation	Cohen, R.J., M.D., Ph.D.	1986 – 89
Regulation of the Human Interleukin-1 Gene	Fenton, M., Ph.D. Auron, P.E., Ph.D.	1986 – 89
Study of Electroporation Using Individual Cells	Weaver, J.C., Ph.D.	1986 – 90
Study of Human Interleukin Gene Expression	Fenton, M., Ph.D. Gehrke, L., Ph.D.	1986 – 90

Title	PI	Years
Expression and Regulation of Human Interleukin 1	Clark, B. Ph.D. / Auron, P.E., Ph.D.	1986 – 90
Gas Scintillation Proport. Camera for Nuclear Cardiology	Lanza, R.C., Ph.D.	1986 – 90
Analysis of Radiopharmaceuticals	Jones, A.G., Ph.D.	1987 – 88
Regulation of Protein Synthesis	London, I.M., M.D.	1987 – 88
Ambulatory Monitoring, Nonlinear Dynamics and Sudden Cardiac Death	Mark, R.G., M.D., Ph.D.	1987 – 88
Olfactory Nerve Microsensors for Detection of Explosives	Sinskey, A.J., Sc.D. / Edell, D.J., Ph.D.	1987 – 89
Cardiac Electrical Instability	Mark, R.G., M.D., Ph.D.	1987 – 89
Biochemical Activity	Weaver, J.C., Ph.D.	1987 – 88
Interfacial Heart Mass Transfer Cryopreservation	Cravalho, E.G., Ph.D.	1987 – 89
Protective Coatings	Edell, D.J., Ph.D.	1987 – 90
Physical Improvements for SPECT Imaging	Lanza, R.C., Ph.D.	1987 – 90
Erythroid Specific Enhancer	London, I.M., M.D.	1987 – 91
Regulation of Growth and Different./Interfer.	London, I.M., M.D.	1987 – 91
Control of Protein Synthesis	Levin, D.H., Ph.D.	1987 – 92
Chondrocyte Biosynthesis	Gray, M.L., Ph.D.	1988 – 89
Implantable Ocular Pressure Transducer	Kamm, R.G., Ph.D.	1988 – 89

Title	PI	Years
Tumor Hyperthermia	Bowman, H.F., Ph.D.	1988 – 89
Studies on the Mechanism of Differential Messgr. RNA	Gehrke, L., Ph.D.	1988 – 89
Lipoprotein Metabolism	Lees, R.L., Ph.D.	1988 – 89
Mechanical Ventilation of Infants	Poon, C.S., Ph.D.	1988 – 90
Beat-to-Beat Blood Pressure	Mark, R.G., M.D., Ph.D.	1988 – 90
Mechanisms in Respiratory Control	Mark, R.G., M.D., Ph.D.	1988 – 89
VA/Q Distribution in the Lung	Mark, R.G., M.D., Ph.D.	1988 – 89
Human B-Globin Gene	Tuan, D.Y., Ph.D.	1988 – 91
Growth of Cartilage *in vitro*, Role of Mechanical Forces	Gray, M.L., Ph.D.	1988 – 91
Cluster-size Distributions	Cohen, R.J., M.D., Ph.D.	1988 – 91
Very Rapid Biodetection: A New Approach	Weaver, J.C., Ph.D.	1988 – 91
A Fundamental Investigation of Electroporation	Weaver, J.C., Ph.D.	1988 – 93
Beat-to-Beat Modulation of Autonomic Function	Cohen, R.J., M.D., Ph.D.	1988 – 93
Analysis of Human Interleukin 1B	Gehrke, L., Ph.D.	1989 – 90
Growth and Differentiation by Interferon	London, I.M., M.D.	1989 – 91
Interactions of Electromagnetic Fields	Grodzinsky, A.J., Sc.D.	1989 – 90
Articular Cartilage and IL-1B	Gehrke, L., Ph.D.	1989 – 90

Title	PI	Years
Cartilage Matrix Metabolism	Grodzinsky, A.J., Sc.D.	1989 – 90
Pre-operative Evaluation System	Rennels, G.D., Ph.D.	1989 – 90
Selective MRNA Translation	Gehrke, L., Ph.D.	1989 – 90
Fabricated Equipment-Cardiac Conduction	Cohen, R.J., M.D., Ph.D.	1989 – 90
Mechanisms in Respiratory Control	Poon, C.S., Ph.D.	1989 – 90
Extracorporeal Removal of LDL	Lees, R.S., Ph.D.	1989 – 90
Regulation of ELF-2 Kinase by HEME	Gehrke, L., Ph.D.	1989 – 91
Fabricated Equipment-tissue Compression System	Gray, M.L., Ph.D.	1989 – 91
Extracorporal Removal of Low Density Lipoproteins	Langer, R.S., Sc.D.	1989 – 92
Pre-operative Evaluation System	Rennels, G.D., Ph.D.	1989 – 92
The Development of Bone-bioerodible Polymer Matrices	Laurencin, C.T., M.D., Ph.D.	1989 – 92
Beat-to-Beat Variability in Hemo-dynamic Parameters	Cohen, R.J., M.D., Ph.D.	1989 – 94
Effects of Gamma Radiation on Biomed. Polymers	Laurencin, C.T., M.D., Ph.D.	1990 – 91
Atherosclerotic Plaque Rupture	Grodzinsky, A.J., Sc.D.	1990 – 91
Immunoassay and Antigen Recognition	Cohen, R.J., M.D., Ph.D.	1990 – 91
Selective MRNA Translation	Gehrke, L., Ph.D.	1990 – 91
Polysomnographic Database	Mark, R.G., M.D., Ph.D.	1990 – 91

Title	PI	Years
The Aberr. Cell: Imp. For Radioph. Design	Jones, A.G., Ph.D.	1990 –
Regulation of FGF by FGF, etc.	Langer, R.S., Sc.D.	1990 – 91
Human Erythroid Specific Enhancer	London, I.M., M.D.	1990 – 91
Biomaterials for Insulation of Implantable Electrodes	Edell, D.J., Ph.D.	1990 – 93
Development of a Polysomno Graphic Database on Colin CD-ROM	Mark, R.G., M.D., Ph.D.	1990 – 91
Mechanism of Adaptation to Dietary Manipulation in Space	Young, V.R., Ph.D.	1990 – 91
Burn Metabolism	Young, V.R., Ph.D.	1990 – 91
A Possible Weak Electromag. Field Interaction	Weaver, J.C., Ph.D.	1990 – 91
Release of Intracellular Interleukin 1B by Membrane	Gehrke, L., Ph.D.	1990 –91
Molecule Counting Immunoassay	Cohen, R.J., M.D., Ph.D.	1990 – 91
Biomaterials	Edell, D.J., Ph.D.	1990 – 92
Tomographic Image Enhance from Degraded Projections	Poon, C.S., Ph.D.	1990 – 93
Osteoblast Growth and Maturation	Laurencin, C.T., M.D., Ph.D.	1990 – 93
Electroporation of Bacteria and Yeast	Weaver, J.C., Ph.D.	1990 – 93
Possible Influence of Weak Electromagnetic Fields	Weaver, J.C., Ph.D.	1990 – 93
Ventilation/Perfusion Distribution in the Lung	Poon, C.S., Ph.D.	1990 – 93
Measurement of Growth and Secretion of Single Cells	Weaver, J.C., Ph.D.	1990 – 93

Title	PI	Years
Basic Issues in the Detection of Electrical Fields by Biological Cells	Weaver, J.C., Ph.D.	1990 – 93
NCSORT-Human Performance in Space	Young, L.R., Ph.D.	1990 – 95
Research and Training Center for Speech and Hearing	Kiang, N.Y.S., Ph.D.	1990 – 97
Horizons in Impedance Imaging	Cohen, R.J., M.D., Ph.D.	1991 – 92
Chondrocytes in Gel Culture	Grodzinsky, A.J., Sc.D.	1991 – 92
Growth and Secretion of Single Cells	Weaver, J.C., Ph.D.	1991 – 92
Cell Interactions with Biomaterials	Cima, L.G., Ph.D.	1991 – 92
Regulation of Protein Synthesis and Erythropoesis	London, I.M., M.D.	1991 – 92
Non Invasive Blood Pressure Monitor	Mark, R.G., M.D., Ph.D.	1991 – 92
Biomedical Research Support Grant	Bowman, H.F., Ph.D.	1991 – 92
Cartilage Degeneration	Grodzinsky, A.J., Sc.D.	1991 – 92
Dietary Protein and Human Protein Metabolism	Young, V.R., Ph.D.	1991 – 92
Post-Transcriptional Regulation	Gehrke, L., Ph.D.	1991 – 94
ELF-2 Alpha Kinase	Chen, J.J., Ph.D.	1991 – 94
Post-Transcriptional Regulation of Interleukin 1 Beta Expression	Gehrke, L., Ph.D.	1991 – 94
Respiratory Assist in Newborns	Poon, C.S., Ph.D.	1991 – 94
Coupled Effects of IL-1B Proteins and Compressive...	Gray, M.L., Ph.D.	1991 – 94

Title	PI	Years
Fall Biomechanics and Hip Fracture Risk	Mark, R.G., M.D., Ph.D.	1991–94
Regulation of Human Beta-globin Gene in Erythroid Cells	Tuan, D.Y., Ph.D.	1991–95
Development of Novel Bone-Bioerodible Polymer Composites	Elgendy, H.M.	1991–95
Tumor Hyperthermia: Science, Technology, and Evaluation	Bowman, H.F., Ph.D.	1991–96
Optimization of Hyperthermia: Biological and Physiological Studies	Herman, T.S., M.D.	1991–96
Basic and Applied Research on Cochlear Prostheses	Eddington, D.K., Ph.D.	1991–96
Regulation and Structure-Function Relationships of Heme-Regulated...	Chen, J.J., Ph.D.	1991–96
Cell Interactions with Resorbable Polymers	Cima, L.G., Ph.D.	1991–
Transdermal Drug Delivery	Weaver, J.C., Ph.D.	1992–92
Gene Therapy for B Thalassemia	London, I.M., M.D.	1992–93
Bioelectromagnetic Mechanisms	Weaver, J.C., Ph.D.	1992–93
Microfabricated Device	Gray, M.L., Ph.D.	1992–93
Cartilage Composition	Gray, M.L., Ph.D.	1992–93
Cloning and Expression of CDI	Langer, R.S., Ph.D.	1992–93
Heme-Regulated EIF-2A Kinase	London, I.M., M.D.	1992–93
Hemodynamic Regulation	Cohen, R.J., M.D., Ph.D.	1992–93
IL-1B and Mechanical Forces on Cartilage	Gray, M.L., Ph.D.	1992–93

Title	PI	Years
Respiratory Assist in Newborns	Poon, C.S., Ph.D.	1992 – 93
Mapping Cardiac Electrical Activity	He, B., Ph.D.	1992 – 93
Neural Optimization Algorithms	Poon, C.S., Ph.D.	1992 – 94
Intraneural Microstimulation	Edell, D.J., Ph.D.	1992 – 94
Cell-Polymer Cartilage Implants	Freed, L.E., M.D., Ph.D.	1992 – 94
Optimization Mechanisms in Respiratory Control	Poon, C.S., Ph.D.	1992 – 95
IL-1 Protein and Mechanical Forces	Gray, M.L., Ph.D.	1993 – 94
Local Vascular Drug Delivery	Edelman, E.R., M.D., Ph.D.	1993 – 94
Proteolytic Fragments of BAPP	Wurtman, R.J., M.D.	1993 – 94
Bioerodible Polymer Matrices	Laurencin, C.T., M.D., Ph.D.	1993 – 94
Kinetics of Epithelial Cell Migration	Cima, L.G., Ph.D.	1993 – 96
Insulating Biomaterials	Edell, D.J., Ph.D.	1993 – 97
NASA Cardiovascular Center	Cohen, R.J., M.D., Ph.D.	1994 – 95
NASA Center Fabricated Equipment	Cohen, R.J., M.D., Ph.D.	1994 – 95
Neural Information Sensors	Edell, D.J., Ph.D.	1994 – 95
Mimic Database Development Consortium	Mark, R.G., M.D., Ph.D.	1994 – 95
Perivascular Drug Delivery	Edelman, E.R., M.D., Ph.D.	1994 – 95

Title	PI	Years
Cartilage Degeneration	Grodzinsky, A.J., Sc.D.	1994 – 95
EIF-2 Alpha Kinase	Chen, J.J., Ph.D.	1994 – 95
Aqueous Pathways in Skin	Weaver, J.C., Ph.D.	1994 – 95
Respiratory Neuroplasticity	Poon, C.S., Ph.D.	1995 – 96
Long Range Detection of Microorganisms	Weaver, J.C., Ph.D.	1995 – 95
Clinical Research	Rubin, R.H., M.D.	1995 – 96
Intelligent Control Paradigms	Poon, C.S., Ph.D.	1995 – 98
Transdermal Drug Delivery	Weaver, J.C., Ph.D.	1995 – 96
Magnetite Mediated Pore Hypothesis	Weaver, J.C., Ph.D.	1995 – 96
Microgravity Tissue Engineering	Freed, L.E., M.D., Ph.D.	1995 – 96
Gene Therapy	London, I.M., M.D.	1995 – 96
Chaos in Cardiac Arrhythmia	Poon, C.S., Ph.D.	1995 – 96

Index

(appendices not included)

A

Abbas, Abul K., photograph, 150e
Abelmann, Walter, 12, 15, 84, 108, 111, 159, 229; "Conclusions/Perspective", 221–223; "Early Collaborative Efforts of Harvard and MIT" (chapter), 1–6; "Evaluation of the M.D. Program" (chapter), 186–200; "The HST Experience" (chapter), 125–150; photographs, ii, 150f
Abrams, Herbert, 40
Adams, Charles Francis, 51
Adelstein, James, 95, 101–106, 110
Administration: Administrative Council, 55–56, 69, 70, 73, 90–92; final proposal, 54–56, 79; planning, 34–35, 54
Administrative Structure, Committee on, 34–36, 68, 70–71, 73, 79
Admissions: affirmative action, 130; to Biomedical Sciences M.D. program, 84–87; Committee, 70, 85–86, 100, 107, 113, 129, 158, 161, 170–171, 174; first class in M. D. program,
49, 51, 84; of M.D. candidates, 70–71; to MEMPS, 160–161, 171–172; of Ph.D. candidates, 71, 154; process, to HST, 128–130
Advisory committee: evaluation of M.D. program, 189–191; membership in 1988, 217–218; membership in 1994, 218–220; review of MEMPS, 201–205; role of, 104–106
Advisory system, 117, 141–142
Affiliated Hospitals Center. See Brigham and Women's Hospital
Aisen, Philip, 65, 72
Albers, Mark, photograph, 150b
Albert Einstein College of Medicine, 62–63, 82
Alberti, Robert, 20
Alpers, Joel, 38
Alter, R., 59
Alumni. See Graduates
Alumni surveys: M.D. graduates, 143–144; MEMP graduates, 205–216
American Academy of Arts and Sciences, 22